Ambulatory Anesthesia

THE REQUISITES IN ANESTHESIOLOGY

SERIES EDITOR   **Roberta L. Hines, MD**
Chair and Professor of Anesthesiology
Yale University School of Medicine
New Haven, Connecticut

OTHER VOLUMES IN
THE REQUISITES SERIES IN ANESTHESIOLOGY:

Adult Perioperative Anesthesia

Cardiac and Vascular Anesthesia

Regional Anesthesia

Pediatric Anesthesia

Obstetric and Gynecologic Anesthesia

Critical Care

Pain Medicine

Ambulatory Anesthesia

THE REQUISITES IN ANESTHESIOLOGY

Scott R. Springman, MD
Professor of Anesthesiology
University of Wisconsin Medical School;
Department of Anesthesiology
University of Wisconsin Hospital and Clinics
Madison, Wisconsin

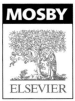

MOSBY

ELSEVIER

MOSBY
ELSEVIER

1600 John F. Kennedy Boulevard
Suite 1800
Philadelphia, PA 19103-2899

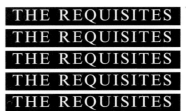
AMBULATORY ANESTHESIA: THE REQUISITES IN ANESTHESIOLOGY   ISBN-13: 978-0-323-03225-4
ISBN-10: 0-323-03225-7

Notice

Knowledge and best practice in this field are constantly changing. As new research and experience broaden our knowledge, changes in practice, treatment and drug therapy may become necessary or appropriate. Readers are advised to check the most current information provided (i) on procedures featured or (ii) by the manufacturer of each product to be administered, to verify the recommended dose or formula, the method and duration of administration, and contraindications. It is the responsibility of the practitioner, relying on his or her own experience and knowledge of the patient, to make diagnoses, to determine dosages and the best treatment for each individual patient, and to take all appropriate safety precautions. To the fullest extent of the law, neither the Publisher nor the Editor assumes any liability for any injury and/or damage to persons or property arising out or related to any use of the material contained in this book.

I most particularly would like to thank Dr. John Kreul for his friendship, teaching, and mentoring over the years. I have looked up to him as a superb clinician and leader. He embodies the combination of intelligence, strength, good-natured spirit, and fairness that serves as an inspiration for all of us. In gratitude, I dedicate this book to him.

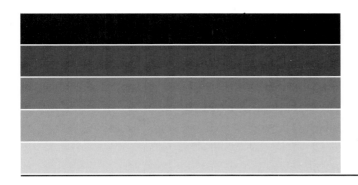

Contributors

George A. Arndt, MD
Professor of Anesthesiology
University of Wisconsin Medical School
Madison, Wisconsin

Joan Benca, MD
Assistant Professor of Anesthesiology
University of Wisconsin Medical School;
Department of Anesthesiology
University of Wisconsin Hospital and Clinics
Madison, Wisconsin

Brian K. Bevacqua, MD
Associate Professor of Anesthesiology
University of Wisconsin School of Medicine;
Chief of Anesthesiology Service
Middleton Veterans Administration Medical Center
Madison, Wisconsin

John Boncyk, MD
Assistant Professor of Anesthesiology
University of Wisconsin School of Medicine;
Department of Anesthesiology
University of Wisconsin Hospital and Clinics
Madison, Wisconsin

Thomas Broderick, MD
Assistant Professor of Anesthesiology
University of Wisconsin Medical School;
Department of Anesthesiology
University of Wisconsin Hospital and Clinics
Madison, Wisconsin

John A. Dilger, MD
Assistant Professor of Anesthesiology
Mayo Clinic
Rochester, Minnesota

Talmage D. Egan, MD
Professor
Department of Anesthesiology
University of Utah School of Medicine
Salt Lake City, Utah

James Fitzpatrick, MD
Associate Professor of Anesthesiology
University of Wisconsin Medical School;
Department of Anesthesiology
University of Wisconsin Hospital and Clinics
Madison, Wisconsin

Michael Ford, MD
Assistant Professor of Anesthesiology
University of Wisconsin Medical School;
Director of Acute Pain Services
Department of Anesthesiology
University of Wisconsin Hospital and Clinics
Madison, Wisconsin

Dorothy S. Fryer, MD
Instructor of Anesthesiology;
Medical Director
Olson Ambulatory Surgery Center
Department of Anesthesia
Northwestern Memorial Hospital
Chicago, Illinois

Tong J. Gan, MB, FRCA, FFARCS(I)
Professor of Anesthesiology
Duke University Medical Center
Durham, North Carolina

Dan Goulson, MD
Medical Director
Center for Advanced Surgery
Department of Anesthesiology
University of Kentucky
Lexington, Kentucky

Ashraf S. Habib, MBBCh, MSc, FRCA
Assistant Professor of Anesthesiology
Duke University Medical Center
Durham, North Carolina

Andrew Herlich, DMD, MD
Professor of Anesthesiology, Otolaryngology,
and Pediatrics;
Medical Director
Human Simulation Center
Temple University School of Medicine;
Staff Anesthesiologist
Temple University Children's Medical Center
Philadelphia, Pennsylvania

Molly Kay Kloosterboer, BS
Administrative Assistant
Department of Anesthesiology
University of Wisconsin Hospital and Clinics
Madison, Wisconsin

Thomas B. Kloosterboer, MD
Assistant Professor of Anesthesiology
University of Wisconsin Medical School;
Department of Anesthesiology
University of Wisconsin Hospital and Clinics
Madison, Wisconsin

Evelyn Loose, MD
Assistant Professor (Clinical)
Department of Anesthesiology
University of Utah School of Medicine
Salt Lake City, Utah

J. Thomas McLarney, MD
Assistant Professor
Department of Anesthesiology
University of Kentucky
Lexington, Kentucky

Hugh M. Smith, MD, PhD
Anesthesiology Resident
Mayo Clinic
Rochester, Minnesota

Michael T. Walsh, MD
Assistant Professor of Anesthesiology
Mayo Clinic
Rochester, Minnesota

Elizabeth S. Yun, MD
Assistant Professor of Anesthesiology
University of Wisconsin Medical School
Madison, Wisconsin

Acknowledgments

I would like to thank my authors for their hard work and my colleagues at the University of Wisconsin–Madison Department of Anesthesiology for their advice and support, as well as Sarah Broderick for assistance in the preparation of the manuscript. Special thanks are in order to my family for their patience, support, and forgiveness during the neglect that book editing often requires.

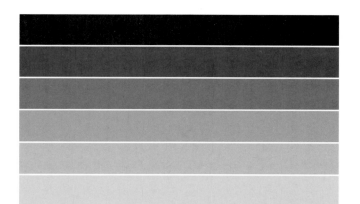

Preface

With the development of modern anesthetic agents, anesthesia machines, monitoring devices, and resuscitative techniques, even the sickest patients can undergo the most complex procedures. Over the last several decades, however, an evolution and transformation of surgery and anesthesia techniques has allowed many procedures to be performed outside the confines of standard operating rooms (ORs). Whether it is in out-of-OR hospital suites, freestanding ambulatory surgery centers, or surgeons' offices, anesthesia is now administered at a wide variety of venues.

Significantly, the majority of procedures performed in the United States today are now done outside the standard hospital setting. Driving forces for this change include economic factors and patient and surgeon demand. Newer, so-called "minimally invasive" techniques continue to be developed and perfected, allowing patients to have extensive procedures done via smaller and smaller incisions. We now have anesthetic agents and adjunctive techniques that afford patients a rapid recovery with fewer side effects, while maintaining the same high safety standards that we have come to expect in a hospital OR suite.

It is with these thoughts in mind that this volume of *The Requisites in Anesthesiology* is offered to anesthesia practitioners and those in anesthesia training. The first chapter describes how ambulatory anesthesia began. Subsequently, the discussion illustrates how current clinical practice is evolving. Patient selection continues to be a challenge as we move "sicker" patients out of the hospital and into the ambulatory arena. We are less commonly asked, "Who *can* have surgery in an ambulatory setting?" Rather, we are now asked, "Is there anyone who *can't* have ambulatory surgery?" We continue to struggle with defining ambulatory standards that will protect our patients' safety.

With safety and satisfaction as our goals, patient assessment and preparation become paramount issues. What really makes a difference in outcomes? It is critical to be mindful of potential perioperative complications and to work diligently to fine-tune our anesthesia techniques. Attention to the details of perioperative management makes the difference between an unexpected hospital admission and a safe recovery and discharge to home.

These authors' chapters will help practitioners review important aspects of anesthesia care, including how inhalation, intravenous, and regional anesthesia can be used to achieve optimum results. While side effects from surgery and anesthesia have been reduced for patients over the last decade, the problems of postoperative nausea/vomiting and pain still deserve close attention. The chapter on anesthesia complications includes suggested prevention and solutions. Two groups of patients—children and the elderly—deserve special attention in this book because many of their needs are unique. A discussion of care of patients during the recovery period and choice of criteria for discharge brings the patient full circle, returning to home.

Although the book primarily focuses on patient care aspects of ambulatory anesthesia, some administrative issues must be mentioned because these are less commonly addressed in standard clinical teaching. Business management is outside the scope of this text, but the basics of planning and building an ambulatory surgery center, along with obtaining accreditation, are described.

Office-based procedures are growing at a rapid rate. Practicing anesthesia in relative "isolation" necessitates the utmost attention to all of the aforementioned aspects of anesthesia care and to other additional issues unique to the peripatetic anesthesia provider. The chapter on office-based and dental anesthesia provides insights into this challenging branch of ambulatory care.

It is my hope that *Ambulatory Anesthesia* will provide the key facts needed to teach the next generation of anesthesia practitioners about maintaining high standards of patient safety and satisfaction in ambulatory settings. I hope it also provides a ready reference and review for current practitioners regarding the art and science of ambulatory anesthesia.

Scott R. Springman, MD

Contents

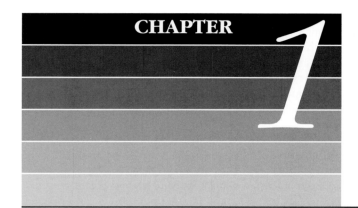

A Short History of Ambulatory Anesthesia

ANDREW HERLICH

THE EARLY DAYS: 1846 AND NITROUS OXIDE

The history of ambulatory anesthesia can reasonably be traced to the history of anesthesiology itself. In the earliest stages of medicine, surgery was performed on a truly outpatient basis, frequently in the home of the patient on the kitchen table or else on the physician's office table, with the patient discharged to be taken home by horse and wagon; surgery might even have been performed under a tree. The surgeon sometimes used any intoxicating substance available, with "able-bodied" assistants helping to "persuade" the patient not to move during the procedure.

Modern ambulatory anesthesia began with dental anesthesia and surgery in Hartford, Connecticut, in 1846. Nitrous oxide was administered as a public demonstration and subsequently was used on Horace Wells himself. About the same time, Gardner Colton, a chemist and public entrepreneur, utilized his marketing skills and relationships with dentists to develop multiple dental offices, wherein nitrous oxide was used to alleviate dental pain. Colton claimed that he had no deaths in over 100,000 patients, using 100% nitrous oxide. One must suspect that

observer bias was present or that the procedures were of such brief duration that recovery would be inevitable in all of the patients. It is noteworthy to remember that the hallmark of great surgeons at that time was the speed with which they completed their procedures and not their gentleness of tissue manipulation: in cases of exodontia, roots were frequently left in the alveolar bone!

THE END OF THE 19TH CENTURY: EARLY DANGERS AND THE BEGINNINGS OF SAFETY

Colton and others administered 100% nitrous oxide. The general belief at that time was that oxygen dissociated from nitrous oxide, and, hence, patients received their oxygen from that particular source. In 1868, Edmund Andrews, a surgeon from Chicago, recognized that hypoxemia resulted from the administration of nitrous oxide alone. He suggested that the addition of oxygen to nitrous oxide would probably result in a safe anesthetic. However, the simultaneous administration of both nitrous oxide and oxygen was, at best, cumbersome. Not until many years later did Thomas Evans realize that nitrous oxide could be compressed into a liquid within a gas cylinder. Subsequently, in the 1880s, the first practical nitrous oxide and oxygen delivery device was made for distribution in the United States. By the last decade of the 19th century and the first decade of the 20th century, a number of dentists and physicians, in conjunction with manufacturers, developed anesthesia machines with both compressed nitrous oxide and oxygen. Despite the availability of oxygen, it was common to induce anesthesia with 100% nitrous oxide until hypoxia occurred. The teeth were quickly removed and 100% oxygen was then administered. This practice continued well into the 1950s. The advent of the interlock chain drive, fail-safe valves, and, most importantly, common sense, in combination with regulatory oversight from the American National Standards Institute in 1979 and the American Society for Testing and Measurements in 1988, brought the end of this dangerous practice. The practitioner was no longer able to purchase anesthesia machines that could deliver hypoxic, or worse, anoxic gas mixtures.

EARLY 20TH CENTURY PIONEERS: NICOLL, WATERS, MCMECHAN, AND CURIOUS DENTISTS

After the turn of the 20th century, outpatient surgery enjoyed increased popularity. Pediatric surgery, especially surgery on infants, was largely performed on an outpatient basis. James Nicoll from Scotland drew attention to the many procedures that could be performed easily with minimal morbidity. They ranged from pyloromyotomies to closure of myelomeningoceles to cleft palate repairs. In his 1909 treatise, however, Nicoll noted that many of his procedures were successful largely due to the fact that there were visiting nurses and facilities for nursing mothers.[1]

The fascinating commentary within the framework of his article drew attention to issues of nosocomial infection and medicolegal consequences of bad outcomes. Nicoll even discussed maternal intelligence and its significance in regards to whether a child should be treated as an inpatient or an outpatient: more intelligent mothers, he thought, should be able to bring their infant children home.[1] To improve efficiency and safety, he suggested that surgical preps should be performed prior to the induction of anesthesia (Fig. 1-1).

In the second decade of the 20th century, as World War I closed, ambulatory surgery made a leap into the office environment in the United States. Ralph Waters wrote a description of his early office anesthesia practice in which he described how he catered to both physicians and dentists.[2] He supplied the operating room, the recovery room, the doctors' "loafing and smoking room," and he personally administered the anesthetics. He used safe techniques for the time, including nitrous oxide-oxygen. He monitored the patient's blood pressure and heart rate frequently. Ill-appearing patients warranted a closer examination prior to the induction of anesthesia. Waters' pioneering concepts emphasized that this office-based practice avoided the obstacles of a hospital operating room and patient and surgeon inconvenience and, in return, offered a pleasant environment for all concerned in an accessible location.

Waters emphasized that it was a financially lucrative situation.[2] The surgeons' satisfaction was his key to financial success. Waters did not trouble the patient or surgeon if the patient could not afford his or her bill. He thought that negative public relations would be a long-term detriment to his practice.

The original account of his experience, related by his own writings, is fascinating and can be found in the chapter appendix.

During the same period, anesthesiologists became more prominent in publishing their techniques and findings. Most medical publications at the time were medical and surgical journals. Many early anesthesia-related publications were supplements to surgical journals. Later, anesthesiologists such as Francis McMechan started separate publications. In his 1915 book, McMechan describes ambulatory anesthesia techniques for the administration of nitrous oxide, including arm and leg grips that the anesthesiologist would use to assist the surgeon during the excitement phases of the anesthetic.[3]

In the 1930s in Great Britain and the United States, several pioneering dentists developed techniques that they had learned during their anesthesia training as oral surgeons. At the same time, John Lundy at the Mayo Clinic introduced the use of thiopental intermittent boluses.[4] The use of intermittent boluses of thiopental seemed appropriate for use in oral surgery outpatients, despite Lundy's objections to any outpatient procedures. Langa used a lower and safer concentration of nitrous oxide in combination with the administration of local anesthesia.[5] During the 1940s, despite the introduction of lidocaine and muscle relaxants such as succinylcholine and d-tubocurarine, ambulatory anesthesia and surgery did not develop markedly. However, Jorgensen, a dentist in Loma Linda, California, used intravenous sedation techniques for office-based ambulatory anesthesia. He combined intravenous pentobarbital, meperidine, and scopolamine for light sedation for oral surgery and general dentistry.[6] These techniques were the forerunners of today's minimal or moderate sedation.

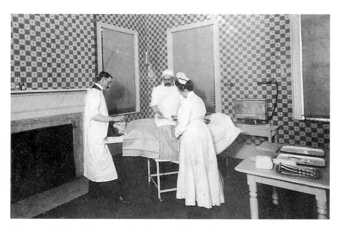

Figure 1-1   Photograph taken in the early 1900s in Massachusetts. This is, perhaps, a hospital ambulatory operating area; it is not an operating room. Surgeon, anesthetizer, and patient appear to have come in off the street. (Photograph courtesy of the Francis A. Countway Library of Medicine, Boston, Massachusetts.)

1950S AND 1960S: IMPETUS FOR MODERN AMBULATORY SURGERY AND ANESTHESIA

In the 1950s, there was increasing interest in outpatient surgery, in large part due to the shortage of hospital beds and the costs of inpatient surgery, especially in Canada. Hernia repair was the most popular procedure for adult outpatient surgery. Advances in outpatient anesthesia were made in the 1960s by John Dillon and David Cohen at the University of California, Los Angeles (UCLA), with the development of their outpatient surgery service.[7] However, unlike the Canadian initiative, which was stimulated by a lack of inpatient beds, Dillon's and Cohen's impetus came from sheer economics: outpatient surgery was dramatically less expensive than inpatient surgery. Slightly later, Levy and Coakley at George Washington University developed a program similar to that at UCLA.[8]

REED AND FORD: THE FIRST FREESTANDING SURGICENTER

The true pioneers of 20th century ambulatory anesthesia and surgery were John Ford and Wallace Reed in Phoenix, Arizona (Figs. 1-2, 1-3). They conceived and implemented the idea of building a freestanding ambulatory surgicenter (Figs. 1-4, 1-5).[9] This concept stemmed from the same issues that confronted Dillon and Cohen at UCLA: cost containment, reimbursement, and efficiency. Additionally, the resulting patient and health care worker convenience was also very appealing. The patients did not have to move a long distance through the health care facility, they could have their loved ones with them until the last possible moment, and they could park their cars close to the entrance. Efficiency, with

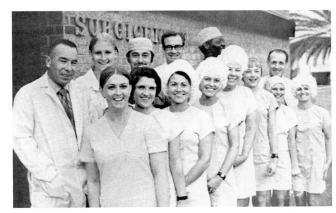

Figure 1-3   The staff of the Phoenix Surgicenter in 1971. (Photograph courtesy of the Wood Library-Museum and Dr. Reed.)

maximal patient throughput, was the top priority, beginning with the architectural design phase and continuing through construction of the new surgicenters. Unnecessary laboratory testing was eliminated, as were unnecessary services such as a cafeteria and transport personnel. As a consequence, the cost to the patient decreased dramatically. Mandatory second surgeons for all procedures were also eliminated. Hence, common procedures such as dilation and curettage (DC), cystoscopy, and eye surgery became much more cost-effective. Most of the surgeries were conducted under general anesthesia. Regional anesthesia and sedation were rarely used. Despite the constraints of older anesthesia agents and techniques, it only took a few more years before much of the country took notice of Ford's and Reed's initiative.

In order for the specialty of ambulatory anesthesia to grow, refinement of older anesthesia techniques, in conjunction with development of newer techniques, had to take place. The addition of newer agents such as propofol, alfentanil, remifentanil, midazolam, sevoflurane, and desflurane improved induction, maintenance, and emergence from general anesthesia. Older medications such as thiopental, halothane, and enflurane were largely eliminated from use in the ambulatory setting. Improved antiemetic therapy, including the use of 5HT3 antagonists, and improved postoperative analgesia, for example, with ketorolac, facilitated patient recovery and home-readiness. Most importantly, these agents improved perioperative patient satisfaction; improved patient satisfaction translated into a better bottom line for both the clinician and the facility. The more liberal use of local and regional anesthesia by the anesthesiologist and the surgeon to supplement or to replace intravenous agents was not new. Waters had cited the use of local anesthetics in his 1919 landmark paper.[2]

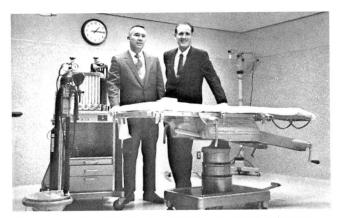

Figure 1-2   Drs. John Ford and Wallace Reed at the Phoenix Surgicenter. (Photograph courtesy of the Wood Library-Museum and Dr. Reed.)

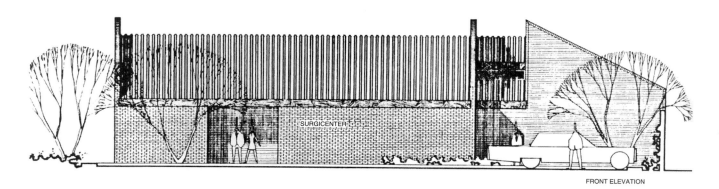

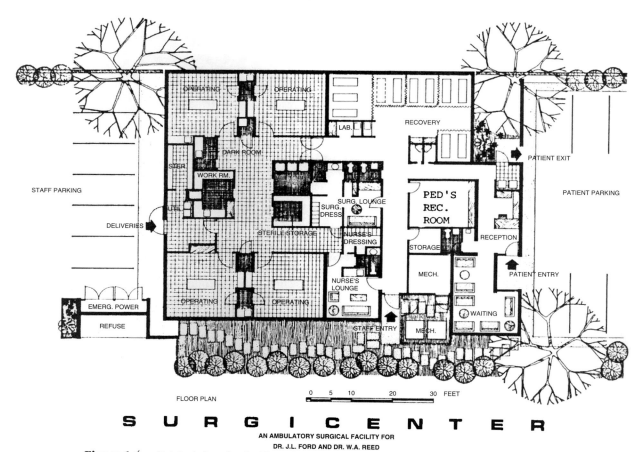

Figure 1-4 Original plans for the Phoenix Surgicenter. (Photograph courtesy of the Wood Library-Museum and Dr. Reed.)

THE SOCIETY FOR AMBULATORY ANESTHESIA

By the 1980s, interest in ambulatory anesthesia took another step in the United States. An annual meeting of an ambulatory anesthesia interest group, headed by Bernard Wetchler, took the initiative to start a subspecialty society. The Society for Ambulatory Anesthesia (SAMBA) was officially founded in 1985. Education and research were its main aims. Annual meetings became quite popular, touching upon all areas of ambulatory anesthesia and surgery.

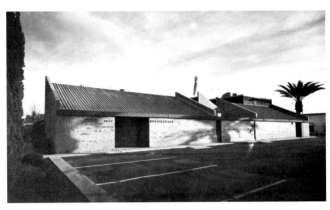

Figure 1-5 The original Surgicenter in Phoenix. (Photograph courtesy of the Wood Library-Museum and Dr. Reed.)

Its growing importance was such that annual meetings of the American Society of Anesthesiologists (ASA) began to include breakfast panels, symposia, and clinical forums discussing ambulatory anesthesia. The educational impact of SAMBA was such that the society was able to implement a midyear meeting immediately preceding the annual ASA meeting. Additionally, the organization developed liaisons with international ambulatory anesthesiology and surgical federations. Within the last several years, SAMBA formed a Latin American Affairs Committee, which has received input from all of Latin and Central America, as well as the Caribbean nations. SAMBA has invested in its future; grants for outcomes research have been made over the past several years. Travel awards have been given to residents who have demonstrated research interest in the area. SAMBA has affiliated with two journals, initially with the *Journal of Clinical Anesthesia* and, more recently, with its official publication, *Anesthesia and Analgesia*. Informative Web sites have also been created for both the general public and SAMBA members.

The impact of ambulatory anesthesia has been such over the past several decades that the American Board of Anesthesiology has mandated education in the discipline. Recognized fellowships are offered at many academic departments. These fellowships have stressed clinical excellence, clinical research, teaching, economics, and the administrative aspects of ambulatory anesthesia.

The most recent leap for ambulatory anesthesia was into its past. During the 1990s, as reimbursement was declining for outpatient procedures at the hospital and surgicenter levels, clinicians recognized the untapped financial source of the office-based environment. Although dentists and plastic surgeons have used office-based practices for many years, general surgeons, ophthalmologists, and many other specialists recently began moving much of their practice away from surgicenters and hospitals to improve reimbursement and to reduce inconvenience. Third-party payers started to reimburse practitioners accordingly.

However, rapid expansion into the office-based environment raised questions of safety. Adverse outcomes became well-known in areas such as pediatric dentistry, liposuction, and endoscopy. Well-publicized deaths of young or influential individuals created sufficient public notice to create changes. State medical and dental boards implemented more stringent regulations or, in many cases, finally enforced regulations that were already in existence. In some states, moratoriums on the use of office-based surgery existed until patient safety could be assured to a wary public. Oversight agencies such as the Joint Commission on Accreditation of Healthcare Organizations (JCAHO), the Accreditation Association for Ambulatory Health Care (AAAHC), and the American Association for Accreditation of Ambulatory Surgical Facilities (AAAASF) assisted in the national effort to promote uniformity and safety for ambulatory procedures, irrespective of where the procedure would be performed.

SUMMARY

As seen in Figure 1-6, the growth of all forms of ambulatory surgery continues. The relatively short history of ambulatory anesthesia parallels the development of anesthesia itself. The applications of techniques that allow rapid and safe patient care, along with improved satisfaction for patients and practitioners, are the result of much effort. Individuals and organizations that promote research, safety, and education will continue to grow and to exert influence over the future of ambulatory anesthesia, ensuring its lengthening history.

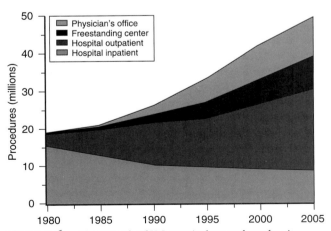

Figure 1-6 The growth of U.S. surgical procedures by site, 1980–2005. (Hospital data through 2001 from the American Hospital Association; freestanding surgery center and physician's office data through 1999 and all estimates after 1999 provided by Verispan, LLC, Chicago. Reprinted from Thomas SK, Orkin FK: Scope of Modern Anesthetic Practice. In Miller RD (ed): Miller's Anesthesia. Philadelphia, Churchill Livingstone, 2005, p 57.)

REFERENCES

1. Nicoll JH: The surgery of infancy. Br Med J 18:753-754, 1909.

2. Waters RM: The downtown anesthesia clinic. Am J Surg (Suppl) 33:71-73, 1919.

3. McMechan FH: The American Year Book of Anesthesia and Analgesia. New York, Surgery Publishing Company, 1915, pp 251-296.

4. Lundy JS, Mousel LH: Recent advances in anesthesia. Surg Clin North Am 19: 1053-1057, 1939.

5. Langa H: Relative Analgesia in Dental Practice: Inhalation and Sedation with Nitrous Oxide. Philadelphia, WB Saunders, 1968.

6. Jorgensen NB, Hayden J: Sedation, Local and General Anesthesia and Dentistry, 2nd ed. Philadelphia, Lea and Febiger, 1972.

7. Cohen DD, Dillon JB: Anesthesia for outpatient surgery. JAMA 196:1114-1116, 1966.

8. Levy ML, Coakley CS: Survey of "in and out surgery"—first year. South Med J 61: 995-998, 1968.

9. Reed WA, Ford JL: Development of an independent outpatient surgical center. Int Anesthesiol Clin 14:113-130, 1976.

SUGGESTED READING

Bennett CR: Conscious-Sedation in Dental Practice, 2nd ed. St. Louis, CV Mosby, 1978, pp 1-203.

Davison MHA: The Evolution of Anaesthesia. Baltimore, Williams and Wilkins, 1965, pp 124-134.

Dorsch JA, Dorsch SE: The Anesthesia Machine. In Understanding Anesthesia Equipment, 4th ed. Baltimore, Williams and Wilkins, 1998, pp 75-120.

Finder RL: The art and science of office-based anesthesia in dentistry: A 150 year history. Int Anesthesiol Clin 41:1-12, 2003.

Fulton JF, Stanton ME: The Centennial of Surgical Anesthesia: An Annotated Catalogue of Books and Pamphlets Bearing on the Early History of Surgical Anesthesia. New York, Henry Schuman, 1946, pp 3-20.

Philip BK: A vision of the future arriving: A history of the Society for Ambulatory Anesthesia. Amb Surg 1:77-79, 1992.

Vandam LD: A history of ambulatory anesthesia. Anesthesiol Clin North Am 5:1-13, 1987.

Webb E, Graves HB: Anesthesia for the ambulant patient. Anesth Analg 38:359-363, 1959.

APPENDIX: RALPH MILTON WATERS' EARLY AMBULATORY ANESTHESIA EXPERIENCE, THE DOWNTOWN ANESTHESIA CLINIC*

Sioux City, Iowa

The subject assigned to me is so foreign to the thoughts uppermost in the minds of us all that I feel almost a slacker in pre-

*Read during the Fourth Annual Meeting of the Interstate Association of Anesthetists with the Indiana State Medical Association, Claypool Hotel, Indianapolis, IN, Sept. 25-27, 1918.
From Waters RM: The downtown anesthesia clinic. Am J Surg (Suppl) 33:71-73, 1919.

senting it. However, in due time, the war will be over and it is possible that many of us may land, thereafter, in new locations. In case we do, I feel sure that a short story of my experiences may be of some value.

In 1915, my practice consisted largely of anesthesia, and I was using my home as telephone headquarters with no office whatever, doing largely anesthetics for major surgery in the various hospitals. An occasional call from a dentist, however, broke the routine, and in many such cases the dentist and patient alike objected to going to the hospital both because of the time and expense involved. It was suggested to me that a downtown office equipped to care for dental and minor surgical cases would be useful as we had no exclusive specialist in exodontia in our town and some surgeons were also anxious to establish extra hospital clinical facilities.

After the Mexican border demobilization in 1916, I made bold to try such a plan, my practice from that time being confined exclusively to anesthesia. An office was equipped with a waiting room and a small operating room with an adjoining room containing a cot on which a patient could lie down after his anesthetic. In due time, the place became popular and we moved. I say we for two reasons. First, it avoids a too egotistical repetition of the pronoun I, and, second, chiefly because my office assistant, a girl of 21, has been more than half responsible for the success of the experiment. Her interest and faithfulness have made it possible to make definite dates and to keep them properly and to see that no dentist or surgeon has felt himself slighted or inconvenienced. I bespeak for any of you who may make a like venture a careful selection of your assistant, and I wish you good luck.

In February 1918, we found ourselves with three units of floor space in the newest and most central office building of our town. The population is 65,000, and we have 100 doctors and 50 dentists in peacetimes. In this building, some 50 doctors and dentists have their offices. We are equipped with a large reception room with easy chairs and reading matter to divert the attention of fond relatives. Our operating room is of ample size, with large south and west windows. In it, we have a modified French chair-table such as you have seen Drs. McKesson and Denman use in Toledo for tonsillectomy and nose work. This we find very convenient for the dentist's use also, as it can be tilted into a half reclining position readily and quickly back to the head-forward position during recovery after bloody extractions. It also makes an excellent flat operating table. We have also a dental engine; a sink with foot pedals to turn on water; a sterilizer for instruments, gauze, towels, gowns, et cetera; and a sterile water tank. In short, the usual equipment for a minor surgery room. The sterilizer, however, we plan to replace with a better one in an adjoining room which we also use for storage of supplies.

To each side of the operating room is a room containing two or three cot-beds; separate doors open into each room through which the operating chair will roll with ease. Thresholds for such a door, we have found, are a nuisance and should be removed. One of these rooms we use for female patients and the other for males. There is running water in each, a mirror, etc. One thing we miss very much is a toilet, and one should not be forgotten when planning such a place in a new building.

In addition, off the men's retiring room, I have a private office with desk and chairs which serves also as a good loafing and smoking room and a place in which doctors can wait when they are early; it has a separate exit to the building corridor.

Our hospital work with major surgery still occupies half our time and makes up half our income, but that is mostly accomplished in the earlier part of the day. The downtown work consists of noontime and afternoon appointments and occupies time which would be otherwise idle.

Dentists bring all sorts of difficult extractions and painful cavity preparations. Surgeons bring circumcisions, abscesses, and fractures and are gradually bringing more minor operations as time goes on. The head specialists bring some work, and they too are gradually bringing more. Some dentists who used to attempt their own anesthesia now bring it to us. Others still do their less difficult cases and bring the more difficult ones to us. We take all sorts of cases, always attempting to give satisfaction regardless of expense. I mean we don't save anesthetic agents and let the patient feel the operation. We make careful physical examination on all suspicious risks. Others are accepted as they come. A sphygmomanometer and stethoscope are constantly present and frequently used. Here again, the well-trained and alert assistant is useful. She often warns me that the next patient is short of breath or shows some other evidence of needing careful examination.

We attempt, as I said, to give satisfaction to operator and patient and charge a fee that will pay expenses and a good profit. We make no fees in advance and have no set prices. Sometimes one tooth extraction takes 10 seconds and sometimes it takes an hour and a half. The cost of materials and the value of our time make it necessary to gauge the fee by the work. Our minimum fee, with present cost of materials, is 7 dollars; the maximum is usually not over 15 dollars. In other words, our fees are considerably less than for similar work in hospitals because less time and trouble is involved.

As to anesthetic agents used, we aim to use N_2O-O as a routine. In particularly nervous patients, we use as preoperative sedatives morphine and scopolamine, sublingually, as a rule. Ether we add very rarely and of course no chloroform for we do not use that even in the hospital.

We keep a card record of every case with physical findings when made, approximate weight, sex, complexion, and other details and also the assistant's estimate, each time, as to the degree of satisfaction of patient, surgeon, and dentist. Also, we record what work was done and the length of time.

As to the satisfaction of my patrons, I think I can say this: there are none who have fault to find with our work. We aim to keep an abundant supply of N_2O-O and use it freely. Many patients and some doctors object to the fees, but they come back and their friends come back. Satisfactory anesthesia and too-large fees work out better than bargain-sale fees and unsatisfactory anesthesia, especially as in open mouth work one cannot wisely be over economical of gases when using N_2O-O anesthesia. People forget the fee, but they never forget the hurt nor fail to tell their friends about it.

We have made no start with local anesthesia as yet but have plans regarding it for the future. I believe it a very useful addition in connection with such an establishment as I am describing. I know that many dentists would appreciate such service greatly as they prefer not to bother with learning the technic of local nerve-blocking and would feel safer in employing one who devotes his time to such work.

As to the preoperative preparation of patients, we worry little about it. We prefer, when possible, a light meal for the last before the operation. Liquids are allowed at all times. Much of our work is done just before or during the noon-hour because patients have then an empty stomach, and, at the same time, we do not disturb the usual routine of the patient in regard to eating. Every patient takes off his or her outer garments above the waist, and corsets are removed by the women. A sheet serves as drapery when coming to the operating room. Every case must go to the toilet before undressing.

As to the aftercare, the only difficulty is to be sure that patients with blood in mouth or nose spit it up and do not swallow it. That we accomplish by using pharyngeal packs during the operation when necessary for dental work and by changing to a head-forward position before removing the pack. The patient is usually awake before the pack is removed in such cases. Then the lateral position in the cot with face turned down by the pillow makes it easy to expectorate without rising up in bed. In this way, we have little swallowed blood and little vomiting. The time required for recovery varies from 1 minute to 3 hours. Occasionally, a woman in poor health who has been nauseated requires help to get home, but this occurs rarely.

As to the success of the venture, I think I can say that the men who are familiar with the place are well-pleased. The place has been running in its present location now for 8 months and is paying my total expenses with a nice profit besides.

I hear objections both from doctors and patients as to prices occasionally. That bothers me not at all. I attempt to pay expenses and a net fair fee for myself in each case. I don't care to work on any other basis. The one thing I do strive for is to satisfy patient and operator. If I fail in that, I wish no fee and I collect none. In the long run, I believe that plan wins out.

As for business-getting activity, it is all with the dentists and physicians. The place is for their use and their convenience, and consideration for them comes first. If Mrs. Jones calls up in regard to an anesthetic because her neighbor Mrs. Brown was pleased, I ask after Mrs. Brown's health and tell Mrs. Jones to make any arrangements she sees fit with her dentist or doctor. His office calls mine and makes the appointment.

One point upon which we lay emphasis and which I think is a business-getter is prompt collection direct from the patient. We never bother a physician or dentist about a patient's bill. A statement is rendered before the patient leaves the office and 75% of patients pay them. If there is to be a loss, we assume it, preferring not to bother the doctor with finances. So we avoid making an enemy of the doctor and patient alike, for every patient who owes you is your enemy.

The future for such a venture, I believe, is bright. I know ours is not yet half-grown. Several additions have been planned for the immediate future; one, a permanent graduate nurse assistant. So far we have only employed the extra assistant as occasions demanded.

We have considered seriously the manufacture of our own N_2O, also. Frequently, other additions suggest themselves or are suggested by physicians and dentists. When the war is over, I trust many of you may develop downtown minor surgery and dental clinics of much larger scope.

Patient Selection for Ambulatory Surgery

DAN GOULSON

J. THOMAS MCLARNEY

PATIENT SELECTION CONSIDERATIONS

General Issues

The number of ambulatory surgery cases has increased rapidly over the last 20 years. It is essential to select appropriate patients in order to maximize the benefits of ambulatory surgery. The benefits of proper patient selection include decreased incidence of adverse outcomes and unplanned admissions, decreased stress on patients and family or caregivers, cost savings for patients and the health care system, and increased efficiency and revenue for the ambulatory surgery center (ASC) or the office-based surgery practice. The only way to determine if our selection criteria are valid is to com-

pare similar groups of patients undergoing the same procedures in inpatient and outpatient care locations. Unfortunately, there is a paucity of large-scale outcomes-based research trials for ambulatory surgery. A contributing factor to this is that economic and medical changes have occurred so quickly that ambulatory surgery scarcely resembles what it was even 5 to 10 years ago.

Decisions about patient selection at an ambulatory facility should involve more than the surgeon's or the surgical scheduler's opinion. The selection process must include the anesthesiologist, the surgeon, and the patient's primary care physician or specialist. Indeed, the decision to care for a specific group of patients should also involve facility nursing staff and facility management. Factors that must be considered in the selection process include the patient's overall health status, psychosocial factors, and individual considerations. Other factors considered should include the type of surgery, the location of the facility, the facility's personnel and equipment resources, and cost-to-revenue estimates.

In order to select appropriate patients for surgery in an ambulatory center or office, it must be recognized that all providers and facilities have limitations regarding the types of patients and procedures that could, or should, be considered. ASCs and, to an even greater degree, office surgery practices usually have a subset of the full health services provided by large acute-care hospitals. Ambulatory providers are justifiably proud of the quality of services rendered to patients, but it is just as important for them to know their limitations as it is for them to know their capabilities.

Facility Limitations

The limitations of a facility are directly related to the facility's location and resources. A continuum exists all the way from hospital-integrated centers, where the operating rooms are located within the hospital, to small freestanding office-based centers. There are some procedures that may be done safely in one type of center but are unlikely to be as safe in another. Adverse events are always possible, and providers must be prepared to manage or to reduce the chance of developing these events. In a hospital-integrated center, there are many more resources readily available to deal with surgical, medical, or anesthetic complications. Hospitals have easy access to medical specialists, such as cardiologists and pulmonologists, and highly specialized care, such as cardiac catheterization labs and intensive care units.

The risk of postoperative hospital admission is often a prime consideration in deciding the location of surgical care. It would be more appropriate to treat patients who have a higher likelihood of requiring admission in a hospital-integrated ambulatory center. Ambulance transport from a freestanding surgery center or office to a hospital can occur from even the most well-prepared and equipped centers; however, the excess costs and time involved for transfer may negate many of the purported advantages of the outpatient experience. Minimizing transfers is much more than a matter of pride for an ambulatory center. The frequent occurrence of transfers can indicate, at best, problems with the selection of procedures or patients and, at worst, true quality-of-care problems.

The need for specialized facility resources may influence the decision to perform specific types of cases. The absence of clinical lab, radiology, or surgical pathology capabilities may exclude certain procedures. For example, highly specialized and expensive equipment such as lasers may not be available for a specific type of case. A cancer procedure that requires frozen sections to demonstrate negative margins may not be possible in a facility without immediate access to surgical pathology.

Patient Characteristics

Other selection factors relate to individual patient characteristics. As a rule, patients should be healthy enough so that the stress of surgery and anesthesia will not preclude returning home and recovering safely. Sometimes special issues are applicable in the selection process. The sections below discuss common patient conditions that should be considered before committing patients to the ambulatory process. In addition, other factors may apply. For instance, some states have requirements that limit certain aspects of adult and pediatric ambulatory surgery.

Psychological and social factors should be considered carefully. For the processes to be successful, patients must be willing to have their procedures performed as outpatients. Postoperatively, patients must have a reliable means of outside communication while at home. A landline telephone or cellular phone is important as a means for receiving preoperative instructions and scheduling information as well as postoperative advice. In addition, immediate communication access is essential if postoperative urgent or emergent medical care is needed. Patients require escorted transportation to return home, and there must be a responsible and competent person to care for the patient in the immediate postoperative period. It is important to remember that even though patients leave the facility after an operation, they are not yet fully recovered and may need further medical care. Patients should have adequate access to an acute care facility that is able to provide urgent and emergent care.

Surgeon and Surgical Procedure

Surgeons must carefully choose an appropriate facility for a specific procedure. In addition, surgeons must consider the complexity of each individual operation and the expected risk of complications. The surgeon should have the most detailed knowledge regarding the extent of the procedure and the recovery impact for the patient. Anticipated difficulties in a prolonged recurrent inguinal hernia case, as an example, may change the decision about the best venue of care. Likewise, some surgical providers are more technically adept than others and are able to minimize surgical duration and tissue trauma, thereby improving recovery.

At one time, only very simple procedures were considered suitable for ASCs and office-based locations. Leaps in technology have allowed extensive procedures to be performed with less tissue trauma and, subsequently, easier recovery for patients. Advances in anesthetic drugs, titration of anesthetics with level-of-consciousness monitoring, more effective antiemetics, and multimodal analgesia have also improved patient comfort and recovery. Ambulatory surgery has not yet found the limits of procedure selection, but it will continue to be true the patient must be appropriately matched with the procedure and the procedure technique in order to achieve acceptable patient satisfaction and safety.

Anesthesia Care Team

The final variable is the anesthesia care team. Anesthesiologists and managers must be aware of the team's limitations as related to the facility, the procedure, and the patient. For example, a specific facility's anesthesia providers may not have adequate clinical experience, skills, and confidence for caring for small infants; therefore, these patients should not be scheduled. Knowledgeable, skillful, and flexible anesthesia providers are able to care for a wider selection of patients. Although flexibility is required for ambulatory anesthesia care, this should not imply omitting limits or standards. Dealing with surgeons, patients, and ASC managers often requires considerable strength of will coupled with superior negotiation skills. In the ambulatory realm, anesthesiologists must truly be complete perioperative physicians. It is essential to effectively coordinate preoperative, intraoperative, and postoperative care, especially for patients who have significant medical problems.

SPECIFIC PATIENT CONSIDERATIONS

Respiratory Disease

Although significant respiratory disease is a risk factor for perioperative complications for inpatient surgery, there is almost no information available about these conditions in the ambulatory surgery setting. Chung reported in 1999 that reactive airway disease, obesity, and smoking are predictors of adverse respiratory events (usually minor ones) in the postoperative time period.[1] Studying a nonambulatory segregated population, Warner reported in 1996 that the risk of adverse respiratory events rises dramatically when patients with asthma have preoperative symptoms and signs of bronchospasm.[2] Although the risk of exacerbating bronchospasm is lowered when propofol is used for induction of anesthesia and when laryngeal mask airways are used for airway management, caution should be used if deciding to anesthetize a patient with active bronchospasm. Moderate to severe bronchospasm should be treated and improved before elective surgery. Issues concerning children with upper respiratory illnesses are discussed in the section "Infected or Colonized Patients."

Obesity

There are no accepted national guidelines related to patient weight restrictions for ambulatory surgery. Facility-specific policies should be developed based on the experience and the equipment available to handle patients at the allowable maximum size and weight. Cardiovascular disease is a leading cause of morbidity and mortality in obese patients. Pulmonary, endocrine, and gastrointestinal disorders are also significant causes of perioperative complications. Important challenges associated with obesity are obstructive sleep apnea and difficult airway access. However, there is little in the literature to indicate that obese patients, in general, have an increased risk of serious perioperative complications. Obese patients have a higher incidence of respiratory problems, but these are usually temporary and uncommonly lead to serious complications. Obesity, by itself, does not appear to lead to unanticipated admission after ambulatory surgery.

Each center might use a different set of criteria for determining weight restrictions. As recently as 1992, a patient with a body mass index (BMI) >30 kg/m^2 was considered unsuitable for ambulatory surgery by the Royal College of Surgeons of England. Other centers have chosen a BMI of 35, the definition of morbid obesity, as a cutoff. Still other facilities have chosen a weight limit because certain equipment, such as operating room (OR) tables, have a maximum weight capacity. Some centers use the patient's weight only in the context of other concomitant medical problems and the proposed procedure. For instance, a center might take care of an otherwise healthy 400-pound patient for a podiatric procedure under peripheral block but decline to care for a 280-pound patient who has diabetes and asthma for laparoscopy. Lastly, facility location should be considered. For example, a center located on an upper level of a multistory building must be concerned about potential emergency evacuation of obese patients, whereas this is much easier in a ground level, freestanding center.

Obstructive Sleep Apnea

In 2000, it was estimated that 40 million Americans had obstructive sleep apnea (OSA). Up to 95% of this group are undiagnosed, and 60% to 90% are obese. These patients are sensitive to respiratory depressant drugs and may be at risk for postoperative respiratory complications.

Anesthetic and opioid medications are central ventilatory depressants and can exacerbate any preexisting tendencies toward airway collapse during sleep. Patients with OSA, predominantly those with obesity, a small lower jaw, and an increased neck circumference, may pose an increased difficulty in viewing laryngeal structures during direct laryngoscopy.

Obstructive sleep apnea in pediatric patients is also a concern. Obese children may have secondary OSA, but the common presence of adenoid and tonsil hypertrophy makes even normal-weight children susceptible to OSA. Most ambulatory surgery centers exclude children under 2 to 3 years of age for tonsillectomy due to a presumed higher risk of severe postoperative obstructive apnea. Parents are specifically questioned about the presence of noisy breathing and apneic spells during sleep in their children coming for adenotonsillectomy, but, in fact, these questions should be used as a screening tool prior to other surgeries as well.

The American Society of Anesthesiologists (ASA) recently approved a set of practice guidelines for the management of patients with OSA.[3] These guidelines identify patients who are at risk for OSA, provide information on perioperative management of these patients to decrease risk, and give guidance on which patients can be safely treated as outpatients. The guidelines state that factors to be considered in determining if outpatient care is appropriate include sleep apnea status, anatomic and physiologic abnormalities, status of coexisting diseases, nature of surgery, type of anesthesia, need for postoperative opioids, patient age, adequacy of post-discharge observation, and capabilities of the outpatient facility.

Infants

Postoperative apnea and bradycardia are risks for young infants. Evidence has shown that this risk is highest in the ex-premature infant, but there is disagreement as to when patients fully outgrow this risk and when to consider it reasonable to discharge an ex-premature infant. "Safe" age recommendations range between 44 and 60 postconceptual weeks, and Coté's work is often cited.[4] Each center should define a minimum age for ex-premature infants based on the resources of the center, the presence of preoperative anemia (i.e., hemoglobin <10 gm/dL) in the patient, and the patient's need for perioperative opioids. Some centers use an observation period of 6 to 8 hours for infants without current preoperative apnea. Some also use caffeine in certain infants to further reduce apnea risk.

It is not clear when healthy term infants are suitable for ambulatory anesthesia. There are no studies as guides. Recommendations range from 42 to 60 weeks postconceptual age, with 44 weeks being a common

---

CLINICAL CONTROVERSY: OBSTRUCTIVE SLEEP APNEA (OSA)

It is not yet known the extent of postoperative risk for patients with OSA. OSA is a clinical spectrum, and risk is further modified by the patient's postoperative opioid requirement and other coexisting disease. Some centers screen patients carefully for undetected OSA. Facility restrictions may vary for patients with known OSA, depending on need for, and use of, CPAP during sleep.

---

requirement. A somewhat extended observation period is often specified, but without supportive data. It is not clear what postoperative analgesic plan is safest.

Elderly

The upper age limit for ambulatory surgery has continued to be extended, and the elderly are increasingly presenting for ambulatory procedures. However, Fleisher showed that age greater than 85 years is a strong predictor of postoperative admission, admission within 1 week of outpatient surgery, and perioperative death.[5] Some feel this suggests that this age range should be cared for in a hospital-associated facility. Other studies have not uniformly confirmed an increased risk based on age alone. Many anesthesiologists and surgeons currently maintain that the type of procedure and anesthetic, as well as the patient's medical condition, functional status, and living situation, should determine ambulatory standing, not an arbitrary age limit. However, because of diminished total body reserve, patients of extreme age may be unsuitable candidates for some of the more extensive procedures conducted at today's surgery centers.

Complex Patients for Simple Procedures

In the early days of ambulatory surgery and anesthesia, it was typical to exclude patients who were designated ASA physical status 3 or 4. As less invasive and improved surgical and anesthetic techniques have been developed, many procedures are now physiologically less stressful than in the past. As techniques have improved, cataract

---

CLINICAL CONTROVERSY: AMBULATORY SURGERY FOR THE ELDERLY

The elderly are a rapidly growing group presenting for ambulatory surgery. Although it is felt that coexisting disease conditions account for most excess risk in the elderly, some clinicians feel that an age of 85 years or older is an independent risk factor.

extraction, for example, is now often performed under no more than topical anesthesia. Even very complex patients can undergo this low-stress procedure with only a small chance for complications. However, other factors, such as the inability of a patient to tolerate the supine position, may yet designate a patient as ineligible.

Patient selection should be made not by using rules dependent only on ASA physical status, but by considering the patient's specific medical conditions and the context of the proposed procedure and the limitations of the facility.

Cardiovascular Disease

Patients who have cardiovascular disease commonly present selection dilemmas. However, patients with unstable ischemic cardiac or cerebrovascular disease are usually considered unsuitable candidates for elective ambulatory surgery, especially in a freestanding location. Although it is known that patients with existing coronary artery disease are at risk for perioperative myocardial infarction, the sensitivity and specificity of screening tests for detecting the magnitude of this risk are relatively poor. Perioperatively, patients may suffer subendomyocardial ischemia when, for example, tachycardia causes coronary oxygen delivery requirements to outstrip supply. However, the majority of transmural infarctions are due to coronary atherosclerotic plaque rupture and subsequent occlusion by clot. These may or may not occur in the immediate operative time and may actually be most likely in the days after the procedure. The American College of Cardiology guidelines on preoperative cardiac evaluation give advice on stratification of patient risk by procedure and patient risk factors. Generally, patients who have only minor clinical predictors and who are scheduled for low- to intermediate-risk procedures may proceed to the operating room without further testing. Major or intermediate clinical predictors should be carefully considered, especially in the context of low activity capacity, when deciding suitability for a particular venue of surgery. Modifications in care, such as perioperative β-blockade and administration of cholesterol-lowering drugs, may be required to reduce cardiovascular risk.

Patients sometimes present for outpatient procedures after relatively recent myocardial infarctions, coronary angioplasty and stenting, or strokes. The absolute minimum time needed to avoid excess risk of further occlusive events has not been determined. Older recommendations to delay for 6 months after myocardial infection may not fit the interventional and risk stratification practices of today. However, even if the patient is asymptomatic, the first several weeks after an event is a higher-risk period due to unhealed tissue and instability of vascular endothelium and plaque. Patients may be taking inhibitors of adenosine diphosphate (ADP) induced platelet aggregation, aspirin, Coumadin, and inhibitors of platelet glycoprotein IIb/IIIa. These drugs may cause significant perioperative bleeding, but discontinuation of these in the first 6 to 8 weeks may cause reinfarction. Furthermore, the activation of clotting pathways in the postoperative period may even overwhelm continued anticoagulation. Therefore, elective surgery in the first 4 to 8 weeks after an ischemic event should be undertaken only after consultation with cardiologists or neurologists and with due consideration of the increased risks. Drug-eluting stents present additional problems in the timing of elective surgery. Risk may be higher for as much as 9 months after placement, and the cardiologist should give advice on when it is safe to proceed. The American College of Cardiology has published guidelines for management of patients with recent percutaneous interventions[6] that suggest that antiplatelet therapy should be administered for as much as 6 months, depending on the type of stent, and ideally, it should continue for 12 months to prevent stent thrombosis.

Pacemakers and Implantable Cardioverter/Defibrillators (ICDs)

Pacemakers and ICDs are complex implanted devices that have significant implications for perioperative care. These small electronic packages are sometimes referred to as "cardiac rhythm management devices" (CRMDs). Patients need these devices for various reasons and often have serious coexisting cardiac problems. Patients with CRMDs may have severe cardiac problems including ongoing ischemic cardiac disease (with previous myocardial infarction) or severe cardiomyopathy. Only minor procedures would seem reasonable in a freestanding center for these types of ASA 3 and 4 patients. The availability of rapid access to cardiology assistance would also be a factor in deciding to care for such patients.

Because of the widely differing features and behaviors of cardiac devices, it is necessary to thoroughly understand the function of the device and its response to electromagnetic interference (EMI)—usually from electrocautery or magnets. Optimally, the patient's cardiologist should provide information that will guide the device's perioperative management in order to avoid complications. If the cardiologist

---

CLINICAL CAVEAT: DRUG-ELUTING CORONARY STENTS

Drug-eluting stents present additional problems in the timing of elective surgery. Risk may be higher for as much as 9 months after placement, and the cardiologist should give advice on when it is safe to proceed.

is not available, it is essential that the anesthesiologist determine the device's features and programming. By contacting the device's manufacturer, the anesthesiologist can determine what issues must be addressed in a given model. The American College of Cardiology states in their guidelines that "patients with implanted ICDs or pacemakers should have their devices evaluated before and after surgical procedures. The evaluation should include determination of the patient's underlying rhythm and interrogation of the device to determine programmed settings and battery status."

The ASA has written in its 2004 "Practice Advisory for the Perioperative Management of Patients with Cardiac Rhythm Management Devices: Pacemakers and Implantable Cardioverter/Defibrillators" that preoperative preparation should include: "(1) determining whether electromagnetic interference (EMI) is likely to occur during the planned procedure, (2) determining whether reprogramming the CRMD pacemaking function to an asynchronous pacing mode or disabling any special algorithms, including rate adaptive functions, is needed, (3) suspending anti-tachyarrhythmia functions if present, (4) advising the individual performing the procedure to consider use of a bipolar electrocautery system or ultrasonic (harmonic) scalpel to minimize potential adverse effects of EMI on the pulse generator or leads, (5) assuring the availability of temporary pacing and defibrillation equipment, and (6) evaluating the possible effects of anesthetic techniques on CRMD function and patient-CRMD interactions."

With many ICDs, it is not possible to know if a magnet has deactivated the device. It is essential to realize that patients who have procedures planned without the use of electrocautery or other EMI can have an ICD left in the "active" mode. However, if a shock is delivered by the device, the patient may move suddenly. If a sudden movement could cause surgical injury during a procedure (e.g., during an eye or middle ear operation), then this plan includes some risk.

CLINICAL CAVEAT: CARDIAC RHYTHM AND MANAGEMENT DEVICES (CRMDS)

The presence of pacemakers and ICDs is not a contraindication to ambulatory surgery per se. However, it is essential to thoroughly understand the device's operational characteristics and the implications of electromagnetic interference (especially electrosurgery) on device performance. Not all devices respond similarly to magnet placement, and this response may be programmable.

Patients with CRMDs take much more time to care for in the perioperative period. Each center should have guidelines about CRMDs to help decide if these patients are appropriate candidates for surgical care in that facility.

Other Implanted Devices

Advances in materials science and microelectronics have helped patients mend or replace a large number of body parts. Some replacement materials are simple, such as metal plates, screws, or prostheses. Others are complex electronic devices that often require consultation with technicians and engineers, not medical providers, to fully understand therapy interactions. The presence of such devices may become a problem while providing ambulatory anesthesia, especially office-based anesthesia, wherein there are limited ancillary technical personnel to help understand the perioperative implications. Anesthesiologists will encounter increasing numbers of patients with microelectronic devices that meet current or future medical needs (Box 2-1).

Any electrical device may interact with an implanted electronic device, even if it is not in direct contact with the patient. Anesthesiologists should check with the external device manufacturer for known EMI problems—the manufacturer may be the most reliable source

---

Box 2-1   Examples of Implanted Electronic Devices

Cardiac pacemakers and cardiac resynchronization therapy (CRT)
Implantable cardioverter/defibrillators (ICDs)
Arrhythmia loop recorders
Cardiac right ventricle pressure transducers (e.g., Medtronic Chronicle)
Spinal cord, deep brain, or peripheral nerve stimulators for pain, movement, and affective disorders
Vagal nerve stimulators for seizure disorders or depression
Cochlear implants
Urinary bladder neuro-control devices
Medication infusion pumps
Diaphragmatic pacemakers
Bone growth stimulators
Gastric stimulation systems (IGSs) for gastroparesis or obesity

of information—but should realize that manufacturers may not have case reports or clinical studies. They may conservatively recommend not using their device in the presence of implanted devices, if only for their own legal protection. Any central nervous system implanted lead or device may be dangerous to patients in the presence of EMI.

Bernards reported on intermittent airway compromise during anesthesia in a patient with a vagal nerve stimulator.[7] This points out that there may be other device-related events yet to be discovered.

Pregnancy

There is no definitive evidence that anesthesia is harmful to the developing fetus. However, health insurance data from Manitoba indicates that there is an increased risk of spontaneous abortion after surgery with general anesthesia, and information from the Swedish National Registry claims an increased risk of low-birth-weight infants and neonatal death. These data do not separate the effects of anesthesia from the effects of surgery. It is known that some surgeries, abdominal and pelvic surgeries in particular, have been associated with spontaneous abortions and preterm labor. Perioperative exposure to x-rays is known to be teratogenic. In addition, exposure to medications in the first trimester is usually considered undesirable, although many practitioners consider brief, short-acting anesthetic exposure to be insignificant. Nonetheless, nonessential surgery and anesthesia during pregnancy is usually avoided, and perhaps this is partly attributable to medico-legal concerns. Because of all of this, some ambulatory centers decline to provide elective surgical care for pregnant patients.

If pregnant patients are accepted, some centers choose to require that pregnancy be near term so that the fetus would be healthy and viable if labor commenced. On the other hand, since ambulatory centers are rarely prepared to deal with fetal monitoring or the precipitous delivery of a potentially viable premature infant, some centers forbid scheduling pregnant patients after the 20th week of gestation.

Malignant Hyperthermia

Since the risk of developing perioperative malignant hyperthermia (MH) is extremely low if a nontriggering anesthetic is given, even freestanding centers should be able to safely take care of patients who either have known MH or are MH-susceptible by family history. This ability presumes that the facility maintains an adequate supply of dantrolene and has the expertise and equipment to treat an MH episode. Prophylactic treatment with dantrolene is not indicated. The Malignant

---

CLINICAL CAVEAT: MALIGNANT HYPERTHERMIA (MH)

A personal or family history of MH susceptibility is not a contraindication to ambulatory surgery if nontriggering anesthetics are used and dantrolene is readily available. Extra time for recovery observation is indicated.

Hyperthermia Association of the United States (MHAUS) recommends an observation period before discharge home of 3 to 5 hours after an uneventful, nontriggering anesthetic. If a patient develops masseter spasm, MHAUS recommends overnight inpatient observation for temperature rise, myoglobinuria, elevated creatine kinase (CK) levels, or progression to an MH episode. Because of the complexity of treatment and the seriousness of an MH episode, there may be some centers that exclude these patients from outpatient surgical care.

Medications

Patients who use some chronic medications have been considered unsuitable for ambulatory surgery. One example is monoamine oxidase inhibitors (MAOIs), which may cause significant interactions with medications including meperidine, cocaine, and indirect-acting vasopressors. It was routine in the past to consider the potential hemodynamic effects as too dangerous for outpatients. It was recommended to discontinue these medications 2 to 3 weeks before surgery. However, the potential benefits of stopping MAOIs, or any chronically administered medication, must be weighed against the risks of discontinuation. For patients who take MAOIs as a last resort for intractable depression, these risks can be considerable. Many anesthesiologists now allow MAOIs to be continued up to the day of surgery for most outpatient procedures and simply avoid the use of drugs with serious interaction potential.

The use of so-called alternative, or herbal, medications continues to increase. Studies have shown that a significant proportion of patients use these nonprescription, nonstandardized drug preparations. In 1997, it was estimated that 12.1% of adults in the United States had used an herbal medicine in the previous year at a total cost of over $5 billion. To make matters more difficult, it may take pointed questioning to determine which patients are taking these drugs. Many patients may be reluctant to admit use of nontraditional substances.

Acute and chronic hepatic or renal toxicity is possible with these agents. Other adverse effects that may complicate the surgical and anesthetic experience include excessive bleeding or sedation. It is often difficult to know if the label completely or accurately indicates the active ingredients. Unknown contaminants or adulterants may complicate resulting physiological effects. Although the magnitude of the risk has not been quantified, most authorities recommend discontinuing alternative and herbal medications for 1 to 2 weeks before elective surgery and anesthesia. Each surgery center must decide what to do if patients arrive on the day of the procedure and admit to continued ingestion of these compounds.

Infected or Colonized Patients

Surgery centers should carefully consider their facility resources before deciding to care for infected patients. Simple incision and drainage of an infected abscess, for example, should not be a problem for an ambulatory center or office. However, patients with contagious illnesses, including diseases such as varicella-zoster, pertussis, influenza, tuberculosis, and viral gastroenteritis, may infect other patients and health care providers at the surgery center. Disseminated infections have caused surgery centers to be severely understaffed or even to shut down for weeks at a time (Table 2-1).

Providers should be aware of local contagious outbreaks and should take into account expected incubation times after patient or provider exposure. It is always useful to quiz patients or parents about recent family illnesses.

After exposure to persons infected with pertussis, the incubation period is usually 7 to 10 days, although it can range from 4 to 21 days before symptoms start.

For varicella-zoster, the incubation period is usually 14 to 16 days; some cases occur as early as 9 or as late as 21 days after exposure. An individual is most contagious 1 to 2 days before the onset of the rash. However, the period of infectivity can last as long as 6 days after the

onset of lesions. Patients with varicella-zoster should have, at a minimum, all lesions dry and crusted over before consideration for surgery.

When infected with influenza, patients can begin spreading the virus 1 day before feeling ill. Adults can continue to infect others for another 3 to 7 days after symptoms start. Children can be contagious for up to 10 days. Patients are symptomatic starting 1 to 4 days after the virus enters the body. Some people can be infected and contagious with influenza but be asymptomatic.

Many different viruses can cause debilitating acute gastroenteritis, including caliciviruses, rotaviruses, adenoviruses, astroviruses, and others. Caliciviruses (including Norwalk agent) account for more than 90% of outbreaks of acute gastroenteritis in the United States for all age groups, whereas rotaviruses are the most common cause in infants and toddlers. These extremely contagious agents should not be taken lightly.

Another common childhood illness, hand-foot-and-mouth disease (HFMD), may be difficult to prevent. Exclusion of ill persons with stomatitis from this coxsackievirus- or enterovirus-caused disease may not totally prevent infection since the virus may be excreted for weeks after the symptoms have disappeared. In addition, some people who excrete the virus, including most adults, may have no symptoms. Postponing patients with active signs of infection is, however, probably beneficial in reducing spread.

This is in contrast to fifth disease (*erythema infectiosum*). Patients infected with this causative agent, parvovirus B19, are contagious during the early febrile illness and before actual signs of rash appear. By the time children have the characteristic "slapped cheek" rash of fifth disease, they are probably no longer contagious and

Table 2-1 Some Endemic Contagious Diseases		
Disease	Incubation Period (days)	Infectious Period
Measles	7–18	5 days after rash appears
Mumps	12–25	Several days before to 9 days after start of parotitis
Pertussis	6–20	21 days after cough starts, or 6 days after start of antibiotics
Rubella	14–23	10 days before to 15 days after rash appears
Varicella-zoster	15 (9–21)	2 days before lesions appear, continuing until lesions are crusted and dry
Hand-foot-and-mouth	3–7	Weeks after start of illness. Adults may excrete virus but be asymptomatic
Fifth disease	4–21	During incubation before rash, but usually not after rash appears
Influenza	1–4	1 day before symptoms appear and up to 7 days after
Calicivirus (including Norwalk agent)	1–2	~3 days (1 day to weeks)
Rotavirus	2	~4 days (2–7 days)

may even return to school or a child care center. Other skin-rash-associated illnesses, such as measles, differ in that they are contagious during the time the patient displays the rash.

Children with an upper respiratory illness (URI) may present with a broad range of signs and symptoms. Common signs of a significant illness include fever, purulent rhinitis, productive cough, and rales or rhonchi on auscultation. These patients should be postponed at least until resolution of lower respiratory signs. Tait et al found that in children with active URIs or recent URIs (i.e., within 4 weeks) and in asymptomatic children, there were no differences in the incidences of laryngospasm and bronchospasm.[8] He did find that children with active or recent URIs had significantly more episodes of breath-holding, major desaturation (oxygen saturation <90%) events, and a greater incidence of overall adverse respiratory events than children with no URIs. Schreiner found that URIs were associated with an increased risk of laryngospasm, especially when cared for by inexperienced anesthesia providers.[9] Several findings (see the Clinical Caveat: Conditions Promoting Respiratory Complications in Children with a URI) are claimed to be predictive of respiratory complications in children with a URI. Unfortunately, postponing a procedure for at least 4 to 6 weeks may be needed to significantly reduce complication risks. Because the respiratory outcomes in most reports did not lead to long-term adverse outcomes, many maintain that otherwise healthy children with mild URIs can be safely managed without the need to postpone many surgeries.

Antimicrobial-resistant organisms, including methicillin-resistant *Staphylococcus aureus* (MRSA) and vancomycin-resistant enterococcus (VRE), have become very difficult clinical management problems. If patients are colonized or infected with these organisms, the Center for Disease Control (CDC) recommends standard procedures to avoid cross-contamination. In addition, they suggest placing a patient with an antimicrobial- resistant infection in a private room to minimize the chance of spread to other patients. Although

---

CLINICAL CAVEAT: CONDITIONS PROMOTING RESPIRATORY COMPLICATIONS IN CHILDREN WITH A URI

Endotracheal intubation
Environmental cigarette smoke exposure
Nasal congestion
Secretions and cough
History of reactive airway disease
History of prematurity (birth <37 weeks)

CLINICAL CAVEAT: THE ANESTHESIOLOGIST'S ROLE IN PATIENT SELECTION

Anesthesiologists are the medical providers best equipped to consider the factors of facility, procedure, patient, and practitioner in order to determine whether surgical patients can be cared for safely in an ambulatory environment. In this situation, anesthesiologists must assume the role of complete perioperative physicians.

---

the CDC maintains that universal precautions to prevent the spread of nosocomial infections should be sufficient, surgery centers may want to consider the OR suite schedule before deciding where to place these patients. It may be more efficient to schedule these patients at the end of the case list.

SUMMARY

Patient selection remains a major factor in preserving the safety of ambulatory surgery and anesthesia. Although surgery centers continue to expand their list of acceptable patient types, careful consideration should be given to patient risks as they relate to the venue of care.

CASE STUDY

A 51-year-old white male presents for right knee arthroscopy for degenerative changes. He has a past medical history significant for chronic stable angina, hypertension, chronic obstructive pulmonary disease (COPD), obesity, and mild sleep apnea without treatment. He had a right inguinal hernia 5 years ago without complications. His medications include oral metoprolol, hydrochlorothiazide, and inhaled albuterol, as needed. He has no allergies. He quit smoking 8 years ago. On exam, his blood pressure is 135/86, his pulse is 70, his respiratory rate is 20, and his room-air oxygen saturation is 95%. He weighs 120 kg and is 70 inches tall. He has a Mallampati class II airway with a thyromental distance of 7 cm and a normal neck range of motion. His chest exam is normal. ECG shows sinus rhythm with nonspecific S-T changes inferiorly. Chest x-ray shows no acute disease but indicates mild cardiomegaly.

On further questioning, you discover he is active and has mild chest pain with moderate exertion about once a week, and this has been occurring for about 3 years, is unchanged, and is relieved by rest. He is followed by his family doctor and a cardiologist on a regular basis; both say that he is medically optimized. Cardiac catheterization 1 year ago showed an occluded right coronary artery with good collateral flow and an ejection fraction of 50%. He rarely uses his nebulizer

(Continued)

CASE STUDY—Cont'd

and has not used it in 3 months. The patient refuses regional anesthesia and desires general anesthesia.

Other Information: The ambulatory facility is a four-OR freestanding surgery center in a small city that also contains a 200-bed community hospital. The patient lives 35 miles away and intends to go home the night following surgery. He will be cared for by his wife and son. You are very familiar with the orthopedic surgeon, and he is someone who you have worked with for many years. The anesthesia care will be provided by an anesthesiologist.

Response: The patient is an ASA 3 with several medical problems. They are all in optimal condition except for mild sleep apnea and obesity. The anesthesiologist could also ask the surgeon to do this procedure with moderate-to-deep propofol sedation and intra-articular local anesthetic. If the patient does well with general anesthesia or sedation and he continues to be asymptomatic and without episodes of airway obstruction during an extended recovery observation, he can be discharged home if opioid requirements are minimal. Femoral nerve block, local anesthesia, and nonsteroidal anti-inflammatory drugs (NSAIDs) are all options to minimize systemic opioids.

Anesthesiologists are the medical providers best equipped to consider the factors of facility, procedure, patient, and practitioner in order to determine whether surgical patients can be cared for safely in the ambulatory surgical environment.

REFERENCES

1. Chung F, Mezei G, Tong D: Pre-existing medical conditions as predictors of adverse events in day-case surgery. Br J Anaesth 83:262–270, 1999.

2. Warner DO, Warner MA, Barnes RD, et al: Perioperative respiratory complications in patients with asthma. Anesthesiol 85(3): 460–467, 1996.

3. Practice Guidelines for Management of Patients with Obstructive Sleep Apena. http://www.asahq.org/publicationsAndServices/sleepapnea103105.pdf

4. Coté, CJ: The upper respiratory tract infection (URI) dilemma: Fear of a complication or litigation? Anesthesiol 95(2):283–285, 2001.

5. Fleisher LA, Pasternak LR, Herbert R, et al: Inpatient hospital admission and death after outpatient surgery in elderly patients: Importance of patients and system characteristics and location of care. Arch Surg 139(1):67–72, 2004.

6. ACC/AHA/SCAI 2005 Guideline Update for Percutaneous Coronary Intervention: Summary article: A report of the American College of Cardiology/American Heart Association Tast Force on practice guidelines. Circulation 113:156–175, 2006.

7. Bernards CM: An unusual cause of airway obstruction during general anesthesia with a laryngeal mask airway. Anesthesiol 100:1017–1018, 2004.

8. Tait AR, Malviya S, Voepel-Lewis T, et al: Risk factors for perioperative adverse respiratory events in children with upper respiratory tract infections. Anesthesiology 95:299–306, 2001.

9. Schreiner MS, O'Hara I, Markakis DA, et al: Do children who experience laryngospasm have an increased risk of upper respiratory tract infection? Anesthesiol 85(3):475–480, 1996.

SUGGESTED READING

Atkins M, White J, Ahmed K: Day surgery and body mass index: results of a national survey. Anaesthesia 57:169–182, 2002.

Benumof JL: Obstructive sleep apnea in the adult obese patient: Implications for airway management. J Clin Anesth 13:144–156, 2001.

Brennan LJ: Modern day-case anaesthesia for children. Br J Anaesth 83:91–103, 1999.

Bryson GL, Chung F, Cox R, et al. (CAARE Group): Patient selection in ambulatory anesthesia—An evidenced-based review: Part I. Can J Anesth 51(8):768–781, 2004.

Bryson GL, Chung F, Cox R, et al. (CAARE Group): Patient selection in ambulatory anesthesia—An evidenced-based review: Part II. Can J Anesth 51(8):782–794, 2004.

Davies KE, Houghton K, Montgomery JE: Obesity and day-case surgery. Anaesthesia 56:1090–1115, 2001.

Friedman Z, Chung F, Wong DT: Ambulatory surgery adult patient selection criteria—a survey of Canadian anesthesiologists. Can J Anesth 51:437–443, 2004.

MacCallum PL, MacRae DL, Sukerman S, et al: Ambulatory adenotonsillectomy in children less than 5 years of age. J Otolaryngol 30:75–78, 2001.

Santos AC, O'Gorman DA, Finster M: "Obstetric Anesthesia." In Barash PG, Cullen BF, Stoelting RK (eds): Clinical Anesthesia, ed. 4. Philadelphia, Lippincott William & Wilkins, 2001, pp 1163–1167.

Stierer T, Fleisher LA: Challenging patients in an ambulatory setting. Anesthesiol Clin North America 21:243–261, 2003.

CHAPTER 3

Preoperative Evaluation of Ambulatory Surgery Patients

MICHAEL T. WALSH

JOHN A. DILGER

The preanesthesia evaluation is an essential aspect of anesthetic care and should be performed on all patients, independent of the type of surgery or the location. Although the extent of the evaluation for a 75-year-old undergoing repair of an aortic aneurysm might differ from that of a healthy 20-year-old having outpatient knee arthroscopy, the basic principles of preoperative evaluation are the same: defining the disease, directing tests and evaluations, optimizing the overall condition of the patient, and providing education and informed consent. The American Society of Anesthesiologists (ASA) has published a practice advisory concerning the preoperative evaluation process. This advisory places considerable emphasis on utilizing the patient's medical history and physical examination as the cornerstone of the preoperative evaluation. With this foundation, decisions can be made concerning needed testing or consultations. This is true for any patient, regardless of venue of anesthetic care.

EVALUATION SYSTEMS

Policy and process are basic issues in the preoperative evaluation of the ambulatory patient. Which patients must be personally evaluated and, importantly, where,

when, and by whom? It is impractical and probably unnecessary for an anesthesiologist to see and evaluate all patients several days prior to their outpatient surgeries. The time, resources, and cost of this approach would be prohibitive, especially since the anesthesiologist's evaluation is usually not reimbursed separately from the global anesthesia fee. Moreover, extensive preoperative evaluation is both inconvenient and unnecessary for healthy patients.

Therefore, patients should first be separated into groups on the basis of expected risk. The ASA evaluation advisory recognizes that healthy outpatients undergoing low-intensity surgery could be evaluated on the day of surgery. Sicker and more complex patients should be evaluated, at a minimum, several days ahead of elective surgery. The primary question is, how do we decide who needs more extensive evaluation? The answer resides in the appropriate use of the preoperative history and physical examination.

All patients scheduled for surgery are required to have a history and physical examination (H&P) prior to surgery. This is often performed by the surgeon, a nonphysician advanced-level provider, or the patient's primary physician. If these clinicians understand the anesthesia provider's guidelines for evaluation, the H&P may serve as an initial screening tool to triage patients into low- or high-risk groups. The utility of this screen is determined by specific provider medical knowledge, consistency of care, and the ability to communicate with anesthesia providers. Although surgeons should be motivated to reduce cancellations and delays on the day of surgery, the motivation to stay current with general medical knowledge varies greatly from surgeon to surgeon. In addition, primary or specialty medicine physicians have variable knowledge of surgical- and anesthesia-related issues. Anesthesiologists may receive medical evaluations ranging from extensive multi-page assessments to a brief (and inadequate) "cleared for surgery" scribbled on a prescription pad.

Only a high-quality preoperative H&P can appropriately guide additional tests and consultations. If anesthesiologists can give specific guidelines, education, and feedback to those performing the preoperative H&P, higher-risk patients can be identified early in the process. To do this well, there must be reasonable agreement and consistency among anesthesia providers at the surgical center in order to avoid large variability in patient evaluation and preparation. If an anesthesia group is not clear about expectations, the product of the process may be unacceptable. Additionally, it is important that anesthesiologists make themselves available to answer questions from medical and surgical personnel during the workup process. When appropriate, anesthesiologists should also take the time to personally examine patients with specific problems prior to the day of surgery. Finally, communication among providers is essential. Anesthesiologists need ready access to the H&P, medical records, and test results. In addition, anesthesiologists must be informed about significant patient issues far enough ahead of time to direct any needed changes in evaluation and preparation.

Unless all medical providers practice under one roof, the preoperative evaluation process may be fragmented over several geographic locations, inconveniencing the patient and making communication among providers more difficult. Traditional preoperative evaluation clinics are usually centralized and often have direct access to an anesthesiologist. These clinics may also be staffed by physician assistants, registered or advanced-practice nurses, internal medicine physicians, or certified registered nurse anesthetists (CRNAs). Preoperative clinics are popular in larger institutions that have the personnel and resources to devote to such an endeavor. Smaller enterprises, especially office-based practices, usually have more informal review mechanisms.

Preoperative Evaluation Clinics

Preoperative evaluation clinics often offer one-stop convenience for the patient and centralized information gathering for the anesthesiologist and surgeon. A clinic such as this greatly increases the likelihood that required testing and consultations are performed and results are available prior to the day of the procedure. Consistent and accurate preoperative information may be distributed to the patient, thereby decreasing tardiness, no-shows, and noncompliance with instructions. Several studies have shown that most day-of-surgery cancellations are due to NPO violations, acute illnesses, no-shows, and other patient-related factors that might be corrected with better patient education and compliance. Although the direct upfront costs of preoperative clinics are considerable, cost savings to the institution and health plans can be generated by decreasing unnecessary tests and minimizing costly delays and cancellations. Several authors have reported a roughly 50% reduction in delays by the use of a preoperative clinic. Cancellation rates also decline significantly after instituting a preanesthesia clinic.

Consistency in requirements and communication among providers are essential. It is critical that health status information and testing reports be available in a timely fashion. When a patient is evaluated and approved for anesthesia and surgery in the preanesthesia clinic, anesthesiologists should, with rare exceptions, be willing to accept the clinic evaluation and to proceed to anesthetize the patient. When anesthesiologists are willing to enter into this type of informal agreement, cancellation and postponement rates can be dramatically reduced—in one study, they were reduced by 87%.

Preanesthesia clinics effectively evaluate patients, but a clinic can be costly to staff and operate. Is there any way to triage patients ahead of time to determine which patients benefit most from the services of a preanesthesia clinic? Can we identify the healthy patient who can arrive on the day of surgery with minimal risk of delay or cancellation? Some maintain that, in the history and physical examination, the history portion is most important. However, there is obviously some information, such as general clinical impressions, undetected heart murmurs, or abnormal lung sounds, that cannot be elicited without an actual examination. How important is an isolated physical finding that is not associated with a symptom reported during an interview? This is not simply an academic question since it would be more efficient to obtain some elements of the history (by questionnaire, for example) prior to determining the need for an actual anesthesia clinic visit. There has been no specific study to answer this question. However, most clinicians find that, for most patients who are reasonably good at communicating symptoms, the history is more useful than the physical examination (Box 3-1).

Box 3-1   Options for Preoperative Patient Evaluation
Preoperative clinic visit Personal patient interview and examination Patient phone interview Hand-written patient questionnaire Review of medical records Internet or intranet patient questionnaire Day-of-surgery medical review

Questionnaires

Several types of questionnaires and different questioning methods have been devised. Written questionnaires are simple and inexpensive but offer no opportunity for individual interaction. Hilditch's group developed a written yes-or-no questionnaire and used it to screen patients for further evaluation.[1,2] Other groups have used a written questionnaire to direct nurse-led interviews. One disadvantage of the paper record is the limited dissemination and availability of the information across care locations. This can be a problem in a noncentralized care system.

Another type of questionnaire uses computer-based interviews, which can use answers to tailor subsequent questions. This can produce sophisticated algorithms and decision-based lines of questioning. Laboratory tests and consultations can then be automatically suggested based on a patient's answers and predetermined criteria. Patient-specific instructions can be programmed to immediately display on a screen at the end of the survey. Using the Internet, a computer-based questionnaire can be completed by the patient and reviewed by caregivers at a remote location. The original computer-based questionnaire was the "Health Quiz" from the University of Chicago. Recent variations on this theme include systems such as "HealthQuest" (Cleveland Clinic), "NetWellness" (University of Cincinnati, Case Western Reserve University, and Ohio State University), and "SmartSleep" (Boston Hospitals). Concerns about encryption and patient confidentiality need to be continually addressed in order to comply with Health Insurance Portability and Accountability Act (HIPAA) requirements.

The final questionnaire method is the phone interview. Although not the same as interviewing in person, it offers human interaction and adaptability. Limitations of the phone interview are the necessities of having the patient's current hard-wire or cellular phone number and contacting the patient at a mutually agreeable time. Patients could be instructed to call for the interview at their own convenience.

Whatever system is chosen, the goal is the same: a focused evaluation to define and optimize patient condition so that anesthesia and surgery can proceed without surprises, delays, cancellations, or unacceptable risk to the patient. Figure 3-1 shows a sample patient questionnaire.

Location of Surgery

What are the preanesthesia evaluation implications of the location of surgery? Is the patient a candidate for out-of-hospital surgical care? This decision is an integral part of the preanesthesia evaluation. Should this case be done in the office, in a freestanding ambulatory surgery center, or in a hospital-based surgery center? There is very little information in the literature to help us decide. Recently published data from Florida showed a tenfold increase in adverse incidents and deaths in the office-based setting compared to ambulatory surgery centers.[3] It is not known if these controversial findings are due to patient health issues, poor patient selection, poor procedure selection, or inadequate anesthetic or surgical care. It seems logical to match specific patients with specific surgical procedures and location resources. However, other inappropriate factors, especially economic ones, may sway the final decision.

Whatever system is used for patient evaluation prior to ambulatory surgery, careful attention to issues identified during the H&P will guide subsequent testing, additional evaluation, and preparation (Box 3-2).

CARDIOVASCULAR EVALUATION

Cardiovascular complications remain the primary cause of serious morbidity and mortality in the perioperative period, even in the ambulatory patient. A number of editorials, guidelines, and original studies on preoperative cardiac evaluation have been recently published. The American Heart Association and American College of Cardiology (AHA/ACC) published guidelines for preoperative cardiac evaluation in 2002. Like most guidelines, the recommendations varied according to the quality of the evidence available. Importantly, the history and physical examination played a central role in determining further workup. The goals of the cardiac evaluation mirror those of the general workup: defining disease, establishing its severity and stability, and documenting prior treatment.

The ACC panel found several other factors important in stratifying cardiac risk such as type of surgery, functional status, and comorbidities. They called these comorbidities "clinical predictors" and divided them into major, intermediate, and minor categories. Decision algorithms were developed based on these interconnected factors. When the issues are clear, decision-making is straightforward.

Box 3-2 ASA Task Force on Preoperative Assessment 2003

"The Task Force believes it is the obligation of the health care system to, at a minimum, provide pertinent information to the anesthesiologist for the appropriate assessment of the severity of medical condition of the patient and invasiveness of the proposed surgical procedure well in advance of the anticipated day of procedure for all elective patients."

Patient's Name _____ Age _____ Sex _____

Planned Operation _____ Date of Surgery _____

Surgeon _____ Primary Doctor _____ Here before: ☐ Yes ☐ No

Cardiologist? _____ When last seen: _____ Is your cardiologist at this institution? ☐ Yes ☐ No

Your height: _____ Your weight: _____ Your weight at age 21: _____

1. Please list **ALL OPERATIONS** (and approximate dates)

a. _____   d. _____

b. _____   e. _____

c. _____   f. _____

2. Please list any **ALLERGIES** to medicines, latex, or other (and your reaction to it)

a. _____   c. _____

b. _____   d. _____

3. Please list **ALL MEDICATIONS** you have taken in the last month (include OVER-THE-COUNTER drugs, inhalers, herbals, dietary supplements, vitamins, and aspirin)

Name of Drug	**Dose & Frequency**		**Name of Drug**	**Dose & Frequency**
a.		f.		
b.		g.		
c.		h.		
d.		i.		
e.		j.		

(Please check YES or NO and circle specific problems)   YES   NO

4. Have you taken steroids (prednisone or cortisone) in the last year?   ☐   ☐

5. Have you ever smoked? (quantify in _____ packs/day for _____ years)   ☐   ☐

    Do you still smoke?   ☐   ☐

    Do you drink alcohol? (if so, when was your last drink? _____)   ☐   ☐

    If so, have you ever had a problem drinking?   ☐   ☐

    Do you use any illegal drugs?   ☐   ☐

6. Can you walk up TWO flights of stairs without stopping?   ☐   ☐

7. When did you last walk up two flights of stairs _____ or walk 6 blocks without stopping _____ ?

8. Have you had any problems with your heart? **(circle)** (chest pain or pressure, heart attacks, abnormal EKG, skipped beats, heart murmur, palpitation, heart failure {fluid in the lungs}, require antibiotics before routine dental care)   ☐   ☐

9. Do you have or have you ever had high blood pressure?   ☐   ☐

10. Have you had any problems with your lungs or your chest? **(circle)** (shortness of breath, emphysema, bronchitis, asthma, TB, abnormal chest x-ray)   ☐   ☐

11. Are you ill or were you recently ill with a cold, fever, chills, flu, or productive cough?   ☐   ☐
    Describe recent changes

12. Have you or anyone in your family had serious bleeding problems? **(circle)** (prolonged bleeding from nosebleed, gums, tooth extractions, or surgery)   ☐   ☐

13. Have you had any problems with your blood (anemia, leukemia, sickle cell disease, blood clots, transfusions)? If yes, when?   ☐   ☐

14. Have you ever had problems with your: **(circle)**   ☐   ☐

    Liver (cirrhosis, hepatitis, jaundice)?   ☐   ☐

    Kidneys (stones, failure, dialysis)?   ☐   ☐

    Digestive system (frequent heartburn, hiatal hernia, stomach ulcer)?   ☐   ☐

    Back, neck or jaws (TMJ, rheumatoid arthritis)?   ☐   ☐

(Continued)

(Please check YES or NO and circle specific problems)	YES	NO
15. Have you ever had: **(circle)**		
Seizures, epilepsy, or fits?	☐	☐
Stroke; facial, leg, or arm weakness; difficulty speaking?	☐	☐
Cramping pain in your legs with walking?	☐	☐
Problems with hearing, vision, or memory?	☐	☐
16. Have you ever been treated for cancer with chemotherapy or radiation therapy? **(circle)**	☐	☐
17. Women: could you possibly (even remotely) be pregnant?	☐	☐
Last menstrual period began:		
18. Have you ever had problems with anesthesia or surgery? **(circle)** (severe nausea or vomiting, malignant hyperthermia (in blood relatives or self), prolonged drowsiness, anxiety, breathing difficulties)	☐	☐
19. Do you have any chipped or loose teeth, dentures, caps, bridgework, braces, problems opening your mouth, swallowing, or choking? **(circle)**	☐	☐
20. Do your physical abilities limit your daily activities?	☐	☐
21. Do you snore?	☐	☐
22. Please list any medical illnesses not noted above:		

_____

_____

23. Additional comments/questions for nurse or anesthesiologist

_____

_____

_____

Figure 3-1   A sample patient preoperative questionnaire. (From Roizen MF: Preoperative Evaluation. In Miller RD (ed): Miller's Anesthesia, 6th ed. Philadelphia, Elsevier/Churchill Livingstone, 2005.)

Patients with major clinical predictors of heart disease, such as unstable coronary syndromes or decompensated congestive heart failure (CHF), should have their surgeries delayed until further evaluation or testing is done. These patients are not candidates for elective surgery, neither as inpatients nor as outpatients. On the other end of the spectrum, patients with only minor (e.g., advanced age, uncontrolled hypertension [HTN], or abnormal electrocardiogram) or no clinical predictors who are undergoing low- or intermediate-risk surgery can go directly to the operating room without further cardiac workup (Figure 3-2).

The situation is more complicated in the group of patients with intermediate clinical predictors. In this group, the type of surgery and functional capacity must be considered in order to determine a course of action. Patients with intermediate clinical predictors such as mild stable angina, diabetes, or compensated CHF may need further noninvasive testing if they have poor functional capacity (<4 metabolic equivalents [METS]), if they are about to undergo high-risk surgical procedures, or both. If the surgical risk is low and the patient reports good exercise tolerance, surgery may proceed without further cardiac evaluation. A number of studies have shown decreased utilization of cardiac consultation and

stress testing when following these guidelines, but validation studies showing overall improved patient outcome are still needed. Several studies have looked at the number of at-risk patients identified during stress tests performed in accordance with AHA/ACC guidelines and have found a relatively low percentage (4.7% to 15%). However, even this low percentage may be worthwhile if serious complications can be avoided.

The updated AHA/ACC guidelines address a number of other areas including coronary revascularization, hypertension, and β-blocker therapy. The indications for preoperative coronary artery bypass grafting (CABG) are said to be independent of the need for elective noncardiac surgery. If a patient needs coronary bypass grafting for long-term improvement, then it should also be undertaken prior to elective surgery. CABG is almost never required solely to get a patient through elective surgery, especially ambulatory surgery.

There are very few data on preoperative percutaneous coronary angioplasty and on stenting being used to reduce perioperative cardiac morbidity. It is important to note that patients are actually at increased perioperative risk during the first 4 weeks post stent placement, when endothelialization of the stent is taking place. Drug-eluding stents may take much longer for endothelialization. Patients may be at increased risk for stent thrombosis up to 9 months after the procedure with these types of stents. Close cooperation with the patient's cardiologist is necessary to plan the safest care.

The AHA/ACC guidelines for hypertension recommend controlling Stage 3 hypertension (i.e., systemic blood pressure [SBP] ≥180 and diastolic blood pressure [DBP] ≥110) prior to elective surgery. They suggest several days to weeks of treatment preoperatively, but they do not specifically say that surgery should be canceled if Stage 3 hypertension exists on the morning of surgery. Recent reviews have noted the lack of strong outcome data to guide decision-making in this area, and several recent small studies suggest it may be safe to proceed. Previous studies supporting postponement suffer from small sample size or surrogate endpoints rather than actual morbidity. More important than the actual blood pressure number are the end-organ effects of hypertension. Common end-organ conditions include the presence of ventricular hypertrophy, diastolic dysfunction, CHF, and occult coronary artery and/or cerebrovascular disease.

Although hypertension itself is only a minor clinical predictor in the AHA/ACC guidelines, a serum creatinine level >2.0 ng/dL is an intermediate predictor. Finally, it is advised to not treat elevated blood pressures over aggressively. Diseased organs such as the kidney, heart, or brain may be used to, and quite dependent on, greater-than-normal perfusion pressure.

Current evidence supports the effectiveness of using β-blocker drugs for patients at risk for cardiac ischemia who are undergoing high-risk surgery. It is not clear, however, how long the therapy should be continued. It is also unclear if ambulatory patients undergoing low- to intermediate-risk surgery would benefit. As Auerbach and Goldman noted, given the overall low rate of events in the ambulatory surgery patient, it would be difficult to conduct a randomized trial to document any benefit, and it is unknown if outpatient β-blockade reduces cardiac risk.[4] Despite these reservations, almost all current recommendations from quality initiatives stress the use of β-blocker medications in patients at risk for cardiac ischemia. Engaging surgeons and internists in developing a workable protocol is essential.

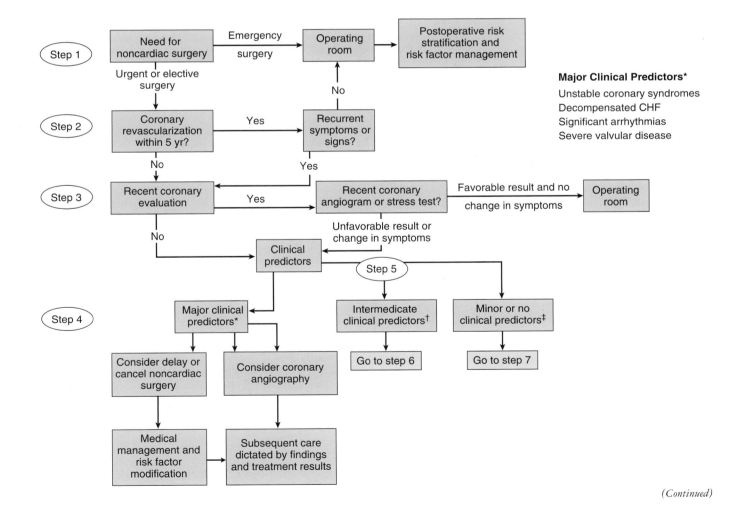

(Continued)

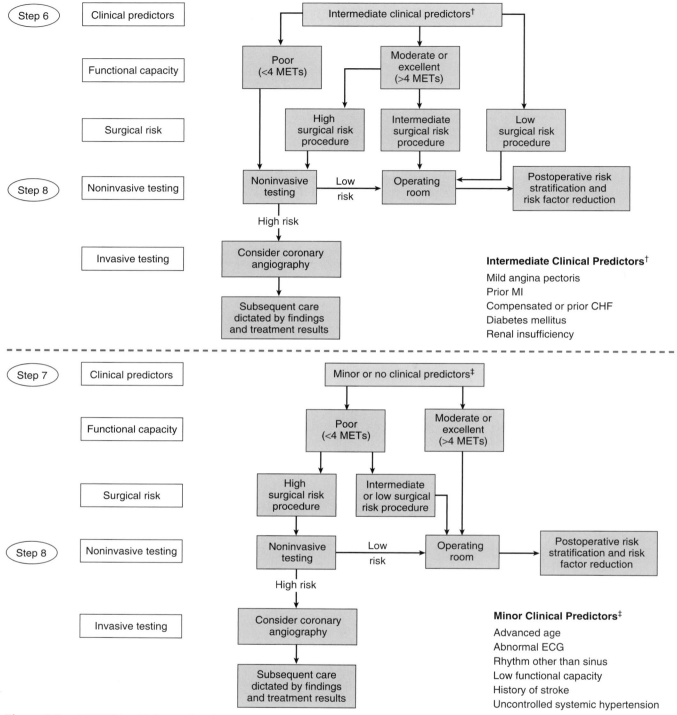

Figure 3-2   ACC/AHA guideline update for perioperative cardiovascular evaluation. CHF, Congestive heart failure; ECG, electrocardiogram; MET, metabolic equivalent; MI, myocardial infarction. (From Roizen MF, Fleisher LA:Anesthetic Implications of Concurrent Diseases. In Miller RD (ed):Miller's Anesthesia, 6th ed. Philadelphia, Elsevier/Churchill Livingstone, 2005. Redrawn from Eagle KA, Berger PB, Calkins H, et al:ACC/AHA guideline update for perioperative cardiovascular evaluation for noncardiac surgery—executive summary:A report of the American College of Cardiology/American Heart Association Task Force on Practice Guidelines [Committee to Update the 1996 Guidelines on Perioperative Cardiovascular Evaluation for Noncardiac Surgery]. J Am Coll Cardiol 39:542-553, 2002.)

PACEMAKERS AND DEFIBRILLATORS

More and more patients with pacemakers and implantable cardioverter/defibrillators (ICDs) are being scheduled for ambulatory surgery. In order to care for these patients, there must exist the capability to electronically interrogate the device during the preoperative and postoperative phases. Pacemaker patients can be operated on safely in a hospital-based facility and may be seen in freestanding ambulatory surgery centers or office facilities under special circumstances. There are wide variations in practice among surgeons and anesthesiologists regarding safe practices for patients with implanted devices. These are complex electronic devices with an increasing number of specialized features, including many that may be confusing. Minute ventilation sensors, rate-adaptive features, auto-capture cycles, and other features may cause what seems to be bizarre, but perfectly predictable, behavior. The facility should have, at a minimum, a way to pace or defibrillate the patient if necessary. If the procedure does not require monopolar electrosurgery, the possibility of electromagnetic interference (EMI) with pacemakers will be minimized. Prospective patients for the ambulatory setting should be otherwise medically stable, preferably not pacemaker-dependent, and should have access to pacemaker interrogation (Box 3-3).

Modern pacemakers are described by the North American Society of Pacing and Electrophysiology/British Pacing and Electrophysiology Group (NASPE/BPEG) codes with a five-letter code indicating chamber-paced, chamber-sensed, response to a sensed electrical activity, rate modulation or responsiveness, and multisite functions. The preoperative evaluation involves identifying the type of pacer, the indication for pacing, the date and status of the last pacer check, and the expected response to magnet placement.

EMI is a considerable concern during surgery. The response of a device can be variable and can include inappropriate inhibition, inappropriate triggering, circuit damage, or asynchronous pacing. Interference is minimized by the device having bipolar leads and the surgeon using bipolar electrocautery or using short bursts of monopolar cautery and placing the return electrode pad as far from the pacemaker as possible. A magnet placed on the pacemaker will usually initiate an asynchronous mode, but it may also result in no change or even loss of pacing altogether. It is critically important to define the magnet response at the preoperative check. Temporary transvenous or transthoracic pacing may be necessary and should be immediately available. Many modern defibrillators are equipped with transthoracic pacing capabilities, and this should be standard equipment in all office-based practices and ambulatory surgery centers. If there has been exposure to electromagnetic interference, the pacemaker should be rechecked postoperatively to ensure that it will function appropriately after the patient leaves the facility.

ICD patients usually have a number of medical problems and may require the immediate presence of a

---

Box 3-3 Preoperative Cardiac Device Questions and Issues

Does the patient have a device ID card, which shows the make, model, and serial number?

When was the last time the device was checked? What is the battery status? Is the device near its replacement time? (Replace it before an elective procedure!)

Why does the patient have the device? How long has it been there?

Identify the number and types of lead wires.

For pacemakers, is patient hemodynamically dependent on device? Is there an underlying cardiac rhythm?

For ICDs, what is the shock history?

What is the hemodynamic response to electrical pacing? (Do all pacing "spikes" on ECG cause peripheral pulses?)

What are the programming parameters? (Usually found on printout from interrogation)

Does the device have rate modulation biosensors?

What will happen when a magnet is applied? Is the response programmable? (e.g., Is the magnet ignored? Is the response a fixed rate? Does the device shut off, and, if so, for how long?)

Should the device be reprogrammed prior to procedure?

What heart rate will be appropriate to meet metabolic demands for the procedure?

Are a defibrillator and an external pacing device available in your facility?

Have you consulted a *knowledgeable* cardiologist and the device manufacturer concerning recommendations?

Reinterrogate the device after the procedure to ensure proper functioning and battery life if electromagnetic interference was present.

ALWAYS consult with a cardiologist if the patient has a device for long QT syndrome or cardiomyopathy or is a pediatric patient.

programmer to turn the ICD off prior to surgery and to restart the ICD immediately following surgery. The ICD should usually be turned off during surgery to prevent inadvertent discharge caused by electromagnetic interference. During this time, an alternative means for defibrillation should be readily available. If there will, with certainty, be no source of EMI, the ICD may be left activated, but thought should be given to possible patient injury if the ICD discharges, causing patient movement, during a critical portion of the surgical procedure.

The use of a magnet to inactivate an ICD is possible, but not without firm knowledge of the magnet's effect on the device and a way to confirm that the magnet is in exactly the correct position throughout the case. A magnet may not be the best solution to many device-related issues without careful consideration of the issues and extensive knowledge of the specific device.

The anesthesiologist or surgeon should always consult with a cardiologist who regularly deals with the device and the device's manufacturer before a planned procedure. In 2004, the ASA published the "Practice Advisory for the Perioperative Management of Patients with Cardiac Rhythm Management Devices (CRMDs): Pacemakers and Implantable Cardioverter/Defibrillators." It recommends that "(1) suspending antitachyarrhythmia functions if present, (2) advising the individual performing the procedure to consider use of a bipolar electrocautery system to minimize potential adverse effects of EMI on the pulse generator or leads, (3) assuring the availability of temporary pacing and defibrillation equipment, and (4) evaluating the possible effects of anesthetic techniques on CRMD function and patient-CRMD interactions are important steps in promoting patient safety and successfully managing patients with CRMDs."

PREOPERATIVE TESTS

Until the 1990s, preoperative laboratory evaluation entailed ordering a wide range of screening tests. This approach was done to ensure that nothing that could delay or cancel the procedure was overlooked. It was expensive but was rationalized by the potential beneficial effects of screening for disease. Currently, this approach has lost favor, and tests are ordered based on the findings of the history and physical examination.

Many studies support this targeted approach. Kaplan's group retrospectively looked at 2236 tests in 2000 patients and found that 65% were not indicated. Although 96 abnormal tests were found, only 10 of these were from the "no indication" group and few were clinically significant.[5]

Narr et al. reviewed screening tests on 3782 healthy patients and found only 4% of tests to be abnormal and none to be clinically significant.[6] After eliminating routine preoperative testing, their follow-up study found no morbidity or mortality in 1044 healthy patients who had been given no lab tests within 90 days of their procedure.

Even advanced age by itself does not appear to be an indication for preoperative laboratory testing. Dzankic et al. studied 544 patients of >70 years of age scheduled for noncardiac surgery with general or regional anesthesia[7] (48% of which were ASA III); 6.8% of all tests were abnormal, and creatinine (12%) and hemoglobin (10%) were most common. After multivariate logistic regression modeling, no abnormal test was a significant predictor of postoperative adverse events.

Schein's group prospectively studied 18,189 elderly patients for cataract surgery and divided them into "screening" tests versus "indicated" tests.[8] They found no difference in intra- or postoperative events or in cancellation rates between the two groups. This study generated considerable discussion and has been used to question the need for any preoperative evaluation for cataract surgery patients. Schein's study did not prove that preanesthesia evaluation is unnecessary in low-risk surgeries. In fact, all patients in the study were evaluated by their primary physician prior to surgery and did receive appropriate testing and evaluation consistent with their current medical condition. Nonspecific screening tests were not done, but appropriately focused medical testing was still performed. It has been stressed in the ASA Practice Advisory on Preoperative Evaluation that, although screening tests are discouraged, "preoperative testing in the presence of specific clinical characteristics" (i.e., symptoms and signs) remains appropriate (Table 3-1).

The elimination of screening preoperative testing has been extensively promoted. The ASA's current practice parameters on preoperative laboratory testing found the current literature ambiguous regarding all testing. Nonetheless, the consensus opinion is that routine pre-

Table 3-1	"Routine" Laboratory Results: Studies Reviewed for the ASA Practice Advisory for Preanesthesia Evaluation

Test	% Abnormal	% Clinically Significant
Hemoglobin	0.5–43.8	0–28.6
Coagulation	0.8–22.0	1.1–4.0
Potassium	1.5–12.8	N/A
Glucose	5.4–13.8	N/A
Urinalysis	0.7–38.0	2.3–100.0
Pregnancy	0.3–2.2	100.0

Routine test: A test ordered in absence of specific clinical indications
Clinical significant: Results of test lead to changes in clinical management

operative testing does not favorably contribute to preoperative assessment and management and, therefore, should be eliminated. Random screening tests may actually do more harm than good. Not only are the direct costs significant, but the indirect cost in repeat testing and further evaluation of false positive tests can be considerable. Some states still require some preoperative tests (e.g., glucose, hemoglobin, and creatinine). A few surgeons and internists still order tests based on misconceptions that they are hospital policy or are always required by the anesthesia group. Clear and consistent guidelines are needed within each organization to reduce unnecessary testing. However, the use of only indication-specific testing has increased the possibility that needed tests may be omitted if systems are not in place to review the evaluation before the day of surgery. Some centers do not rely on outside testing and instead use point-of-care laboratory testing done on the day of surgery.

One area of controversy is preoperative screening for pregnancy. Positive test results are uncommon, but not rare, with most studies quoting rates of 0.30% to 2.2%. The cost for screening is considerable, with estimates of $1050 to $7750 to detect each unsuspected positive result. Some anesthesiologists justify always obtaining a pregnancy test because a positive result may have profound effects on anesthetic management and, more importantly, even the decision to proceed with surgery.

Further controversy involves mandatory testing, especially in adolescents who may be afraid to admit the possibility of pregnancy or may not understand the implications. A 1995 study demonstrated no positive tests in patients less than 15 years of age and recommended testing only menstruating women greater than age 15. With a higher proportion of today's adolescents engaging in sex at younger ages, this study may not be valid. There are significant medicolegal implications to testing minors; state laws differ on who should get the results (i.e., patient vs. parent). The medical provider should involve social services since the pregnancy may be the result of child abuse.

A medical and legal issue is fetal teratogenicity or fetal wastage as the result of exposure to perioperative medications or radiologic tests. Although there is no compelling evidence that anesthesia by itself is harmful to the fetus, most would delay elective surgery, especially in the first trimester. In most studies, elective surgery was cancelled upon discovery of a positive pregnancy test. Mandatory testing was often done in the past without the patient's knowledge. This is probably an unethical practice. Today, most anesthesiologists feel that, at the least, selective testing is warranted for some patients. There remain institutions that feel more comfortable requiring mandatory preoperative pregnancy testing for all females of childbearing years. It should be noted that the ASA practice advisory found insufficient evidence for universal testing on all premenopausal women and recommended considering testing in all female patients of childbearing age. They later clarified their position after concerns by the ethics committee to say that pregnancy tests should be offered but not required.

An interesting alternative to the ASA's practice recommendations is the United Kingdom's National Institute for Clinical Excellence (NICE) preoperative guideline. NICE (http://www.nice.org.uk) works on behalf of the United Kingdom National Health Service to develop practice consensus guides. Their guidelines and recommendations are more extensive and specific regarding patient condition and case type than are the ASA's guidelines. The NICE guidelines rely extensively on UK provider input (Box 3-4).

MORBID OBESITY AND OBSTRUCTIVE SLEEP APNEA

The alarming rise in obesity in the United States has had profound effects on the health of the population. According to the 2000 National Health and Nutrition Examination Survey, 30% of U.S. adults (59 million people) have a body mass index (BMI) >30. The anesthetic effects of obesity are profound, and preoperative evaluation should focus on the airway and any comorbid conditions. Obesity, especially around the face and neck, is associated with an increased incidence of difficult

---

CLINICAL CONTROVERSY: AGE AS A SOLE INDICATION FOR ECG?

Pros:
- Cardiac complications are the leading cause of serious morbidity and mortality
- Incidence of cardiac disease and abnormal ECGs increases with age
- Establishes baseline for comparison
- AHA/ACC guidelines recommend ECGs for males >45 and women >55 years of age
- ASA practice advisory makes no age-based recommendations

Cons:
- No evidence that screening ECG makes a difference in outcome
- No evidence that screening ECG makes a difference in clinical decision making
- Cost

Box 3-4 Considerations in Preoperative Testing Guidelines

ASA Practice Advisory
AHA/ACC Guidelines
NICE UK Guidelines
Consensus among anesthesia providers
Written (and disseminated) guidelines
Anesthesia/surgical service review of results of ordered tests ahead of surgery

---

CLINICAL CAVEAT: POTENTIAL PERIOPERATIVE PROBLEMS FOR THE MORBIDLY OBESE PATIENT

Difficult airway
Obstructive sleep apnea
Systemic and pulmonary hypertension
Congestive heart failure
Diabetes mellitus
Ischemic cardiac and vascular disease
Restrictive respiratory disease
Postoperative atelectasis
Deep vein thrombophlebitis and pulmonary emboli
Facility equipment inadequate for patient size and weight

---

intubations. In the ASA Closed Claims Data, obesity was a factor in 31% of difficult intubation claims (as opposed to only 14% of all other claims). Perhaps more important is an increased likelihood of difficult mask ventilation, increasing the possibility of the dreaded "can't intubate, can't ventilate" scenario. Difficulty with ventilation could lead to gastric insufflation and secondary pulmonary aspiration. Because of a greatly reduced functional residual capacity, apnea causes a rapid drop in oxygen saturation, which decreases available laryngoscopy time. Preoperative evaluation should also focus on common associated comorbidities such as hypertension, diabetes, asthma, and obstructive sleep apnea. There are no large controlled studies on same-day surgery and obesity. Early recommendations suggested limiting outpatient surgery to BMI <35, but a recent controversial small study reported no difference in complication rates or unplanned admissions between non-obese and obese patients. Except for specific limitations on equipment, carts, and operating tables, total weight or BMI may not be limiting factors for some day surgery centers. However, the presence of comorbid conditions such as coronary artery disease, chronic obstructive pulmonary disease (COPD), obstructive sleep apnea, and difficult airway may, by their presence, disqualify many obese patients. The morbidly obese patient will certainly be more labor intensive postoperatively, and office-based and freestanding surgery centers may elect to limit care to these patients on that basis alone.

Anesthesia for patients with obstructive sleep apnea (OSA) primarily involves airway concerns, and there is very little literature to guide recommendations. It is estimated that up to 5% of male adults in the United States have significant OSA, although most are undiagnosed. The workup begins with a history and physical examination and a high index of suspicion. Signs and symptoms of occult OSA include snoring, excessive daytime somnolence, and obesity. Many patients with sleep apnea are obese. However, whereas a BMI >35 increases the likelihood of sleep apnea, not all obese patients have sleep apnea. A sleep partner may observe episodes of choking and airway obstruction. It has been noted that a neck circumference >17 inches also has good prognostic value for OSA.

The gold standard for diagnosing OSA is the overnight sleep study or polysomnography. Ventilation sensors in pacemakers have recently been reported to record significant airway obstructive episodes and may be useful in diagnosis. The recorded number of apnea and hypoapnea episodes help stratify patients as mild, moderate, or severe. Episodes with cardiac arrhythmias and oxygen desaturation are also noted. Moderate to severe OSA patients may be referred for corrective airway surgery or may be given a trial on continuous positive airway pressure (CPAP), which can be titrated during polysomnography. The sleep test is time-consuming and expensive, however, and is not always covered by insurance. Most patients present with symptoms suspicious for OSA and have no documented sleep study.

It is not known if formally diagnosing and treating patients with OSA before outpatient surgery affects outcome. It may influence patient selection. Some centers will not perform surgery on severe OSA patients on an outpatient basis, but there are no controlled studies to support this policy. It is known that OSA is associated with several conditions of concern, including obesity, hypertension, congestive heart failure, arrhythmias, and gastroesophageal reflux. OSA may increase the likelihood of difficult intubation, but it is not clear if this increased risk is due solely to OSA or if obesity, a large tongue, or a thick neck plays the predominant role. The ASA has formed a task force to examine the issues surrounding OSA and anesthesia with the goal of providing practice recommendations.

PEDIATRIC PREOPERATIVE EVALUATION

Preoperative evaluation of the ambulatory pediatric patient follows the same basic process as exists for adult patients (i.e., a history and physical followed by directed laboratory testing and consultations) with the same caveats and limitations. A preoperative clinic strategy may be useful in identifying high-risk patients for further evaluation. Issues of particular importance in pediatric ambulatory anesthetic evaluation are upper respiratory tract infections, heart murmurs, and the lowest safe-age limit for ambulatory surgery. The risk of apnea following anesthesia in former premature infants has been well-described, and current recommendations for overnight observation range from 50 to 60 weeks postconceptual age. The "safe" age for any individual patient will depend on the postconceptual age at birth, perinatal medical problems, postbirth intubation and ventilation, subsequent growth, the presence of anemia, and any history of apnea-bradycardia.

The pediatric perioperative cardiac arrest (POCA) data suggest an increased risk of anesthesia for children less than 1 year of age, and limiting selection to children over 1 year of age may be a reasonable policy for centers in which care of children is not a routine practice. Whatever the cutoff policy, it is important that age-appropriate equipment and personnel are available. Although most accrediting bodies require such age-specific equipment and personnel, not all ambulatory or office-based surgery facilities are required to be accredited in all states.

In 1979, McGill's group reported on pediatric airway complications, and found that 10 of 11 of their cases had experienced a recent upper respiratory tract infection (URTI).[9] Other studies in the 1980s echoed these findings and saw increased complications for up to 4 weeks after a URTI. It became common practice to cancel surgery and to wait 4 to 6 weeks after a URTI. This was often a problem because by then the odds were good that the child would have acquired another URTI. It was important to reexamine this practice because many practitioners did not believe it added safety. In addition, cancellations are the bane of an ambulatory surgery center's existence. They disrupt the family's schedule and the surgery schedule, and they create great inefficiencies in the system.

Tait and Knight were the first to challenge the URTI dogma when they prospectively studied 489 children scheduled for myringotomy who had a current or recent URTI.[10] They found no increased airway complications, but, importantly, these patients were not intubated. The authors went on to study those factors that increased airway complications during or immediately following a URTI. Not surprisingly, the presence of an endotracheal tube, a history of asthma, home smoke exposure, and copious secretions were risk factors. Children with medical conditions, OSA, or underlying airway surgery also seem to be at increased risk. Most airway complications (e.g., cough, bronchospasm, and blood oxygen desaturation) were relatively mild and easily treated. Other studies have confirmed these findings.

The current practice for a mild URTI, therefore, is to inform the patient or parent of the issues, to proceed with minor to moderate surgery, to avoid an endotracheal tube when possible, and to treat complications as they arise. If the child is acutely ill with signs and symptoms of purulent rhinitis, a fever, a productive cough, or evidence of lower respiratory tract involvement (including wheezing), surgery should be postponed and rescheduled in several weeks, depending on the duration and severity of illness.

Heart murmurs in children are common and are usually innocent flow murmurs. Innocent murmurs are typically medium-pitched in quality and systolic in timing. They may be vibratory but should not radiate. These murmurs are completely normal in children and usually do not require further evaluation. Pathologic murmurs, on the other hand, are usually harsh, loud, and are associated with other abnormal heart sounds. They may occur during systole; however, diastolic or constant murmurs should always be considered pathologic. Previously undiagnosed pathologic murmurs need further evaluation and require postponement of elective surgery. How easy is it to tell the difference? In one study, Canadian academic pediatricians missed 18% of pathologic murmurs. U.S. community pediatricians and pediatric residents fared even worse. Pediatric cardiologists are very accurate in their assessments and likely could eliminate the need for an echocardiographic study. Indications to delay surgery and to request consultation include, in children, easy fatigability, failure to thrive, poor feeding, and age of less than 1 year, and, in adolescents, palpitations during exercise.

PREOPERATIVE INSTRUCTIONS

A thorough preoperative evaluation does more than generate information about patients for use by physicians. It also offers an opportunity to convey information to the patient. A preoperative interview and educational session can help allay anxiety and set the foundation for informed consent. Information should include instructions about preoperative eating and drinking (i.e., nothing by mouth [NPO]) rules, medications to continue or hold, and important safeguards such as driving prohibition and adult supervision. The ASA has published guidelines for oral intake. These recommend withholding clear liquids for 2 hours, breast milk for 4 hours, light meals for 6 hours, and heavy and fatty meals for at least 8 hours prior to surgery. These guidelines are intended for otherwise healthy patients and have become generally accepted minimum times. For a busy outpatient facility, the NPO policy may include an hour or so of buffer in order to increase scheduling flexibility. Including a buffer time allows the option to move up scheduled cases and to avoid the inefficiencies of an empty operating room. For most healthy adult patients, the practice of allowing clear liquids up to 3 hours and solids up to 8 hours is neither unrealistic nor punitive.

In general, patients are encouraged to take their usual medications with small sips of water on the morning of surgery. Several medications have a significant impact on anesthesia and surgery and deserve special emphasis. Most antihypertensive drugs, β-blockers in particular, should be continued until surgery. There is controversy regarding continuing day-of-surgery angiotensin-converting enzyme inhibitor (ACEI) and angiotensin receptor blocker (ARB) drugs. There are anecdotal reports of refractory hypotension after induction of anesthesia in patients taking these medications on the day of surgery. Although there is little evidence-based consensus, it is common to hold ACEIs and ARBs on the morning of surgery. Monoamine oxidase inhibitors (MAOIs) are no longer routinely discontinued prior to surgery. Although the possibility of interaction with anesthetic and vasopressor medications still exists, the risks of withholding these medications for 2 to 4 weeks prior to surgery may outweigh the risks of continuation. The indication for the MAOI should be carefully considered before discontinuation.

Patients with diabetes mellitus need special attention to avoid the consequences of hypo- or hyperglycemia. In general, oral hypoglycemic agents are held the morning of surgery and are restarted once the patient resumes oral intake. Insulin-dependent diabetics have several choices, depending on time of surgery and overall glycemic control. One approach is to hold all short-acting insulin and to administer half of the dose of intermediate-acting insulin on the morning of surgery. Administering insulin without eating can result in hypoglycemia, especially if surgery is scheduled in the afternoon. Hypoglycemia can be minimized by offering a light meal 6 hours prior to surgery. Another option is to hold all insulin on the morning of surgery. The patient's blood glucose is then checked upon arrival to the facility and either half the usual neutral protamine Hagedorn (NPH) insulin dose or incremental amounts of regular insulin are administered subcutaneously as needed. This approach may increase the risk of hyperglycemia, or even ketosis, on occasion. Some patients may be instructed to take their usual amount of basal long-acting insulin glargine the night before or the morning of surgery.

Ultimately, the choice of preoperative insulin management will depend on physician preference, tailored to the individual patient and also to the brittleness of the disease. Whatever approach is chosen, every effort should be made to schedule diabetic patients early in the morning and to return them to regular oral intake and their usual insulin regimen as soon as possible.

Patients on insulin pumps are usually keenly aware and highly involved in all aspects of their diabetic care. Patients usually decrease their basal rate during fasting hours according to their endocrinologist's instructions. Frequent measurements and glucose-containing intervenous (IV) maintenance fluids may be all that are necessary for most patients.

Diabetes is associated with a number of comorbid conditions including cardiovascular, renal, gastrointestinal, and neuropathic diseases. Preoperative evaluation of the diabetic patient should focus on these areas.

HERBAL MEDICATIONS

A number of recent reviews have outlined the issues in the perioperative use of herbal medications. Herbal medicine consumption has expanded tremendously within the last several years, with recent estimates of 32% to 37% of Americans using some sort of herbal therapy, with a 10% to 26% incidence of herbal use in preoperative patients. Crowe et al. found that 12% of their ambulatory surgery patients were taking herbal medications.[11] Most patients were unaware of any potential side effects, and 83% had not informed the surgical team. Other studies support this poor disclosure rate. In the United States, except for ephedrine-containing compounds, herbal medications are classified as dietary supplements and are not regulated by the Food and Drug Administration (FDA).

The quality and potency of the ingredients in each preparation varies from manufacturer to manufacturer and from batch to batch. Many incidents of adverse reactions and hundreds of deaths from the use of these preparations have been reported to the FDA. However, there are no controlled studies of anesthesia complications caused by herbal medicines. Most side effects and interactions can be divided into cardiovascular problems, bleeding, and prolongation of anesthesia. The ASA has published a pamphlet for patient and physician education on the interactions of herbal products and anesthesia. It advises patients to withhold herbals for 2 to 3 weeks before surgery, although some practices find that 1 week is just as effective and more practical. Some common herbal medications are discussed below.

Ephedra (ma huang), commonly used to promote weight loss, contains multiple drugs such as ephedrine, norephedrine, pseudoephedrine, and methylephedrine. Like ephedrine, it acts at β_1-, α_1-, and β_2-receptors by both direct and indirect stimulation. Perioperative use of ephedra can cause hypertension and tachycardia and may lead to myocardial infarction, stroke, or both. Long-

CASE STUDY

An anesthesiologist is considering entering the exciting world of office-based anesthesia. She is concerned about being pressured to do cases even when the patient is a poor candidate for outpatient surgery or was inadequately evaluated. She wants to develop a system to evaluate patients preoperatively in order to avoid inappropriate patients from presenting the day of surgery. Her strategy includes:

1. Educating the surgeons: She makes up a list of contraindications to surgery (AHA/ACC major clinical predictors) as well as potential red-flag conditions that she would like to know about ahead of time.

2. Collaborating with primary physicians: She tries to assemble a select group of internists and cardiologists with a particular interest in preoperative evaluation. She communicates her concerns and encourages smooth exchange of information.

3. Instituting a screening questionnaire: She implements a paper questionnaire consisting of 20 yes-or-no questions exploring exercise tolerance, anesthetic history, and systems review. After being scheduled for surgery, patients fill out the questionnaire, and it is faxed to the anesthesia office for review.

4. Using telephone interviews: Higher-risk patients, identified by screening methods above, are phone interviewed by the anesthesiologist prior to surgery.

5. Encouraging communication: She gives the surgery offices her cellular phone and pager numbers and encourages anyone with questions to call her. On specific occasions, arrangements can be made for her to personally see and evaluate the patient as needed.

By using these techniques, problems on the day of surgery are greatly reduced. It is essential to document and review the inevitable incidents of system failures for quality improvement efforts.

term therapy can cause sympathetic nervous system down-regulation, causing hemodynamic instability during surgery. If hypotension occurs, direct-acting sympathomimetic drugs may be more effective than indirect-acting drugs due to chronic depletion of norepinephrine stores. Finally, ephedra should not be used in conjunction with MAOIs since hypertension and hyperpyrexia may result, ultimately leading to coma. Although late in 2003 the FDA issued a rule banning manufacturers from distributing ephedrine-containing compounds in the United States, consumers may have stockpiled considerable amounts or may continue to import the drug.

Ginseng is another compound that can cause tachycardia or hypertension in the perioperative period.

Garlic has been shown to inhibit platelet aggregation, especially when combined with other platelet-inhibitor drugs.

The herb ginkgo inhibits platelet-activating factor, and there have been multiple reports attributing bleeding to its use.

Kava, an anxiolytic and sedative, and valerian, used to treat insomnia, have both been associated with potentiation of anesthetic and sedative effects.

Patients with mild to moderate depression taking Saint-John's-wort may experience delayed emergence. Saint-John's-wort has been shown to induce cytochrome P450, altering the metabolism of many perioperative medications including alfentanil, midazolam, lidocaine, warfarin, and calcium channel blockers.

Echinacea, a member of the daisy family, is used for prophylaxis and treatment of infections including the common cold. A number of studies have shown immunostimulation with echinacea. Patients on long-term therapy may be at increased risk for poor wound healing. Allergic reactions have been reported, with one case of anaphylaxis (Table 3-2).

SUMMARY

The timing and depth of the preoperative evaluation depend on the patient's overall health and the planned surgery. Most healthy outpatients can be evaluated by the anesthesiologist on the day of surgery. Each ambulatory surgery center needs to develop a system to identify patients who can safely have surgery and those patients with comorbidities who might benefit from more intensive evaluation and testing. The key to the evaluation process is the history and physical examination. The H&P is used to direct further testing and consultation. Further goals of an effective preanesthesia evaluation include preparing patients for anesthesia and surgery, avoiding surprises on the day of surgery, and identifying those patients who are inappropriate ambulatory surgery center or office surgery candidates.

Table 3-2   Drug Interactions: Herbal Medicine Side Effects

Herbs (Common Names)	Important Pharmacologic Effects	Perioperative Concerns	Preoperative Discontinuation
Echinacea Purple coneflower root	Activation of cell-mediated immunity	Allergic reactions Decreased effectiveness of immunosuppressants Potential for immunosuppression with long-term use	No data
Ephedra (ma huang)	Increased heart rate and blood pressure through direct and indirect sympathomimetic effects	Risk of myocardial ischemia and stroke from tachycardia and hypertension Ventricular arrhythmias with halothane Long-term use depletes endogenous catecholamines and may cause intraoperative hemodynamic instability Life-threatening interaction with MAO inhibitors	At least 24 hours before surgery
Garlic (ajo)	Inhibition of platelet aggregation (may be irreversible) Increased fibrinolysis Equivocal antihypertensive activity	May increase risk of bleeding, especially when combined with other medications that inhibit platelet aggregation	At least 7 days before surgery
Ginkgo (duck-foot tree, maidenhair tree, silver apricot)	Inhibition of platelet-activating factor	May increase risk of bleeding, especially when combined with other medications that inhibit platelet aggregation	At least 36 hours before surgery
Ginseng (American ginseng, Asian ginseng, Chinese ginseng, Korean ginseng)	Lowers blood glucose Inhibition of platelet aggregation (may be irreversible) Increased PT/PTT in animals Many other diverse effects	Hypoglycemia May increase risk of bleeding May decrease anticoagulant effect of warfarin	At least 7 days before surgery
Kava (awa, intoxicating pepper, kawa)	Sedation Anxiolysis	May increase sedative effect of anesthetics Ability to increase anesthetic requirements with long-term use unstudied	At least 24 hours before surgery
Saw palmetto (dwarf palm, sabal)	Inhibition of 5-α reductase Inhibition of cyclooxygenase	May increase risk of bleeding	No data
St. John's wort (amber, goat weed, hardhay, hypericum, Klamath weed)	Inhibition of neurotransmitter reuptake MAO inhibition is unlikely	Induction of cytochrome P450 enzymes, affecting cyclosporin, warfarin, steroids, and protease inhibitors and possibly affecting benzodiazepines, calcium channel blockers, and many other drugs Decreased serum digoxin levels Delayed emergence	At least 5 days before surgery
Valerian (all heal, garden heliotrope, vandal root)	Sedation	May increase sedative effect of anesthetics Benzodiazepine-like acute withdrawal May increase anesthetic requirements with long-term use	No data

MAO, Monoamine oxidase; PT, prothrombin time; PTT, partial thromboplastin time.

From Ang-Lee M, Yuan C, Moss J: Complementary and Alternative Therapies. In Miller RD (ed): Miller's Anesthesia, 6th Edition. Philadelphia, Elsevier/Churchill Livingstone, 2005, p 607.

REFERENCES

1. Hilditch WG, Asbury AJ, Crawford JM: Pre-operative screening: Criteria for referring to anaesthetists. Anaesthesia 58:117-124, 2003.

2. Hilditch WG, Asbury AJ, Jack E, McGrane S: Validation of a pre-anaesthetic screening questionnaire. Anesthesia 58:874-910, 2003.

3. Auerbach AD, Goldman L: β-blockers and reduction of cardiac events in noncardiac surgery, JAMA 287(11): 1435-1444, 2002.

4. Vila H, Soto R, Cantor AB, Mackey D: Comparative outcomes analysis of procedures performed in physician offices and ambulatory surgery centers. Arch Surg 138:991-995, 2003.

5. Kaplan EB, Sheiner LB, Boeckmann AJ, et al: The usefulness of preoperative laboratory screening, JAMA 253: 3576-3581, 1985.

6. Narr BJ, Hansen TR, Warner MA: Preoperative laboratory screening in healthy Mayo patients: Cost-effective elimination of tests and unchanged outcomes. Mayo Clinic Proceedings 66:155-159, 1991.

7. Dzankic S, Pastor D, Gonzalez C, Leung JM: The prevalence and predictive value of abnormal preoperative laboratory tests in elderly surgical patients. Anesth Analg 93:301-308, 2001.

8. Schein OD, Katz J, Bass EB, et al: The value of routine preoperative medical testing before cataract surgery. New Eng J Med 342:168-175, 2000.

9. McGill WA, Coveler LA, Epstein BS: Subacute upper respiratory infection in small children. Anesth Analg 58: 331-333, 1979.

10. Tait AR, Knight PR: The effects of general anesthesia on upper respiratory tract infections in children. Anesthesiol 67:930-935, 1987.

11. Crowe S, Fitzpatrick G, Jamaluddin MF: Use of herbal medications in ambulatory surgical patients. Anaesthesia 57:203-204, 2002.

SUGGESTED READING

American Society for Anesthesiologists Taskforce on Preanesthesia Evaluation: Practice advisory for preanesthesia evaluation. Anesthesiology 96:485-496, 2002.

Chung F, Mezei G, Tong D: Pre-existing medical conditions as predictors of adverse events in day-case surgery. Br J Anaesth 83:262-270, 1999.

Davies KE, Houghton K, Montgomery JE: Obesity and day-case surgery. Anaesthesia 56:1112-1115, 2001.

Eagle KA, Berger PB, Calkins H, et al: ACC/AHA guideline update for perioperative cardiovascular evaluation for noncardiac surgery—executive summary: A report of the American College of Cardiology/American Heart Association Task Force on Practice Guidelines (Committee to Update the 1996 Guidelines on Perioperative Cardiovascular Evaluation for Noncardiac Surgery). Anesth Analg 94:1052-1064, 2002.

Ferrari LR: Preoperative evaluation of pediatric surgical patients with multisystem considerations (Review Article). Anesth Analg 99:1058-1069, 2004.

Fleisher LA, Pasternak LR, Herbert R, Anderson GF: Inpatient hospital admission and death after outpatient surgery in elderly patients: Importance of patient and system characteristics and location of care. Arch Surg 139:67-72, 2004.

Flowerdew RM: Preanesthetic evaluation in private practice. Anesthesiol Clin North America 22:141-153, 2004.

Howell SJ, Sear JW, Foëx P: Hypertension, hypertensive heart disease and perioperative cardiac risk. Br J Anaesth 92:570-583, 2004.

Kam PCA, Liew S: Traditional Chinese herbal medicine and anaesthesia. Anaesthesia 57:1083-1089, 2002.

Loadsman JA, Hillman DR: Anaesthesia and sleep apnoea. Br J Anaesth 86:254-266, 2001.

Park KW: Preoperative cardiology consultation. Anesthesiology 98:754-762, 2003.

Salukhe TV, Dob D, Sutton R: Pacemakers and defibrillators: Anaesthetic implications. Br J Anaesth 93:95-104, 2004.

Stevens RD, Burri H, Tramèr MR: Pharmacologic myocardial protection in patients undergoing noncardiac surgery: A quantitative systematic review. Anesth Analg 97:623-633, 2003.

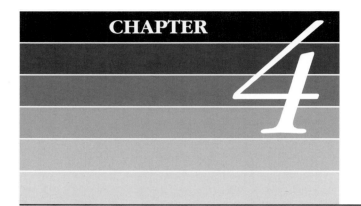

Short-Acting Intravenous Anesthetics

EVELYN LOOSE

TALMAGE D. EGAN

The outpatient anesthesia revolution of the last several decades was driven initially by economic concerns and, more recently, by advances in minimally invasive surgery. Perhaps the most important implication of the outpatient revolution for anesthesia practice has been the necessity to render patients "street ready" as soon as possible after the operation and anesthetic. For an outpatient procedure, the anesthetic technique should promote the rapid recovery of psychomotor function and the resumption of the activities of everyday living with a low incidence of adverse events that might delay or prevent discharge. Important primary goals are avoiding pain and postoperative nausea and vomiting (PONV).

The goal of this chapter is to review the use of total intravenous anesthesia (TIVA) techniques in outpatient anesthesia, with special emphasis on the clinical pharmacology of the short-acting intravenous agents remifentanil and propofol.

CLINICAL PHARMACOLOGY OF REMIFENTANIL

Remifentanil is the newest member of the fentanyl family of opioids. Remifentanil was approved by the U.S. Food and Drug Administration in 1996 and is now in widespread use internationally for a variety of anesthetic applications. In general, it shares most of the therapeutic and adverse effects of other fentanyl congeners, including analgesia and respiratory depression. Remifentanil's unique feature is its rapid onset of effect (i.e., rapid blood-brain equilibration) and similarly rapid offset. The pharmacokinetic and pharmacodynamic profile of this opioid makes it especially useful in situations in which rapid titration and predictable offset are essential.

METABOLISM

Remifentanil's short duration of action is a function of its esterase-based metabolism. Remifentanil is metabolized by nonspecific blood and tissue esterases. It is the rapid hydrolysis of the ester structure that leads to the fast dissipation of remifentanil's effects. Within the bloodstream, the main location for remifentanil's metabolism is inside the erythrocyte. The primary product of remifentanil's de-esterification is the acid metabolite GI 90291. Ninety percent of the drug is excreted in the urine in the form of this metabolite. Although the metabolite has very weak μ-agonist activity, for practical purposes, the metabolite is inactive even in patients with renal failure, in whom the metabolite accumulates.

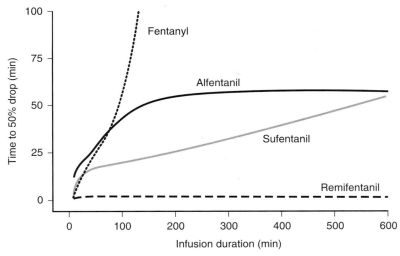

Figure 4-1   Context-sensitive half-times (CSHTs) of the fentanyl congeners. The CSHT is the time necessary to achieve a 50% decrease in plasma concentration after termination of a continuous infusion; see text for details. (Redrawn from Egan TD, Lemmens HJ, Fiest P, et al: The pharmacokinetics of the new short-acting opioid remifentanil (GI87084B) in healthy adult male volunteers. Anesthesiology 79:881–892, 1993.)

Pharmacokinetics

Remifentanil's rapid clearance and short duration of action are its distinguishing features. Remifentanil clearance is substantially greater than hepatic blood flow. This is consistent with extrahepatic metabolism. Perhaps the best way of contrasting remifentanil's pharmacokinetic profile with the previously marketed fentanyl congeners is by examining the context-sensitive half-time (CSHT) of this drug class. The CSHT is the time required to achieve a 50% decrease in plasma or effect-site concentration after termination of a steady-state infusion. Remifentanil's CSHT is approximately 4 to 5 minutes and is independent of the duration of infusion as shown in Figure 4-1. This is in contrast to the other fentanyl congeners, which exhibit much longer context-sensitive half-times. Therefore, even when administered at doses that produce profound opioid effect, remifentanil's effects will dissipate rapidly despite prolonged administration.

Pharmacodynamics

In terms of its therapeutic and adverse effects, remifentanil is indistinguishable from the other fentanyl congeners, with only a few exceptions. As shown in Table 4-1, remifentanil, like all other fentanyl congeners, can produce analgesia, sedation, respiratory and hemodynamic depression, pruritus, and muscle rigidity. Remifentanil's potency appears to be comparable to that of fentanyl, based on studies examining the ventilatory response to the rebreathing of carbon dioxide, the reduction of minimal alveolar concentration, and electroencephalographic slowing.

There are a few adverse effects that are unique to remifentanil when compared to the other fentanyl congeners. Perhaps the most important is the rapid dissipation in analgesia that occurs when a remifentanil infusion is terminated. For example, if a remifentanil infusion pump malfunctions or if the syringe supply of remifentanil runs dry without prompt detection, the opioid contribution to the anesthetic will quickly decline. Prevention of this potential problem requires careful diligence regarding the integrity of the remifentanil delivery system.

A related concern is the controversy surrounding acute opioid tolerance and hyperalgesia. This issue applies to all opioids but is likely more of a concern with opioids like remifentanil, which are typically used at higher concentrations.

Another important and unique adverse effect of remifentanil is a function of its formulation. Remifentanil is formulated with glycine, an important inhibitory neurotransmitter in the central nervous system of mammals. When remifentanil is introduced into the spinal fluid or epidural space of rodents, a reversible motor weakness occurs, which is thought to be due to the inhibitory neurotransmission effect of the glycine formulation. Therefore, neuraxial administration of remifentanil is contraindicated.

Because of remifentanil's esterase-dependent metabolic pathway, questions inevitably arise about prolonged effect in patients with pseudocholinesterase deficiency. Recent *in vitro* studies, as well as clinical reports, have confirmed that pseudocholinesterase deficiency does not affect the rate of remifentanil metabolism and, thus, dosage adjustment is unnecessary.

Table 4-1   Remifentanil Effects by Organ System

Organ System	Therapeutic Actions	Nontherapeutic Actions
Central nervous system	Analgesia, sedation, pain-related anxiolysis, and cough suppression	Lethargy, dysphoria, pruritus, dose-dependant muscle rigidity, and rare neuroexcitatory phenomena
Respiratory system	Depression of the upper airway and tracheal reflexes	Dose-dependant respiratory depression
Cardiovascular system	Blunting of hemodynamic reflexes to noxious stimulation	Bradycardia and hypotension
Endocrine system	Blunting of hormonal perioperative stress response	
Gastrointestinal system		Nausea and vomiting and delayed gastric emptying

Special Patient Populations

Knowledge of drug disposition and effect in special populations, such as patients with metabolic organ failure or the extremes of age or body habitus, is typically important in formulating optimal dosage strategies. For remifentanil, the main issues are body weight and age. Although patients with severe liver failure may exhibit greater effect from a given level of remifentanil, the drug's pharmacokinetics are not appreciably altered by hepatic insufficiency. Similarly, although remifentanil's acid metabolite accumulates in patients with impaired renal function, the metabolite is nearly 5000 times less potent than remifentanil and can be considered essentially inactive.

Remifentanil's central clearance and volume of distribution are decreased in the elderly population, and its potency increases with advancing age. Senior adults should generally receive one-half of the bolus dose and one-third of the infusion rate of younger individuals.

Remifentanil's pharmacokinetics do not appear to be appreciably different in children compared to those of adults. Remifentanil has been successfully used as a component of general anesthesia for a variety of pediatric anesthesia procedures. For example, it has been used during tonsillectomies to allow rapid tracheal extubation. It also has gained popularity in the setting of moderate and deep sedation, particularly in areas remote from the operating room in which intravenous anesthesia techniques are required.

Body weight is also an important consideration in the formulation of remifentanil dosage regimens. Absolute distribution volumes and clearances are similar in lean and obese patients. This means that dosing regimens based on total body weight (TBW) for obese patients will result in much higher remifentanil concentrations than regimes based on lean body mass (LBM). Obese patients do indeed require more remifentanil than lean patients, but they do not require nearly as much as would be suggested by TBW-based dosing.

Drug Combinations

There is a tremendous synergistic pharmacodynamic interaction between remifentanil and propofol (as well as other sedatives or hypnotics and volatile anesthetics) in terms of therapeutic actions and side effects. The quantitative and qualitative nature of this opioid-hypnotic interaction is perhaps the most important issue to consider when using these drugs in combination. In practical terms, the powerful pharmacodynamic synergism between remifentanil and propofol translates into a very substantial dosage reduction for both drugs.

For example, as shown in Figure 4-2, adding moderate levels of remifentanil (e.g., 5 ng/mL, which equates to a continuous infusion of about 0.2 μg/kg/min in a healthy adult) to levels of propofol that would normally be considered typical for sedation (e.g., 2 μg/mL, which equates to an infusion rate of about 70 μg/kg/min) dramatically changes the nature of the anesthetic, making the probability of no response to laryngoscopy shift from about 10% to nearly 100%. This powerful pharmacodynamic synergy means that relatively small doses of propofol and remifentanil, when combined, will produce general anesthesia, even though these doses of remifentanil and propofol, if used alone, would not produce a significant depth of anesthesia. Capitalizing on this pharmacodynamic synergy makes it possible to achieve general anesthesia with a very rapid recovery time. Small doses of the individual drugs are used so that concentrations of each drug fall to minimal levels very quickly.

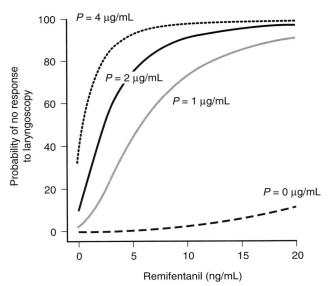

Figure 4-2 The remifentanil-propofol interaction: the probability of preventing movement or hemodynamic response to laryngoscopy. Relatively low concentrations of remifentanil substantially reduce the probability of responding to laryngoscopy at any given concentration of propofol. P, Propofol concentration. (Redrawn from Kern SE, Xie G, White JL, Egan TD: Opioid-hypnotic pharmacodynamic synergy: A response surface analysis of propofol-remifentanil pharmacodynamic interaction in volunteers. Anesthesiology 100:1373–1381, 2004.)

CLINICAL PHARMACOLOGY OF PROPOFOL

Perhaps more than any other innovation in this area, propofol revolutionized total intravenous anesthesia. Its popularity in clinical anesthesia is due to both pharmacokinetic and pharmacodynamic features. Whereas propofol is thought to share its primary mechanism of action (i.e., enhancement of the inhibitory effects of γ-aminobutyric acid [GABA] receptor activation) with many of the other intravenous induction agents, its pharmacodynamics are somehow different, for reasons that are not understood. Perhaps chief among these desirable pharmacodynamic properties are clearheadedness upon emergence from anesthesia and the antiemetic effect.

Metabolism

Propofol is primarily cleared by biotransformation in the liver to essentially inactive metabolites (e.g., glucuronides and sulfates). The observation that propofol's clearance is higher than hepatic blood flow provides evidence of extrahepatic metabolism, perhaps in the lung.

Pharmacokinetics

Propofol exhibits rapid blood-brain equilibration after bolus injection. The clinical implication of this rapid equilibration is that the onset of therapeutic effect after a propofol bolus is also very rapid (i.e., within 60 to 90 seconds). For sustained effect, propofol must be administered by continuous infusion. Its pharmacokinetic profile in this context is quite favorable compared to many of the other sedative-hypnotics, such as thiopental and methohexital. Its context-sensitive half-time is less than 15 minutes for infusions lasting less than 5 to 6 hours. This relatively short context-sensitive half-time is another reason for propofol's clinical popularity (Fig. 4-3).

Pharmacodynamics

Propofol's favorable pharmacodynamic profile is well known to clinicians and is probably the single biggest factor explaining its clinical popularity in ambulatory surgery. From a marketing perspective, propofol has been a remarkable success in anesthesia, and this is why there has been so much interest in the development of generic propofol formulations. Propofol is associated with less residual sedation than other sedative-hypnotic drugs. This type of recovery is especially useful after outpatient anesthesia. In addition to dose-related effects on consciousness (ranging from anxiolysis to general anesthesia), propofol has a number of nonhypnotic actions. For example, propofol has been used successfully as an antiemetic in subanesthetic doses. This feature is particularly appealing for outpatient anesthesia because the antiemetic properties persist even after the profound effects on consciousness have dissipated. In addition, propofol is known to have considerable antipruritic effects.

Propofol shares many of the adverse effects that are typical of the other sedative-hypnotics that act at the GABA receptor. For example, propofol produces dose-dependent hemodynamic and ventilatory depression. It is also occasionally associated with a variety of abnormal involuntary movements such as opisthotonos, choreoathetosis, and myoclonus.

The currently marketed propofol formulation has a number of undesirable properties that are, in part, a function of the lipid emulsion formulation and that deserve special mention. This lipid-based formulation frequently produces pain on injection and has also been associated with serious allergic reactions. In addition, because the lipid formulation supports rapid microbial growth, inadvertent contamination of the formulation can be a cause of life-threatening postoperative sepsis. There is substantial interest in the development of new formulations of propofol that are devoid of the undesirable features of the current formulation. A variety of alternative formulations, including a water-soluble prodrug, a water-soluble

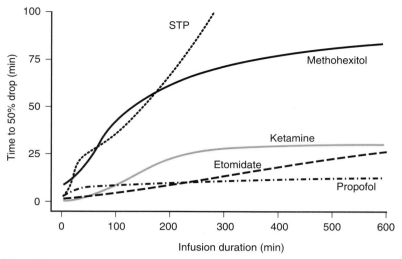

Figure 4-3   The context-sensitive half-times (CSHTs) of the common sedative-hypnotics. STP, Sodium thiopental. (Redrawn from Egan TD: Pharamacokinetics and Rational Intravenous Drug Selection and Administration in Anesthesia. In Lake CL, Rice L J, Sperry R J[eds]: Advances in Anesthesia, vol 12. St. Louis, Mosby, 1995, pp 363–388.

cyclodextrin-based formulation, and other lipid-based formulations, are under investigation.

Since propofol contains soybean oil, glycerol, and egg lecithin, a history of egg allergy has to be carefully considered but does not necessarily contraindicate its use. Most egg allergies involve reactions to the proteins in egg white, whereas egg lecithin is a phospholipid extracted from egg yolk.

Special Patient Populations

For propofol, the main issues of importance with regard to special populations are body weight and age. Moderate hepatic failure does not appear to alter dosing significantly, although reduced dosages are prudent in severely debilitated patients. Propofol metabolites accumulate in renal failure. However, evidence suggests that accumulation of metabolites is of little clinical significance.

The extremes of age, on the other hand, do play a prominent role in the formulation of rational dosing strategies for propofol. Elderly patients require less propofol, for both pharmacokinetic and pharmacodynamic reasons. The disposition and the potency of the drug are different in older adults. Pediatric patients, in contrast, require higher doses to achieve a given effect, at least in part because the clearance of the drug is greater.

Interestingly, propofol sedation of pediatric patients (and, rarely, of adults) in the intensive care unit has been associated with severe lactic acidosis (i.e., the so-called "propofol infusion syndrome"). Recognition of this problem has substantially curtailed the enthusiasm for propofol in prolonged pediatric sedation.

Similarly, as is true for most drugs, body habitus is also an important factor in the determination of propofol dosage. Propofol kinetics appear to be more closely related to lean body mass than to total body mass. This means that propofol dosing schemes should not be based on total body weight in the morbidly obese patient.

TOTAL INTRAVENOUS ANESTHESIA FOR AMBULATORY SURGERY

Total intravenous anesthesia (TIVA) using short-acting hypnotics and opioids has emerged as an attractive alternative to inhaled anesthesia in the setting of ambulatory anesthesia. It allows for rapid control of intraoperative stresses in a variety of surgical procedures as well as for faster recovery and less toxicity than when the individual drugs are used alone in higher doses. Although opioids are not a necessary component of TIVA, they provide analgesia and reduce the dose of the hypnotic, thereby improving hemodynamic stability and the speed of recovery. Several different combinations of hypnotic-analgesic agents have been used for TIVA, but remifentanil and propofol have emerged as a popular choice.

Propofol-Opioid Infusion

It is well known that opioids produce a marked reduction in the level of propofol required, and vice versa. This interaction is highly nonlinear. When the two drugs are combined, the clinical effect is greater than the sum of the effect of each drug alone. This is often termed "pharmacodynamic synergy." The substantial synergy that results when remifentanil and propofol are combined is the primary foundation for the formulation of rational dosing schemes. Practically speaking, loss of consciousness with propofol alone occurs at blood levels of about 3.5 μg/mL, versus levels as low as 1 μg/mL in the presence of moderate levels of opioids (i.e., a propofol dosage reduction of more than 50%).

Initial management of a total intravenous anesthetic will usually require bolus administration of the desired opioid to achieve adequate plasma levels. In the case of remifentanil, it is advisable to begin a continuous infusion before inducing general anesthesia to avoid inadequate levels of anesthetic depth during the critical time of induction and airway management. In the same manner, propofol will be initially administered as a bolus and then will be maintained as an infusion.

For TIVA, the literature suggests using remifentanil in a range between 0.2 and 0.4 μg/kg/min when combined with propofol. Although potent opioids will reduce the amount of propofol required for TIVA, the infusion rate of propofol should rarely be less than 75 μg/kg/min. Such low doses should be applied cautiously to assure adequate hypnosis and amnesia. Intraoperative noxious stimuli should be anticipated, requiring titration of the anesthetic agent. Changes in drug infusion rate and administration of additional boluses are often necessary.

An attempt should be made to find the lowest appropriate opioid/hypnotic concentration and to reduce infusion rates gradually toward the end of the anesthetic by 10% to 25%, without compromising anesthetic depth. Dosage reduction can usually be accomplished during skin closure because the prevailing surgical stimulus is typically less than it is earlier in the procedure.

With TIVA, muscle relaxation with neuromuscular blockers is often avoided unless it is required to facilitate the surgical procedure. Purposeful movement can then be used as a sign of inadequate anesthesia.

Higher opioid concentrations may be needed in hemodynamically unstable patients, whereas higher propofol concentrations may be beneficial to prevent nausea and vomiting postoperatively.

Emergence time from TIVA will depend on several factors, including the length of the surgery, the context-sensitive half-time of the drugs involved, and patient-specific covariates that affect drug disposition and effect.

When long-acting opioids are combined with propofol, the opioid concentration decay curve will be the major rate-limiting step in determining the speed of recovery. However, when propofol is used with the short-acting opioid remifentanil, propofol's pharmacokinetic profile plays a more prominent role in the speed of recovery. Emergence from anesthesia using a TIVA technique is usually characterized by excellent wake-up conditions. Patients are tolerant of the endotracheal tube, have clear senses, and have good analgesia. The patients usually experience minimal nausea and vomiting and appear to have the mild euphoria that is typical of propofol sedation.

Because of its short duration of action, the analgesic effect of remifentanil will have dissipated within 10 to 15 minutes after termination of the infusion, making the addition of longer-lasting opioids necessary to provide postoperative analgesia for moderately painful procedures. Establishment of postoperative analgesia should occur before the case is finished and could consist of longer acting opioids, nonopioid analgesics, peripheral nerve blocks, and infiltration of the surgical site with local anesthetic. A summary of a typical approach to TIVA in terms of dosing strategy can be found in Table 4-2.

Propofol-Ketamine Infusion

As an alternative to the combination of the propofol-opioid mixture, some practitioners have adopted the practice of using a propofol-ketamine mixture. Ketamine, used as a sole anesthetic, has strong analgesic and hypnotic properties. The analgesic effect is apparent at much lower concentrations than is its hypnotic effect. Ketamine can be used as an alternative to an opioid during a balanced anesthetic or propofol sedation. In order to avoid ketamine's undesirable effects of excessive sedation, increased postoperative nausea and vomiting, and adverse psychomimetic effects, it is important to use the lowest total dose necessary. When mixing the two drugs for an infusion, a final concentration of ketamine (1 to 1.8 mg/mL) in propofol appears to provide an optimum level of analgesia and sedation. When ketamine is used as a separate infusion, appropriate dosing is 15 to 45 μg/kg/hr. Psychomimetic emergence reactions can be greatly reduced by the concomitant use of benzodiazepines. Using subhypnotic concentrations of ketamine in combination with propofol can provide excellent analgesia without opioid-induced respiratory depression.

Economic Issues

Concerns regarding the cost of TIVA techniques inevitably arise. This is an area of considerable controversy. Drug acquisition costs for a TIVA technique are certainly higher than those associated with an inhalation

Table 4-2	**A Practical Approach to TIVA Dosing of Remifentanil and Propofol for General Anesthesia in Ambulatory Surgery**	
Induction	**Maintenance**	**Postoperative Pain**

Remifentanil:
• Bolus: 1-3 µg/kg
  or
• Infusion at higher rate:
  0.5-1 µg/kg/min during
  preoxygenation
	Remifentanil:
	• Continuous infusion:
	  0.1-0.3 µg/kg/min
		• 5-10 minutes before the end of surgery:
		  Fentanyl, 50-200 µg IV
		• 20-30 minutes before the end of surgery:
		  Morphine, 5-15 mg IV

Propofol:
• Bolus: 1.5-2 mg/kg
	Propofol or volatile gas:
	• Continuous infusion:
	  50-125 µg/kg/min
	• Volatile anesthetic:
	  0.5-0.8 MAC
		• Patients feasible for epidural anesthesia:
		  Epidural anesthesia and NSAIDs

anesthetic using generic anesthetic vapor and generic opioids. The advent of generic propofol formulations has mitigated the cost disadvantage associated with TIVA to some degree, especially when compared to newer inhaled anesthetics with low solubility (e.g., desflurane and sevoflurane). With TIVA, the typical patient will receive about 1 mg/hr of remifentanil. This equates to just under $10/hr for remifentanil, based on current average U.S. pricing.

Whether the additional cost connected with TIVA is cost-effective depends on how costs are computed and which clinical outcome priorities are deemed most important. If the only goal is to reduce drug acquisition costs, TIVA is typically inferior to inhaled techniques. If indirect costs are considered, a strong argument in support of TIVA can be made. In addition, if high patient satisfaction is a primary goal, TIVA may be very cost-effective.

Target-Controlled Infusion

Until recently, the most sophisticated delivery device for the administration of intravenous anesthetics was the standard calculator infusion pump, a device that enabled an accurate and precise delivery of fluid per unit of time. Used in both clinical and research settings, the physician operator of these devices simply specifies a delivery rate in terms of mg/hr or µg/kg/min. The patient-controlled analgesia machine is a hybrid of the calculator pump that permits patient control of opioid administration within physician-constrained parameters. The limitation of these calculator pumps is that they cannot predict drug pharmacokinetics.

Advances in pharmacologic modeling and infusion pump technology have now made it possible to administer injectable anesthetics by a computer-controlled infusion pump. By coding a pharmacokinetic model into a computer program and linking it to an electronic pump modified to accept computerized commands, the delivery of drugs is done according to specific pharmacokinetic parameters. The physician operating a target-controlled infusion (TCI) system designates a target blood concentration rather than specifying an infusion rate. The TCI system then calculates the necessary

---

CLINICAL CAVEAT: PROTOTYPE CASES FOR TIVA

• Orthopedic and general surgery procedures: offers required rapid progression of discharge eligibility (i.e., "street readiness")
• Plastic surgery: emphasizes reduced postoperative nausea and vomiting
• Brief deep sedation or general anesthesia for ophthalmologic procedures: promotes rapid return of patient cooperation after retrobulbar block placed

---

CLINICAL CONTROVERSY: COST-EFFICIENCY OF TIVA VERSUS INHALED TECHNIQUE

• Drug acquisition cost of TIVA techniques are higher as compared to inhaled techniques.
• TIVA may reduce staffing requirements in the postanesthesia care unit if fast-track clinical pathways are established to enable primary recovery bypass.
• TIVA may reduce the number of unanticipated admissions due to uncontrolled nausea and vomiting.
• Patient satisfaction with a TIVA technique is usually very high.

infusion rates to achieve the targeted concentration, as shown in Figure 4-4.

Borrowing from inhalation anesthesia concepts, TCI pumps make progress toward the concept of a vaporizer-like system for intravenous drugs. TCI addresses the fundamental limitation associated with delivering drugs directly into the circulation. Constant-rate infusions result in continuous drug uptake. TCI systems, in contrast, gradually decrease the rate of infusion based on the drug's known pharmacokinetic properties. The bolus, elimination, and transfer (BET) method used by a TCI pump takes into account the initial blood concentration after a bolus dose and the subsequent drug distribution and clearance during an infusion.

The TCI system changes the infusion rates at frequent intervals, sometimes as often as every 10 seconds.

Successful use of a TCI pump requires knowledge of the therapeutic concentrations appropriate for a specific clinical indication.

Computer-controlled drug delivery in the operating room is an exciting area with promising potential, particularly in ambulatory anesthesia. TCI systems are used in North America for research purposes. Sadly, unlike much of the world, they are not yet commercially available in the United States for routine clinical use.

SUGGESTED READING

Cox EH, Langemeijer MW, Gubbens-Stibbe JM, et al: The comparative pharmacodynamics of remifentanil and its metabolite, GR90291, in a rat electroencephalographic model. Anesthesiology 90:535–544, 1999.

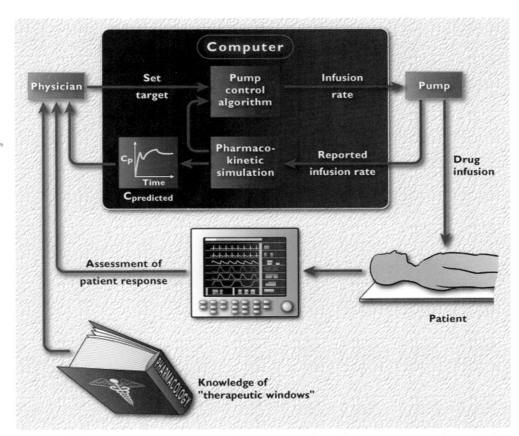

Figure 4-4   A schematic representation of a target-controlled infusion (TCI) system for anesthetic drugs. Based on knowledge of therapeutic windows, patient response, and the current prediction of drug concentration ($C_{predicted}$), the physician sets the anesthetic drug concentration target. Using a pharmacokinetic model for the drug, the computer calculates the appropriate infusion rates over time to achieve and maintain the target concentration, and then it directs the infusion pump to administer the appropriate amount of drug. The pump reports to the computer the amount of drug administered to the patient so that the computer's pharmacokinetic simulation of the current drug concentration can be updated and confirmed. (See text for details.) (Redrawn from Egan TD: Target-controlled drug delivery: Progress toward an intravenous "vaporizer" and automated anesthetic administration. Anesthesiology 99:1214–1219, 2003.)

Dexter F, Tinker JH: Comparisons between desflurane and isoflurane or propofol on time to following commands and time to discharge. A meta-analysis. Anesthesiology 83:77–82, 1995.

Egan TD: Target-controlled drug delivery: Progress toward an intravenous "vaporizer" and automated anesthetic administration. Anesthesiology 99:1214–1219, 2003.

Egan TD, Huizinga B, Gupta SK, et al: Remifentanil pharmacokinetics in obese versus lean patients. Anesthesiology 89:562–573, 1998.

Egan TD, Lemmens HJ, Fiset P, et al: The pharmacokinetics of the new short-acting opioid remifentanil (GI87084B) in healthy adult male volunteers. Anesthesiology 79:881–892, 1993.

Egan TD, Minto CF, Hermann DJ, et al: Remifentanil versus alfentanil: Comparative pharmacokinetics and pharmacodynamics in healthy adult male volunteers. Anesthesiology 84:821–833, 1996.

Egan TD, Shafer SL: Target-controlled infusions for intravenous anesthetics: Surfing USA not! Anesthesiology 99:1039–1041, 2003.

Fisher DM: Propofol in pediatrics. Lessons in pharmacokinetic modeling. Anesthesiology 80:2–5, 1994.

Hoke JF, Shlugman D, Dershwitz M, et al: Pharmacokinetics and pharmacodynamics of remifentanil in persons with renal failure compared with healthy volunteers. Anesthesiology 87:533–541, 1997.

Kern SE, Xie G, White JL, Egan TD: Opioid-hypnotic pharmacodynamic synergy: A response surface analysis of propofol-remifentanil pharmacodynamic interaction in volunteers. Anesthesiology 100:1373–1381, 2004.

Litman RS: Conscious sedation with remifentanil during painful medical procedures. J Pain Symptom Manage 19:468–471, 2000.

Manullang J, Egan TD: Remifentanil's effect is not prolonged in a patient with pseudocholinesterase deficiency. Anesth Analg 89:529–530, 1999.

Minto CF, Schnider TW, Shafer SL: Pharmacokinetics and pharmacodynamics of remifentanil. II. Model application. Anesthesiology 86:24–33, 1997.

Minto CF, Schnider TW, Egan TD, et al: Influence of age and gender on the pharmacokinetics and pharmacodynamics of remifentanil. I. Model development. Anesthesiology 86:10–23, 1997.

Nieuwenhuijs DJ, Olofsen E, Romberg RR, et al: Response surface modeling of remifentanil-propofol interaction on cardiorespiratory control and bispectral index. Anesthesiology 98:312–322, 2003.

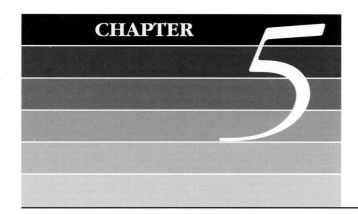

CHAPTER 5

Advances in General Anesthesia Techniques for Ambulatory Anesthesia

ELIZABETH S. YUN

GEORGE A. ARNDT

Over the past 20 years, ambulatory surgery has grown immensely in popularity, allowing patients to undergo many surgical procedures as outpatients. The challenge for the anesthesiologist is to plan a technique that allows patients to recover quickly with minimal side effects, thereby maintaining efficiency in the ambulatory setting. When general anesthesia is required, careful attention to each phase is important. The key steps of a successful general anesthetic technique are smooth induction, optimal surgical conditions with or without muscle relaxation, rapid emergence, and fast recovery with minimal side effects. Other important issues include safe control of the airway, amnesia during surgery, and postoperative analgesia management.

Several major advances in the past decade have helped anesthesiologists provide improved anesthesia conditions in the ambulatory setting. Two important advances include the development of drugs with short elimination half-lives and the introduction of new supraglottic airway management devices. Controversial issues,

such as the utility of depth-of-consciousness monitors, continue to be debated by anesthesia providers and the general public (Box 5-1).

INHALED VAPOR AGENTS

For the outpatient anesthetic practice, an ideal inhaled agent should have a rapid onset, should maintain patient cardiovascular stability, and should provide for rapid recovery. With these goals in mind, desflurane and sevoflurane were introduced in 1992 and 1994, respectively. Because of their low blood solubility, these drugs produce quick onset, rapid changes in depth of anesthesia, and short duration. Both have unique properties tailored to specific needs. Sevoflurane is often utilized for inhalation induction because of its relatively pleasant and nonirritating odor. Desflurane, as the most insoluble potent vapor, allows for the most rapid onset and emergence from anesthesia. Nitrous oxide, a gas that has

---

Box 5-1   Basic Goals of Outpatient Anesthesia

Management of preoperative anxiety
Airway management
Maintenance of anesthesia
Monitoring
Need for muscle relaxation balanced against potential complications
Rapid recovery from anesthesia
Prevention of postoperative nausea and vomiting
Management of minor and major side effects and complications
Providing good service to the patient and surgeon

been used for many years, is still popular in the ambulatory setting. It has a very low blood solubility, a low cost, and a long record of safety. Modern anesthesia machines (Figs. 5-1, 5-2) provide for compact and safe use of inhaled anesthetic agents in outpatient surgery centers and office-based practices. Yokes for two vaporizers are common on smaller machines.

The important choice often faced by anesthesiologists is which agent vaporizers to choose. Some practitioners choose to have both sevoflurane and desflurane vaporizers, with a spare isoflurane vaporizer available. Alternatively, either sevoflurane or desflurane may be the standard, and isoflurane may or may not be available.

Desflurane

Desflurane is a methyl ethyl ether. Because of fluorination, this drug has an increased vapor pressure that contributes to its low solubility and low potency. However, it would be unusable as an inhalation agent at room temperature. Therefore, a special vaporizer was designed to

heat and pressurize desflurane. The vapor can then be titrated precisely at room temperature. An undesirable property of desflurane is a pungent odor that may cause coughing and airway irritation. Because of this, desflurane is unlikely to be used for an inhalation induction.

The cardiovascular properties of desflurane are similar to isoflurane; desflurane causes a dose-dependent increase in heart rate and a dose-dependent decrease in mean arterial pressure and systemic vascular resistance. Sympathetic nervous activity may suddenly rise if the concentration of desflurane is rapidly increased. Degradation products are a concern with desflurane. When desflurane passes through a CO_2 absorbent, carbon monoxide may be formed when the CHF_2 group of desflurane reacts with high-pH material. Inhaled carbon monoxide may then produce carboxyhemoglobin. Factors that can influence this reaction in the absorber are dryness of the absorber, a high temperature of the absorber, a barium hydroxide lime absorber (recently withdrawn from the U.S. market), and a high gas flow. To prevent this breakdown process from occurring,

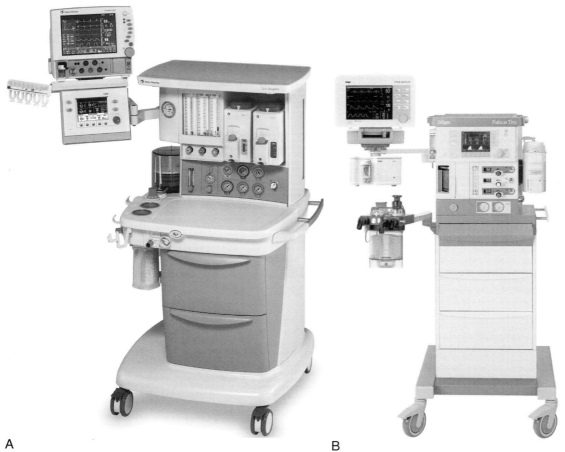

A   B

Figure 5-1   Modern compact anesthesia machines (not to equivalent scale). **A,** Aestiva. (Courtesy of Datex-Ohmeda GE, Madison, WI.) **B,** Fabius Tiro. (Courtesy of Dräger USA, Telford, PA.)

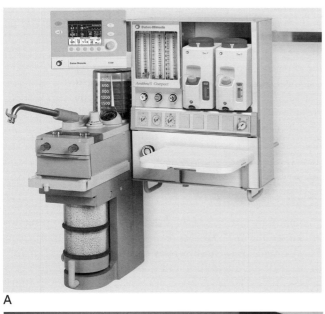

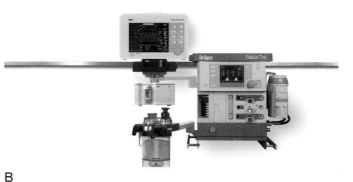

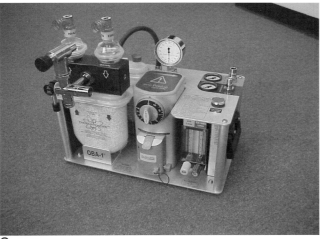

Figure 5-2   Wall-mounted or portable anesthesia machines for small operating rooms or offices. **A**, Aestiva. (Courtesy of Datex-Ohmeda GE, Madison, WI.) **B**, Fabius Tiro. (Courtesy of Dräger USA, Telford, PA.) **C**, OBA-1. (Courtesy of OBAMED, Inc., Louisville, KY.)

measures must be taken to prevent CO_2 absorbers from becoming desiccated, especially if the anesthesia machine is not used for several days (Table 5-1).

Sevoflurane

Sevoflurane is a fluorinated methyl isopropyl ether. Like desflurane, it shares a similar property of low solubility, thus allowing for rapid onset and rapid emergence. Unlike desflurane, its vapor pressure is similar to enflurane, and it

is delivered with a conventional vaporizer. Clinically, however, it is possible for end-tidal agent concentration to fall unexpectedly when the vaporizer is only one-third full.

Sevoflurane's clinical effects are more similar to those of isoflurane and halothane than to desflurane's. Like desflurane, sevoflurane causes a dose-dependent increase in heart rate and a dose-dependent decrease in mean arterial pressure and in systemic vascular resistance. Coronary vasodilation and sympathetic nervous system activation do not occur. Sevoflurane

Table 5-1 Advantages and Disadvantages of Desflurane	
Advantages	**Disadvantages**
1. Most rapid onset and emergence from general anesthesia	1. Requires an expensive heated vaporizer
2. Low cost at low flow	2. Pungent smell inappropriate for inhalation induction
3. Low solubility of all volatile agents	3. Potential airway irritant
	4. CO formation by reactive CO_2-absorbing material

Table 5-2 Advantages and Disadvantages of Sevoflurane	
Advantages	**Disadvantages**
1. Reliable inhalation and induction agent	1. Production of inorganic compounds from metabolism
2. Nonpungent odor	2. Need for minimal 1 L/min flow, not to exceed 2 MAC hours
3. Low solubility	3. Need to keep vaporizer full to work properly
4. Rapid onset and offset	
5. Does not cause arrhythmias	

CLINICAL CAVEAT: DESFLURANE

- A poor choice for inhalation induction due to its pungency
- May react with CO_2 absorbent to form carbon monoxide

also produces bronchodilation and a decrease in airway reactivity. Sevoflurane does not share halothane's tendency, especially in the presence of epinephrine, to cause cardiac arrhythmias. Unlike halothane, sevoflurane does not degrade to an acyl halide intermediate, an intermediate that has been implicated in an immune-mediated hepatotoxicity. Therefore, because of its inherent safety and its nonirritating odor, sevoflurane has become very popular for inhalation inductions in the pediatric population.

Sevoflurane is unique among inhalation agents in its metabolism and breakdown products. It is metabolized in the kidney into inorganic fluoride at higher concentrations than seen with other modern agents. Despite these higher levels, prolonged sevoflurane exposure does not lead to impaired renal function in patients. Sevoflurane has been safely administered to patients with chronic renal disease. Of more concern is the formation of Compound A as a result of the breakdown of sevoflurane. Compound A develops when sevoflurane reacts with CO_2 absorbers. Studies in rats have shown that Compound A is a dose-dependent nephrotoxin. However, in human studies, the amount of Compound A that formed with prolonged sevoflurane exposure was much less than the amount that caused nephrotoxicity. To help minimize the concentration of Compound A and to minimize the effect of fluoride metabolism, it is currently recommended (in the United States, but not in the United Kingdom) that sevoflurane not be used at less than 1 L/min flow for more than 2 MAC-hours (Table 5-2).

Nitrous Oxide

Nitrous oxide is an odorless gas. It has low potency and low blood solubility. Potent vapor concentrations may be reduced when nitrous oxide is also used because of its additive anesthetic effects. Nitrous oxide also possesses analgesic properties. Nitrous oxide, when used for extended periods of time, may inactivate vitamin B_{12}, leading to inactivation of enzymes including methionine synthetase and thymidylate synthetase. Reduced levels of these enzymes may impair myelin formation and deoxyribonucleic acid (DNA) repair, in addition to potentially causing bone marrow suppression and adverse neurologic effects. However, for routine surgical procedures, these are not likely to be a problem. Nitrous oxide also can cause the expansion of closed air spaces, including the inside of the gut. Nitrous oxide has been reported to increase the incidence of postoperative nausea and vomiting (Box 5-2).

INDUCTION OF ANESTHESIA

For adult outpatients, intravenous induction of anesthesia with propofol is common. Propofol offers rapid onset and emergence and has antiemetic properties. In contrast, inhalation induction has been less favored for adult patients due to concerns about patient acceptance

Box 5-2 Properties of Nitrous Oxide

Low potency requires a concentration of 70% nitrous oxide for clinical effect
Low solubility for rapid induction and emergence
Expansion of closed air space
Low cost

and duration of induction. Despite this, sevoflurane's low solubility makes it an acceptable agent for inhalation inductions. Some anesthesiologists favor inhalation inductions with this vapor versus an intervenous (IV) induction for all age groups.

During an inhalation induction, the concentration of sevoflurane can be progressively increased, or the single breath technique may be used. The anesthesia circuit is primed with 8% sevoflurane in nitrous oxide with oxygen at fresh gas flows of 8 L/min. This is sometimes called the "Eight and Eight technique." Patients are then coached to take a vital capacity breath: to exhale fully, then to inhale fully, and finally to hold their breath as long as possible. Loss of consciousness occurs in the first or second breath. Adverse airway events such as coughing or laryngospasm are risks of an inhalation induction. There were few airway events in a study examining airway insertion (of an endotracheal tube or a laryngeal mask airway) in healthy volunteers after sevoflurane induction. Breath-holding constituted the majority of undesirable events.

Several studies have compared an inhalation induction with sevoflurane to an IV induction using propofol for speed of induction, side effects, and patient satisfaction. In a study by Phillips et al. in 1999,[1] 56 patients were randomized to receive either an intravenous propofol induction or a sevoflurane inhalation induction. The results indicated that the inhalation induction was faster than the intravenous induction. During the inhalation induction, side effects included cough and hiccough. During intravenous induction, patients experienced more movement and hemodynamic changes. Recovery was about the same for both techniques, but patients who underwent an inhalation induction had a slightly higher incidence of postoperative nausea and vomiting. Patient satisfaction was the same for both groups. In terms of cost, using sevoflurane was less expensive than propofol, especially if fresh gas flows were kept at or below 4 L/min.

A meta-analysis by Joo et al. in 2000,[2] examining 12 studies from 1992 to 1999, compared propofol versus sevoflurane induction and time to insertion of a laryngeal mask airway. Both propofol and sevoflurane had no severe complications during induction. Sevoflurane had a higher first-time laryngeal mask insertion success rate and had fewer episodes of apnea compared to propofol.

CLINICAL CAVEAT: SEVOFLURANE

- Allows rapid and smooth inhalation induction of anesthesia
- Similar clinical properties to halothane, without many of halothane's side effects

---

Table 5-3	Advantages and Disadvantages of Sevoflurane-Inhaled Induction	

Advantages	Disadvantages
1. Rapid induction compared to halothane	1. Need to place an intravenous line after induction before airway is secured
2. No need for intravenous access for induction	2. May not be appropriate for claustrophobic patients
3. Low cost	3. Higher patient dissatisfaction

However, although no major statistical difference was noted, there was a higher trend of patient dissatisfaction with the sevoflurane technique. The reason for this difference is unclear; although inhalation inductions may be associated with patient claustrophobia from the mask, propofol inductions may be accompanied by significant pain on injection.

Another issue with sevoflurane is the higher incidence of postoperative nausea and vomiting. This complication would occur regardless of the induction technique used. All of the above studies conclude that although sevoflurane has potential issues that make it a less desirable induction agent compared to propofol, an inhalation induction with this drug is a safe alternative to IV induction. Other potential uses for inhalation inductions in the ambulatory setting could be sedation of a needle-phobic patient or of a patient with difficult intravenous access (Table 5-3).

MAINTENANCE AND RECOVERY

The key to a successful anesthesia plan in the ambulatory setting is to select the drug for maintenance of general anesthesia that will also produce a rapid emergence. For most practitioners, inhaled vapors remain a popular technique because of the ease of titration and monitoring compared to total intravenous anesthesia (TIVA).

There are many studies in the literature comparing sevoflurane, desflurane, and propofol for maintenance and emergence. The results have varied as to the drug that provides the fastest emergence and postoperative recovery. The most recent study to attempt to answer this question was a 2004 meta-analysis by Gupta et al. of articles from 1996 to 2002.[3] The analysis compared isoflurane, propofol, sevoflurane, and desflurane as individual agents and inhaled anesthetics versus TIVA as groups. Sevoflurane and desflurane were faster in terms of early recovery (defined as eye opening and following commands) compared to isoflurane and propofol. Desflurane had a more rapid early-recovery profile than sevoflurane. The statistical difference was small, however. This result might be surprising, considering the properties of sevoflurane and desflurane. It is possible that other drugs, such as neuromuscular blockers and opioids, delayed recovery.

Late recovery or "home-readiness" is defined as the time when patients are ready to be discharged home based on standard postanesthesia discharge criteria. In the Gupta paper, sevoflurane had an earlier home-readiness compared to isoflurane.[3] Home-readiness with propofol TIVA was not different compared with isoflurane. When comparing "home discharge" (the actual time patients left the hospital), patients receiving propofol infusion left the earliest. Despite this finding, it is true that many nonmedical factors, such as waiting for transportation home, affect real-world discharge times.

In a study comparing sevoflurane, desflurane, and propofol TIVA recovery profiles, patients receiving sevoflurane or desflurane for maintenance of anesthesia were eligible for discharge earlier from Phase 1 recovery compared with those patients receiving propofol. Despite this, patients receiving vapor agents did not actually leave the Phase 1 recovery area sooner than patients receiving propofol because of minimum stay rules. This indicates that patient discharge time depends not only on anesthetic technique but also on other unrelated issues.

Other factors need to be considered in selecting an anesthetic. The incidence of postoperative complications may vary with technique. The Gupta meta-analysis showed few side effects with either inhaled or intravenous techniques, but the major complication was postoperative nausea and vomiting.[2] In this report, propofol caused significantly less postoperative nausea and vomiting, and, not surprisingly, patients receiving inhaled agents needed more antiemetic therapy. However, there was no significant difference in nausea and vomiting between the propofol and the sevoflurane/desflurane groups in the time of discharge.

Cost is another important factor that must be taken into account during anesthetic technique selection. Whereas newer inhaled agents are expensive compared to older agents, the cost of their use is still less than that of propofol. A report by Visser in 2001[4] compared TIVA with propofol versus inhaled isoflurane/nitrous oxide. The authors noted that the cost of propofol was three times that of isoflurane. Although propofol did decrease the incidence of postoperative nausea and vomiting and patient recovery times, these benefits did not translate into economic savings for the patient and hospital. It was found that the major expense in postoperative recovery—personnel costs—was not affected. Thus, the cost of propofol may be relevant in the total cost of an outpatient surgery.

Therefore, in terms of anesthetic maintenance and recovery, both inhaled anesthetics and TIVA with propofol are equally safe and are equally associated with good outcomes. Inhaled anesthesia has a slightly faster recovery and a lower cost, but it has a higher incidence of postoperative nausea and vomiting. Total intravenous anesthesia with propofol is associated with less nausea and vomiting but has a slower recovery profile and a higher cost. The decision on technique will depend on cost-value judgments, available resources, training and experience, and the specific needs of the patient (Boxes 5-3, 5-4).

NEUROLOGIC MONITORING DURING MAINTENANCE OF AND EMERGENCE FROM ANESTHESIA

A major goal of ambulatory anesthesia is to provide rapid emergence and recovery without compromising patient care. However, determining the minimum amount of drug needed to provide anesthesia without risking intraoperative recall remains a challenge. Neuromonitors, such as the BIS (bispectral index) monitor and newer devices, are supposed to measure the level of CNS (central nervous system) depression by drugs. These monitors may be utilized by anesthesiologists to titrate anesthetic dosing during maintenance of and emergence from anesthesia.

The BIS monitor processes EEG (electroencephalogram) signals using a proprietary system. The BIS is designed as a monitor of the patient's responsiveness and explicit recall. It does not necessarily correspond with MAC or predict patient movement. The monitor generates a number between 0 and 100 to designate depth of anesthesia and is claimed to predict the

---

Box 5-3 Characteristics of Anesthesia Maintenance with Inhaled Agents

Lower drug costs
Faster recovery from anesthesia
Higher incidence of postoperative nausea and vomiting

Box 5-4 Characteristics of Anesthesia Maintenance with Intravenous Agents

Lower incidence of postoperative nausea and vomiting
Higher drug costs
Slower early recovery

possibility of awareness. This BIS number is generated from a proprietary algorithm using bispectral, power-spectral, and time-domain analysis. The algorithm was reportedly developed by monitoring sedation and anesthesia in patients receiving medications such as propofol, midazolam, isoflurane, midazolam-alfentanil, and propofol-nitrous oxide. It is claimed that a BIS number of 75 or less should predict lack of explicit recall in most patients.

In the ambulatory anesthesia setting, the BIS monitor has been used as a depth-of-anesthesia monitor to assist in titration of anesthetic agents. In a study by Song et al. in 1997, the amount of sevoflurane or desflurane was administered to patients based either on clinical signs or by maintaining the BIS number at 60. Both groups had no recall, but the BIS group used less anesthetic agent.[5]

Possible disadvantages with using the BIS monitor include issues of cost and efficacy. The monitor and electrodes add cost to each case; the company states that their proprietary disposable electrodes must be used with each patient. (An agreement to use these electrodes can reduce the initial acquisition price of the device.) A justification often given for using the BIS monitor is that it allows anesthesiologists to conserve propofol, sevoflurane, and desflurane by allowing precise titration. However, using generic propofol or achieving low fresh gas flows for vapor agents may produce considerable cost savings alone.

Also controversial is the device's efficacy. Although this monitor appears to decrease the already low rate of intraoperative recall, there is considerable interpatient variation in monitor readings. Additionally, the BIS does not reliably predict when the patient will respond to noxious stimuli. Monitor readings may vary depending on which anesthetic agent is used. Therefore, although the BIS monitor may have some role in the ambulatory anesthesia setting in terms of drug savings, its use as a depth-of-anesthesia monitor is not, as yet, universally accepted.

However, in 2004, the Joint Commission on Accreditation of Healthcare Organizations issued a safety alert and warned of possible patient awareness during general anesthesia, especially during outpatient anesthesia. What effect this will have on the spread of depth-of-anesthesia monitoring is unknown. Other newer neuromonitors, including the Everest Biomedical SNAP II, the Datex ABM Anesthesia and Brain Monitor, the Physiometrix 4000, and the Alaris Auditory Evoked Potential (AEP) monitor, have also been used to gauge intraoperative depth of anesthesia.

The newer SNAP II uses a range of standard EEG frequencies, as well as higher frequencies not usually recorded by the EEG. The company reports that this lowers response latency and improves accuracy over the use of standard EEG frequencies alone (Figs. 5-3, 5-4).

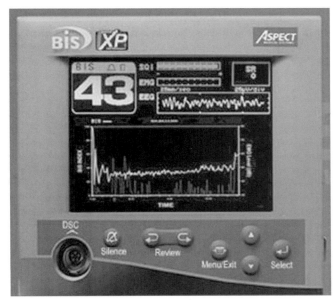

Figure 5-3   The Aspect BIS level-of-consciousness monitor. (Courtesy of Aspect Medical Systems, Inc.)

In a 2004 meta-analysis,[6] Liu concluded that the use of the BIS "modestly reduced anesthetic consumption, risk of nausea and vomiting, and recovery room time." However, there was no improvement in discharge time, and Liu felt that the cost of using this monitor more than offset any cost savings.[6]

On October 25, 2005, the American Society of Anesthesiologists (ASA) House of Delegates approved the *Practice Advisory for Intraoperative Awareness and*

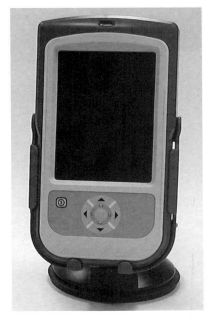

Figure 5-4   Everest Biomedical SNAP II level-of-consciousness monitor. (Courtesy of Everest Biomedical Instruments.)

CLINICAL CONTROVERSY: DEPTH-OF-ANESTHESIA MONITORS

- Used to titrate anesthetic drug dose
- May indicate risk of intraoperative awareness
- Individual variations exist in readings

CLINICAL CAVEAT: THE LARYNGEAL MASK AIRWAY (LMA)

- Possibly the most important development in airway management of the normal and the difficult airways
- Provides a conduit to the lung by the supraglottic airway, making an abutment joint with the glottic aperture

Brain Monitoring.[7] The advisory focuses on four areas of management: the preoperative evaluation, the preinduction phase, the use of intraoperative monitoring, and the postoperative care of a patient with intraoperative recall. The preoperative evaluation recommends screening for potential risk factors for intraoperative awareness, such as previous episodes of awareness, type of surgery (e.g., Cesarean section, trauma, cardiac surgery), history of substance abuse, possible difficult intubation, and ASA 4 and 5 status. Patients with these risk factors should be informed of the possibility of intraoperative awareness when circumstances permit. Before induction of anesthesia, the anesthesia delivery systems, especially infusion pumps and tubing, should be checked for proper function. The utility of using prophylactic amnesic medications, such as benzodiazepines, depends on the case and the patient. Detection of intraoperative awareness may be based on monitoring purposeful or reflex movement and conventional physiologic monitoring (e.g., electrocardiogram, blood pressure, heart rate). At this time, the advisory states that brain function monitors (BFMs) are not required during routine general anesthesia. Whether to use BFMs for specific cases or patients is left to the discretion of individual practitioners. If awareness does occur, the advisory recommends discussing the event with the patient, offering psychological support and counseling, and completing an occurrence report for quality improvement review. It should be noted that this advisory is a synthesis of opinion and consensus surveys. It is not considered standard of care or even a practice guideline. Therefore, it can be adopted, changed, or rejected by clinicians.

SUPRAGLOTTIC AIRWAY DEVICES

One of the most significant innovations over the past 20 years for outpatient anesthesia practice has been the invention and the widespread use of the laryngeal mask and other supraglottic airways. These have become a popular alternative to the use of an endotracheal tube or facemask ventilation for many types of cases. In this section, three common types of the laryngeal mask airway (LMA), the LMA Classic, the LMA ProSeal, and the LMA Fastrach, are described, as is their use in the ambulatory setting (Table 5-4).

The Classic Laryngeal Mask Airway

The LMA Classic was developed in 1983 as an alternative to the endotracheal tube. The inventor, Archie Brain, noted that an airway with a similar diameter to the trachea would provide better gas flow with less turbulence compared to two tubes of dissimilar diameters connected by inserting one inside the other. With this engineering principle in mind, the LMA consists of three parts: a large-bore airway tube with a standard 15-mm airway connector, a specially designed airway cuff with aperture bars and an inflation indicator balloon, and a valve that is used to inflate the cuff. The LMA is made of a silicone rubber material that is reusable and latex-free (Fig. 5-5).

The insertion of the LMA is simple. With one hand, the head is extended and the neck is flexed, thus opening the mouth. With the index finger of the other hand, the LMA is inserted so that the black line on the tube faces the upper lip and the mask aperture bars are face-forward. The index

Table 5-4	Types of Reusable LMAs and Uses			
LMA Airway Type	**Primary Use**	**PPV Limits**	**Adult Sizes**	**Pediatric Sizes**
LMA Classic	For routine cases	<20 cmH$_2$O	4, 5, 6	1, 1.5, 2, 2.5, 3
LMA ProSeal	For cases needing higher seal pressures, especially with PPV	<30 cm H$_2$O	4, 5	1.5, 2, 2.5, 3
LMA Flexible	For head and neck cases, especially eyes, ears, nose, and throat	<20 cmH$_2$O	4, 5, 6	2, 2.5, 3
LMA Fastrach	To facilitate endotracheal intubation	<20 cmH$_2$O	4, 5	3

PPV, Positive pressure ventilation. (Courtesy of LMA North America, Inc.)

finger guides the LMA in cranial direction along the hard and soft palate until resistance is felt. The cuff is then inflated to achieve an airtight seal (Figs. 5-6, 5-7, 5-8).

Because of its design, the LMA lies above the vocal cords, with its distal tip in the inferior recess of the hypopharynx, and is surrounded by the piriform fossa and the base of the tongue. It is usually easy to insert without muscle relaxation or laryngoscope blade. LMAs are usually associated with less postoperative sore throat than endotracheal tubes. Patients also tolerate an LMA at lower concentrations of anesthesia compared to an endotracheal tube.

An endotracheal tube (ETT) functions differently than the LMA. An ETT provides an airway by forming a coaxial joint within the trachea (i.e., a tube within a tube). This provides a very reliable and secure airway and acts as a stent to hold the vocal chords open. It has the inherent disadvantage of requiring, at times, considerable skill for placement. It requires instrumentation of the sensitive airway mucosa with a rigid laryngoscope and an ETT. Finally, placement of an ETT usually requires either a deep-plane anesthesia or muscle relaxation.

In contrast, an LMA works by forming an abutment connection. The LMA mask reliably places the airway tube

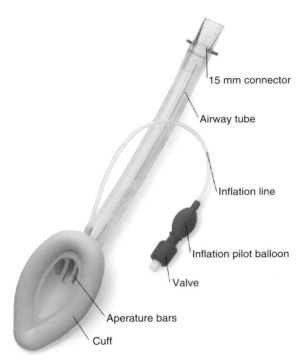

15 mm connector

Airway tube

Inflation line

Inflation pilot balloon

Valve

Aperature bars

Cuff

Figure 5-5   The LMA Classic. (Courtesy of LMA North America, Inc.)

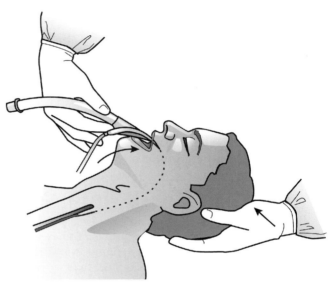

Figure 5-7   Initial insertion of the LMA Classic. (Courtesy of LMA North America, Inc.)

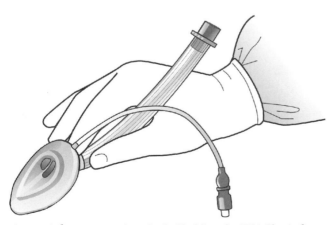

Figure 5-6   Suggested method of holding the LMA Classic for insertion. (Courtesy of LMA North America, Inc.)

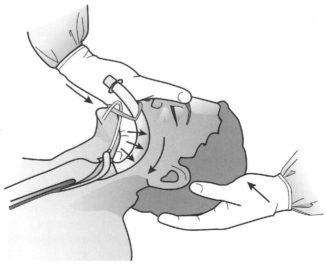

Figure 5-8   Final insertion of the LMA Classic. (Courtesy of LMA North America, Inc.)

Table 5-5	Advantages and Disadvantages of Supraglottic Airways
Advantages	**Disadvantages**
1. Easy to insert without special instrumentation	1. Gastrointestinal tract and airway are not separated as well
2. No muscle relaxants needed for insertion	2. Increased risk of aspiration
3. Maintenance of spontaneous ventilation	3. Less overall clinical utility than endotracheal tube in some clinical situations
4. Minimal instrumentation of the airway	
5. Excellent rescue airway for the difficult airway	

in proximity to the glottis, thereby making a continuous passage for respiratory gas into the trachea. This does not require use of muscle relaxant, and the plane of anesthesia is not quite as deep. Not only does it reduce stimulation of the airway, there is evidence that use of the LMA reduces the increase in postoperative laryngeal resistance that occurs with routine endotracheal intubation (Table 5-5).

Clinical Issues with Laryngeal Mask Airways

Some clinicians prefer not to use desflurane with LMAs. LMAs do not prevent laryngospasm or provide airway protection, as does an endotracheal tube, so an airway irritant such as desflurane may cause coughing or laryngospasm. However, in a study by Eshima et al. in 2003 that compared airway responses to sevoflurane and desflurane, both agents worked equally well with LMAs.[8]

Relative or absolute contraindications to the use of the LMA exist. Because the LMA does not isolate the trachea from the esophagus, patients are at a higher risk for the aspiration of gastric or oropharyngeal material. Many clinicians prefer not to routinely use the LMA in morbidly obese patients, in patients with delayed gastric emptying, in patients who have not fasted, and in pregnant patients over 14 weeks gestation. Additionally, the LMA creates a low-pressure seal with the trachea. Consequently, patients with decreased pulmonary compliance may not be successfully ventilated with an LMA. These disadvantages need to be considered when deciding to use an LMA.

It has been suggested that the LMA may provide major advantages over the endotracheal tube in terms of decreased anesthetic requirements and postoperative complications. A prospective randomized multicenter study by Joshi et al. from 1997 compared these two airway techniques in various outpatient surgeries.[9] The authors found that although volatile anesthetics requirements were similar

in both groups, less fentanyl was used in the LMA group. Postoperative complications were also similar in both groups, although there were significantly fewer sore throats among patients with the LMA than among those in the endotracheal group. Although LMA patients had a shorter stay in the recovery room, home-readiness was, again, similar for both groups. By avoiding nondepolarizing muscle relaxants, the use of the LMA proved to be less costly.

The ProSeal Laryngeal Mask Airway

Although the LMA Classic has many advantages, it is possible to have a malpositioned LMA and still to be able to provide adequate gas exchange. However, despite adequate ventilation, there may be an increased risk of regurgitation and aspiration. To address this problem, the LMA ProSeal (LMA PS) was created. Its most important feature is a drainage tube integrated into the LMA. This tube has its opening at the distal end of the cuff. When positioned properly, the drain tube sits above the upper esophageal sphincter and provides, if necessary, for venting of the stomach. An oral gastric tube can also be placed through the drain tube blindly, thus allowing for suctioning of gastric contents. Other features of the

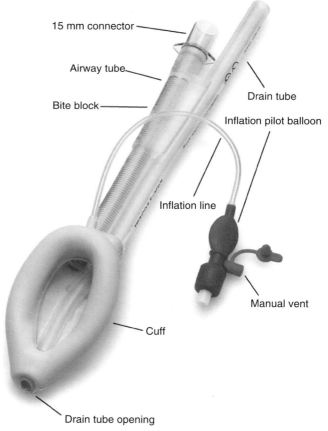

Figure 5-9   The LMA ProSeal. (Courtesy of LMA North America, Inc.)

LMA PS include a low profile, a bite block to prevent tube damage, a softer cuff that creates a better seal, a double-tube arrangement that provides extra stability to the LMA PS, and a double cuff to make a more reliable seal. The posterior surface of the LMA PS also inflates, pushing the mask forward. Contraindications to the use of the LMA PS are the same as those of the LMA Classic; namely, the LMA PS should not be used in those patients at risk of aspiration or with very poor pulmonary compliance (Fig. 5-9).

There are several techniques available to place an LMA PS. The first technique is the finger technique, in which the index finger is placed into the introducer strap and the LMA PS is held like a pencil. Under direct vision, the LMA PS is inserted into the mouth and is pressed up against the hard palate. The index finger is extended, pushing the mask forward into the hypopharynx, and the other hand holds the head and exerts counter-pressure. When firm resistance is felt, the LMA PS is in the right place.

The second technique involves the use of a specially designed introducer tool. This tool is placed into the introducer strap, and the LMA PS is fitted around the introducer. The tip of the cuff is pressed against the hard palate and is slid further toward the back of the soft palate with an arc motion into the hypopharynx until resistance is felt. The introducer is then removed from the LMA PS (Figs. 5-10, 5-11).

Recently, the bougie method, a new technique to place the LMA PS, has been described. It requires gentle laryngoscopy. A lubricated bougie is preloaded with the LMA PS through the gastric tube, and the bougie is deliberately placed into the esophagus. The LMA PS is advanced into the airway over the bougie, and the bougie is removed. The advantage of this technique is the ability to align the distal gastric port of the LMA PS with the upper esophageal sphincter. This allows the LMA PS to meet its optimal design proportion and to offer easy passage of an oral gastric tube. Once the LMA PS is positioned, it is then inflated to a maximum pressure of

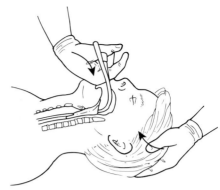

Figure 5-11   Final insertion of the LMA ProSeal. (Courtesy of LMA North America, Inc.)

60 cmH$_2$O. Many clinicians now recommend the use of a pressure manometer to check intracuff pressures, especially if nitrous oxide is used or for longer-duration cases.

A test to confirm the proper position of the LMA PS involves placing a small amount of lubricant gel on the top of the drain tube. In a well-positioned LMA PS, the gel moves slightly up and down with each respiration. If gel does not move or is ejected, the LMA PS must be repositioned.

Several studies have compared the use of the LMA Classic and the LMA PS in paralyzed and unparalyzed anesthetized patients. All show that the LMA Classic was easier and faster to place than the ProSeal. In addition, the LMA PS needed a deeper plane of anesthesia for insertion and also had a slightly higher incidence of complications, including blood on the LMA PS after insertion, cough, and laryngospasm. However, the LMA PS had a higher laryngeal seal pressure compared to the LMA Classic. This feature allows for more reliable positive pressure ventilation with the LMA PS. When the LMA PS was properly positioned, it isolated the glottis from the esophagus better than the LMA Classic, and the drain tube provided a conduit away from the oropharynx for any refluxed gastric fluid (Box 5-5).

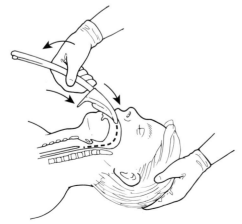

Figure 5-10   Initial finger insertion of the LMA ProSeal. (Courtesy of LMA North America, Inc.)

Box 5-5   **Characteristics of the ProSeal Laryngeal Mask Airway**
Double cuff that creates a low pressure airway seal Built-in bite block Better separation of the gastrointestinal trunk and the airway than a classic LMA The ability to place an oral gastric tube to decompress the stomach Flexible tube for a lower profile More difficult to place compared to the LMA Classic

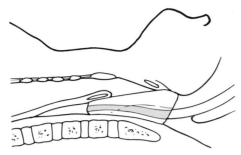

Figure 5-12 Correct LMA ProSeal placement with good seals at the glottis and the upper esophageal sphincter. (Courtesy of LMA North America, Inc.)

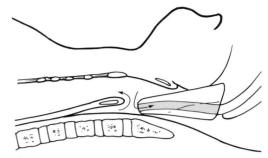

Figure 5-13 Incorrect ProSeal placement. The device is placed too high in the pharynx, with a poor seal allowing gas and fluid to pass in directions shown by arrows. (Courtesy of LMA North America, Inc.)

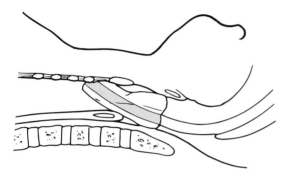

Figure 5-14 Incorrect LMA ProSeal placement. The device is placed with the tip in the laryngeal vestibule; ventilation is obstructed and deteriorates if the mask is pressed in. (Courtesy of LMA North America, Inc.)

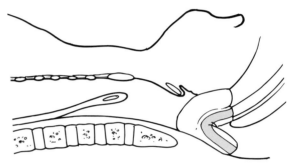

Figure 5-15 Incorrect LMA ProSeal placement. The mask is folded back on itself in the hypopharynx, causing the drain tube to become obstructed. (Courtesy of LMA North America, Inc.)

Despite several potential advantages of the ProSeal, malplacement can occur, and it is important for the clinician to understand how to diagnose and treat these potential problems. Figures 5-12 through 5-15 show correct and incorrect cuff positions, and Table 5-6 lists most of the possible malpositioning issues.

The Fastrach Laryngeal Mask Airway

The LMA Fastrach (LMA FT) was invented to allow intubation using a new LMA and a special endotracheal tube. The LMA FT differs from conventional LMAs as it has a large-bore stainless-steel C-shaped airway conduit that will direct an endotracheal tube blindly through the glottis when the LMA FT is correctly placed. The LMA FT is designed to use a special bullet-tipped endotracheal tube: the Euromedical endotracheal tube. The bullet tip facilitates intubation by easily passing through the glottis. The LMA FT allows airway management in patients with known and unexpected difficult airways. It has the ability to maintain spontaneous or controlled ventilation with an LMA (Fig. 5-16).

A new modification of the LMA FT is the LMA CTrach. This is a refinement that incorporates a fiberop-

tic system in the LMA FT design. It uses two fiberoptic bundles opening on the ventral mask aspect to illuminate and visualize the glottis. This interfaces with a removable monitor that clips onto the LMA CTrach. The monitor is composed of a video screen, a video chip, and a light scope to view the glottis during intubation. The LMA CTrach was introduced into the U.S. market in 2005.

Use of the Laryngeal Mask Airway During Laparoscopy

Commonly, surgeries in the ambulatory operating room involve laparoscopy. Using an LMA as the airway in this situation is still very controversial. Because many laparoscopic procedures are short in duration, the LMA might appear to be a good choice. It can be inserted without muscle relaxation, and less initial anesthesia may be required. However, lower esophageal pressure is often increased during laparoscopy due to the required pneumoperitoneum. When coupled with the head-down position during the procedure, aspiration may occur. Studies looking at the use of the LMA Classic in short-duration diagnostic laparoscopy showed that the

Table 5-6 Troubleshooting LMA ProSeal Placement

Problem After Insertion	Possible Causes	Possible Solutions
Poor airway seal or air leak (i.e., an audible air leak or poor ventilation)	Mask is seated too high in the pharynx	Advance mask in further and resecure the airway tube
	Inadequate anesthesia	Deepen anesthesia
	Poor fixation of the tube	Ensure palatal pressure and proper fixation
	Overinflation of the cuff	Check cuff pressure
	Herniation of the cuff	Check cuff integrity before placement
Gas leakage up the drain tube	Mask is seated too high in the pharynx	Advance mask in further and resecure the airway tube
	Incorrect placement in the laryngeal vestibule	Remove and reinsert
	Open upper-esophageal sphincter	Monitor
Airway obstruction (i.e., difficult ventilation, phonation, or stridor)	Incorrect placement in the laryngeal vestibule	Remove and reinsert
	Distal tip of the mask is pressing on the glottic inlet with mechanical closure of the vocal cords	Ensure adequate anesthesia and correct cuff inflation
		Place patient's head and neck in the sniffing position
		Try PPV or add PEEP
	Folding of cuff walls medially	Consider insertion of a ProSeal that is one size smaller
		Ensure correct cuff inflation pressure, especially if using N_2O
Gastric insufflation	Distal tip of the mask is folded backward	Remove and reinsert or sweep behind the tip with a finger
	Mask is seated too high in the pharynx	Advance the mask in further and resecure the airway tube
Migration and rotation, or the mask pops out of the mouth	Overinflation of the cuff	Check cuff pressure at the start and periodically during the case, especially if using N_2O
	Herniation of the cuff	Confirm cuff integrity prior to use
	Accidental displacement	Ensure proper fixation
	Distal tip of the mask is folded backward	Remove and reinsert or sweep behind the tip with a finger
	Poor fixation	Ensure palatal pressure and proper fixation
Resistance to OG tube insertion	Insufficient lubrication	Add lubricant and reattempt passing the OG tube
	Distal tip of the mask is folded backward	Remove and reinsert or sweep behind the tip with a finger
	Mask is seated too high in the pharynx	Advance mask in further and resecure the airway tube
	Incorrect placement in the laryngeal vestibule	Remove and reinsert
	Gross overinflation of the cuff	Ensure correct cuff inflation pressure, especially if using N_2O

OG, Orogastric; PEEP, positive end-expiratory pressure; PPV, positive pressure ventilation. (Courtesy of LMA North America, Inc.)

risk of adverse events and aspiration was low. Still, it is not the universal practice in the United States to routinely use LMAs for these cases.

The use of LMAs for laparoscopic cholecystectomy is even more controversial. Since the patient is head-up during the surgery, this position might be more favorable from a ventilatory standpoint. But the procedure may be lengthy, and the upper gastrointestinal tract might be more disturbed by the surgery and the pneumoperitoneum. This may lead to a higher risk of aspiration compared to a diagnostic laparoscopy. There have been several studies showing that the Classic and ProSeal LMAs can be used successfully for laparoscopic cholecystectomies, although the sample sizes involved were too small to draw any firm conclusions about safety. In 2002, Lu et al. compared the Classic and

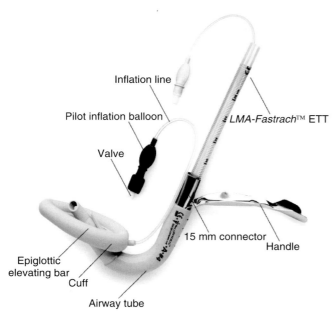

Figure 5-16 The LMA Fastrach and Euromedical endotracheal tube. (Courtesy of LMA North America, Inc.)

ProSeal for positive pressure ventilation in this surgery.[10] Although the LMA Classic was easier to insert, it became difficult to ventilate the patient when the pneumoperitoneum was begun. In contrast, patients with the LMA ProSeal tolerated the pneumoperitoneum better, and ventilation was adequate. When a gastric tube was placed through the drain tube and the contents were examined, a large percentage of patients had fluid that was bile-stained or semisolid, despite the fact that these patients had no risk factors for aspiration preoperatively. Therefore, it appears that although the LMA ProSeal would be the best LMA choice for laparoscopic procedures, the role of these devices in this situation is still not defined.

Alternative Supraglottic Airway Devices

Disposable versions of the Classic and flexible LMA have been released. Depending on shelf life of the reusable versions and other reprocessing issues, these may be economical alternatives. At least two other airway devices have been developed as possible alternatives to the original LMA. These include the cuffed oropharyngeal airway (COPA) and the laryngeal tube. The COPA is shaped like a Guedel airway with an attached inflatable cuff. When this cuff is inflated, it displaces the tongue and holds the device in place. Similarly, the laryngeal tube is a variation of the esophageal obturator airway. It is a silicone tube with two inflatable cuffs: a proximal cuff that pushes on the base of the tongue and lifts the epiglottis, and a distal cuff that occludes the esophagus. The patient is venti-

lated from an opening between the two cuffs. Whereas both airways are relatively easy to place, their failure rate is higher compared to the LMA. It is assumed that additional supraglottic airways will be introduced. At this time, the role of these airways in the ambulatory anesthesia setting remains undefined.

SUMMARY

In the ambulatory practice, we intend for the patient to undergo a successful general anesthetic with minimal side effects and to have a rapid discharge home. Various forms of supraglottic airways and the newer inhaled agents, sevoflurane and desflurane, are major advances for ambulatory anesthesia. Together, they facilitate a more rapid recovery. Each provides improvement over older techniques in the management of patients for outpatient surgery. In addition, newer level-of-sedation monitoring may become routine if more studies confirm its utility and device refinements occur. General anesthesia will continue to be a very popular technique for outpatient anesthesia care.

REFERENCES

1. Philips BK, Lombard L, Roaf, ER, et al: Comparison of vital capacity induction with sevoflurane to intravenous induction with propofol for adult ambulatory anesthesia. Anesth Analg 89:623–627, 1999.

2. Joo HS, Perks WJ: Sevoflurane versus propofol for anesthetic induction: A meta-analysis. Anesth Analg 91:213–219, 2000.

3. Gupta A, Stierer T, Zuckerman R, et al: Comparison of recovery profile after ambulatory anesthesia with propofol, isoflurane, sevoflurane and desflurane: A systematic review. Anesth Analg 98:632–641, 2004.

4. Visser K, Hassink, EA, Bonsel GJ, et al: Randomized controlled trial of total intravenous anesthesia with propofol versus inhalation anesthesia with isoflurane-nitrous oxide; postoperative nausea with vomiting and economic analysis. Anesthesiology 95:616–626, 2001.

5. Song D, Joshi GP, White PF: Titration of volatile anesthetics using bispectral index facilitates recovery after ambulatory anesthesia. Anesthesiology 87:842–848, 1997.

6. Liu SS: Effects of bispectral index monitoring on ambulatory anesthesia: A meta-analysis of randomized controlled trials and a cost analysis. Anesthesiology 101:311–315, 2004.

7. American Society of Anesthesiologists: Practice Advisory for Intraoperative Awareness and Brain Monitoring. Approved October 25, 2005. Available at http://www.asahq.org/publicationsAndServices/AwareAdvisoryFinalOct05.pdf

8. Eshima RW, Maurer A, King T, et al: A comparison of airway responses during desflurane and sevoflurane administration via a laryngeal mask airway for maintenance of anesthesia. Anesth Analg 96:701–705, 2003.

9. Joshi G, Inagaki Y, White P, et al: Use of the laryngeal mask airway as an alternative to the tracheal tube during ambulatory anesthesia. Anesth Analg 85:573–577, 1997.

10. Lu PP, Brimacombe J, Yang C, et al: ProSeal versus the classic laryngeal mask airway for postive pressure ventilation during laparascopic chlecystectomy. Br J Anaesth 88:824–827, 2002.

SUGGESTED READING

American Society of Anesthesiologists: Practice Advisory for Intraoperative Awareness and Brain Function Monitoring. http://asahq.org/publicationsAndServices/AwareAdvisoryFin alOct05.pdf

Brimacombe J, Keller C: The ProSeal laryngeal mask airway: A randomized, crossover study with the standard laryngeal mask airway in paralyzed anesthetized patients. Anesthesiology 93:104–109, 2000.

Chikungwa M, Smith I: Controversial issues in ambulatory anesthesia. Anesthesiology Clin N Am 21:313–327, 2003.

Joshi G: Inhalational techniques in ambulatory anesthesia. Anesthesiology Clin N Am 21:263–272, 2003.

Maltby JR, Beriault MT, Watson N, et al: The LMA-ProSeal is an effective alternative to tracheal intubation for laparoscopic cholecystectomy. Can J Anesth 49:857–862, 2002.

Maltby JR, Beriault MT, Watson N, Fick GH: Gastric distension and ventilation during laparoscopic cholecystectomy: LMA-Classic vs. tracheal intubation. Can J Anesth 47: 622–626, 2000.

Muzi M, Robinson BJ, Ebert TJ, O'Brian TJ: Induction of anesthesia and tracheal intubation with sevoflurane in adults. Anesthesiology 85:536–543, 1996.

Song D, Joshi GP, White PF: Fast track eligibility after ambulatory anesthesia: A comparison of desflurane, sevoflurane, and propofol. Anesth Analg 86:267–273,1998.

Stoelting RK: Inhalational Anesthetics. In Stoelting RK (ed): Pharmacology and Physiology in Anesthetic Practice, 3rd ed. Philadelphia, Lippincott-Raven, 1999, pp 36–77.

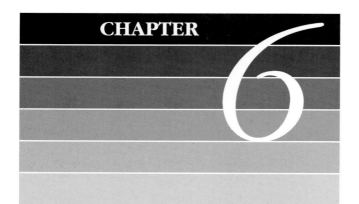

CHAPTER 6

Regional Anesthesia and Analgesia for Ambulatory Surgery

MICHAEL FORD

THOMAS BRODERICK

The majority of surgeries in the United States are performed on an outpatient basis. Cost savings associated with avoiding hospitalization are substantial, driving health care providers to demand that surgical procedures be completed in the ambulatory setting. Subsequently, the frequency, diversity, and complexity of the operations undertaken have continued to rise, and outpatient surgery on patients with significant comorbid medical conditions has become common. Procedures associated with patients experiencing moderate to severe pain postopera-

tively are frequent. Multimodal perioperative analgesia, which may include regional anesthesia and analgesic techniques, is necessary to achieve satisfactory pain control at the facility and after discharge.

Unfortunately, many ambulatory surgical patients still experience moderate to severe pain after discharge from the facility, suggesting that achieving pain control within the outpatient facility is not a sufficient goal. Developing and adhering to surgical-procedure-specific multimodal analgesic pathways at best achieves an analgesia continuum. Surgeons, nurses, and anesthesiologists must collaborate to develop effective pathways for controlling pain during recovery from anesthesia at the facility and after patient discharge. Education regarding the analgesic care plan is critical for both the patient and the health care provider. Regional anesthetic and analgesic techniques are often vital and integral components of these pathways. For example, use of continuous local anesthetic infusion into surgical wounds, in proximity to peripheral nerves or a plexus of nerves, can extend analgesia for 2 to 3 days. Coadministration of a nonsteroidal anti-inflammatory drug, acetaminophen, or both, on a scheduled basis, along with the availability of an oral opiate for breakthrough pain, completes the multimodal analgesic strategy.

In 2001, the Joint Commission on Accreditation of Healthcare Organizations (JCAHO) released standards for pain management (Box 6-1). In particular, the standards urge that pain should not inhibit the patient taking part in his or her rehabilitation and recovery, most of which occurs at home after ambulatory surgery. Implementing effective pain management after the patient is discharged from the surgical facility is crucial. Patients have to know how and when to take their pain medicines, and they have to be able to contact a health care provider if pain control is inadequate or if analgesic side effects are troublesome. Adhering to the JCAHO pain standards should improve the management of pain in the outpatient surgery patient.

All patients have the right to receive appropriate assessment and management of pain.

Screen for the presence of pain.

Assess the nature and degree of pain.

Pain intensity should be assessed. Use a standard scale such as the 0 to 10 pain scale.

Reassess pain on a regular ongoing basis.

Document the pain assessment in a manner that enables reassessment and follow-up.

Measure staff competency in pain assessment and treatment.

Orient new health care providers to the methods of pain assessment and treatment.

Set policies and procedures that support appropriate ordering and prescribing of analgesics.

Ensure pain does not inhibit the patients from taking part in rehabilitation and recovery.

Educate patients and their families about the importance of adequate and effective pain management.

Address the need for patient symptom management, and make the necessary arrangements in the discharge planning process from the health care facility.

Include pain management measures, including effectiveness and appropriateness in continuous quality improvement processes of the institution.

Prior to discharge after outpatient surgery, patients must be ambulatory, mentally alert, tolerating oral intake, and they must have pain satisfactorily controlled. Inadequate analgesia and postoperative nausea and vomiting (PONV) are two major factors that contribute to a prolonged length of stay at outpatient surgical facilities and unplanned hospital admission.

Obtaining adequate analgesia when pain is moderate to severe typically requires the administration of an opiate. Unfortunately, opiates contribute to PONV. Utilizing nonopiate analgesics, local anesthetic infiltration or instillation, or peripheral nerve blockade, or a combination thereof, as first-tier multimodal analgesic therapies reduces opiate use. Decreased opiate dosage lessens opiate-mediated side effects, including PONV. Regional anesthetic and analgesic techniques, when used as part of a multimodal perioperative analgesic strategy, reduce the incidence of PONV by minimizing opiate analgesic administration or by avoiding general anesthesia entirely.

Surgeon acceptance of regional anesthetic and analgesic techniques for outpatient surgeries is growing, but reluctance to utilize these techniques is still widespread. Some surgeons worry that the time needed to perform the regional anesthetic or nerve block can slow operating room turnover or may delay the actual surgical start time. Utilizing a separate block room staffed by a dedicated anesthesiology block team addresses this concern. The regional anesthetic technique can be performed in a centralized area with all the desired equipment and supplies readily available without the hovering and impatient crowd watching. The patient is subsequently transported to the operating room on schedule with a functioning sensory block. The regional anesthesia team is also available postoperatively to troubleshoot analgesia, to initiate and optimize local anesthetic infusions, and to perform regional techniques during recovery.

Some surgeons will wish to perform a neurologic examination after the surgical procedure is complete. Performance of a preoperative block could preclude this exam. In facilities without this block-team and room capability, patients deemed likely candidates for a regional anesthetic technique could be scheduled as first cases. The anesthesiologist can begin early, increasing the likelihood of a successful regional anesthetic technique and an on-time start. Another area of concern by surgeons is the occasional inadequate regional anesthetic or a failed block. Regional anesthesia is not always completely effective, and the anesthesiologist may need to move on to an alternative plan, usually general anesthesia, in a timely fashion, but have confidence that, the next time, the regional technique will likely be successful.

Patient acceptance of regional anesthetic techniques is higher if the surgeon has informed the patient that the technique is available and desirable. The surgeon and the anesthesiologist must not be contradictory in regards to the anesthetic plan. Patient education is best started in the surgeon's office and should include the surgeon's endorsement of regional anesthesia as a primary anesthetic option or as a component of general anesthesia. It is helpful if the surgery's electronic or paper scheduling system has fields for the surgeon's and patient's regional anesthesia preferences so that cases can be flagged appropriately.

Since outpatient anesthesiologists do not usually see most outpatients until the day of the procedure, a phone call to the patient the night prior to the procedure by the anesthesiologist is often helpful in assisting an ambivalent or uninformed patient in choosing a regional anesthetic technique. The phone information can be reinforced during the preoperative evaluation and anesthetic plan discussion on the day of the procedure. Anesthesia providers should also pay particular attention to the patient's desired level of consciousness during performance of the regional anesthesia procedure and during the surgery itself.

OPIATE ANALGESICS

Relieving moderate to severe postoperative pain commonly requires an opiate. Undesired opiate-mediated side effects may delay discharge from the ambulatory surgery center and lead to a less-than-ideal recovery at home. Patients take their prescribed opiate to diminish pain, but the opiate may make them sick, so they discontinue taking the opiate and, therefore, have increased pain, catching the patient between the postoperative Scylla and Charybdis. Multimodal perioperative analgesic strategies are needed to reduce and eliminate opiate dosing while providing at least equivalent, and perhaps superior, pain relief.

Opiate medications continue to play an important role in perioperative analgesia. Intravenous opiates are utilized as components of general anesthesia, as part of intraoperative sedation and analgesia for monitored anesthetic care and primary regional anesthetic techniques, and for analgesia during initial recovery at the facility. Because of its fast onset, ease of titration, and low cost, fentanyl continues to be commonly used for outpatient surgery. Prior to patient emergence from general anesthesia, many anesthesiologists give small doses of intravenous morphine or hydromorphone to patients who are likely to experience moderate to severe postoperative pain.

Meperidine, at a dose of 0.25 to 0.5 mg/kg, administered toward the end of a general anesthetic, may contribute to initial analgesia and decrease the incidence of shivering during emergence.

Some anesthesiologists use remifentanil, administered by continuous intravenous infusion, to provide profound intraoperative analgesia. The analgesia quickly dissipates due to rapid metabolism by blood and tissue esterases, with termination of the infusion regardless of the length of administration. Patients likely to experience moderate to severe postoperative pain will require analgesics very soon after the remifentanil is stopped, however.

In ambulatory patients, spinal anesthesia can be performed with a mixture of fentanyl and a reduced-dose local anesthetic. Recovery from this bimodal spinal anesthetic can be as rapid as recovery from general anesthesia. Epidural fentanyl can also be administered to outpatients, but using neuraxial hydrophilic opiates such as morphine is relatively contraindicated in the ambulatory patient secondary to the risk of delayed respiratory depression. Intra-articular injections of morphine or meperidine may lead to slightly improved analgesia after orthopedic procedures.

After general anesthesia or during Phase 1 recovery, intermittent doses of intravenous opiates supplement further analgesia. Once fluid intake begins, oral opiates are started. Some physicians prefer to use single-drug opiate preparations instead of acetaminophen and opiate combinations. This allows opiate dose adjustments without exceeding daily maximum acetaminophen dosage recommendations (approximately 4 gm/day for adults). Acetaminophen can then be prescribed on a scheduled basis, and the patient can take the immediate-release opiate on an as-needed basis.

In outpatient procedures associated with several days of moderate to severe postoperative pain, such as open shoulder or reconstructive knee surgeries, sustained-release oral opiate preparations can be given on a scheduled basis. Immediate-release opiate preparations are also prescribed for rescue analgesia or breakthrough pain. In opiate-naïve adults, sustained release oxycodone, 10 to 20 mg every 12 hours, may provide better analgesia with less sedation, sleep disturbance, and postoperative nausea, at a lower total daily dose when compared with immediate-release oxycodone, taken on either a timed or an as-needed schedule.

Giving a preoperative dose of the oral sustained-release opiate may shorten patient discharge time, lower postoperative pain scores, decrease opiate requirements during recovery, and lessen nausea and vomiting. Some providers hesitate to use sustained-release opiates in outpatients because of the potential for abuse or high drug levels (if the tablets are chewed). Preoperative patient assessment is crucial in patients considered for controlled-release oral opiates. Oral morphine is also available in a sustained-release formulation, including a recently released lower-cost generic preparation.

CURRENT CONTROVERSY: USE OF SUSTAINED-RELEASE OPIATES IN OUTPATIENTS

- Some providers hesitate to use sustained-release opiates in outpatients because of abuse potential or danger of high drug levels if the tablets are chewed.
- In opiate-naïve adults undergoing procedures associated with several days of moderate to severe pain, sustained-release oral opiates may provide better analgesia with less sedation, sleep disturbance, and postoperative nausea at a lower total daily dose when compared with immediate-release opiates taken on either a timed or as-needed schedule.
- Preoperative patient education regarding pain management is crucial in patients who are prescribed controlled-release oral opiates.

New opiate agonists, selective antagonists of opiate-mediated side effects, and novel opiate delivery systems are under study. A metabolite of morphine, morphine-6-glucuronide, demonstrates analgesia with less respiratory depression and a milder extent of opiate-mediated side effects than is observed after administration of a parent compound. Peripheral opiate antagonists designed to preserve central-mediated pain relief while attenuating peripheral-mediated side effects are undergoing clinical trials. Drugs in this class, such as alvimopam, can be administered orally; methylnaltrexone can be given both orally and intravenously. What role these opiate agonists and peripheral opiate antagonists will play in ambulatory surgery patients has not yet been determined.

Patient-controlled analgesia utilizing fentanyl delivery by an iontophoretic mechanism is currently undergoing clinical trials. A self-adhesive credit-card-sized device is attached to the skin on the chest or upper arm. After a button is pressed twice within a short defined time period, a low-intensity electric current moves a fixed dose of fentanyl from the device reservoir to the surface in contact with the skin, from where it is systemically absorbed. A lockout interval is preset and only a finite number of doses can be released during the 24 hours that the device is active. Administration of fentanyl in this manner may prove to be effective in treating moderate to severe pain following discharge from the ambulatory care facility. Transcutaneous sustained-release fentanyl patches and oral "lollipop" immediate-release fentanyl preparations are neither recommended nor approved for treating acute postoperative pain in opiate-naïve patients. Table 6-1 lists common opiates used to treat acute pain in the ambulatory surgery setting.

NONSTEROIDAL ANTI-INFLAMMATORY DRUGS AND ACETAMINOPHEN

Nonsteroidal anti-inflammatory drugs (NSAIDs) can provide significant analgesia and, when coadministered with opiates, decrease patient opiate consumption and improve pain control, particularly lessening pain with movement. Reducing patient opiate requirements postoperatively lowers opiate-mediated side effects, facilitating discharge from ambulatory surgery centers. In cases in which pain is expected to be mild in nature, or as pain subsides, NSAIDs may be sufficient for analgesia when administered alone. When postoperative pain is moderate to severe, however, analgesia using only NSAID therapy is usually inadequate. Scheduled dosing of NSAIDs should be considered as an integral component of multimodal analgesia for treating postoperative pain in the ambulatory patient, including pain management at home during convalescence. Incorporating NSAIDs into multimodal analgesic pathways must be individualized for each patient and for each surgeon, considering the potential adverse effects of NSAID administration, such as impaired platelet function, gastrointestinal irritation, renal dysfunction, impaired osteogenesis, and hypersensitivity reactions.

There are two forms of the cyclo-oxygenase (COX) enzyme that are present in many tissues. COX-1 and COX-2 are induced in response to tissue injury, inflammation, and pain, producing prostaglandins that activate and sensitize nociceptors. The COX-1 and COX-2 enzymes also produce eicosanoids, including prostacyclin and thromboxane A_2, which mediate the interactions between platelets and blood vessel walls. Prostaglandins also help regulate blood flow to the gastric mucosa and the kidneys. Selective COX-2 inhibitors appear to have less gastrointestinal side effects and no adverse effect on platelet function, making them more attractive as analgesics in the perioperative setting. Preoperative NSAID administration may provide preemptive analgesia and may have a greater opiate sparing effect compared to postoperative administration. COX-2 inhibitors have equal analgesic efficacy when compared to nonselective COX inhibitors.

Table 6-1 Common Opiate Analgesics Used in Outpatient Surgery

Opiate	Route	Dosage	Comments
Fentanyl	IV	0.5–1 µg/kg	• Rapid onset and short-acting • Used in the operating room and during Phase 1 recovery
Hydromorphone	IV	10–20 µg/kg	• Used in the operating room and during Phase 1 recovery
Meperidine	IV	0.25–1 mg/kg	• Primarily used to treat shivering, but may be useful in some patients for acute pain in limited doses.
Morphine	IV	50–100 µg/kg	• Used in the operating room and during Phase One recovery • Parenteral opiate favored for pediatric patients
Codeine	Oral	0.5–1 mg/kg	• 50-kg patient dose is 30–60 mg • 10% of patients cannot convert pro-drug to active form
Hydrocodone	Oral	135 µg/kg	• Similar to, but more potent than, codeine • Oral preparation is only available in combination with acetaminophen, which can limit maximum dosing based on the acetaminophen component
Oxycodone	Oral	100–200 µg/kg	• 50-kg patient dose is 5–10 mg • Immediate-release form available alone or in combination with acetaminophen • Sustained-release preparation available • Sustained-release preparation use in opiate-naïve outpatients is controversial

Table 6-2	COX-2 Inhibitors for Treating Acute Pain in Adults			
COX-2 Drug	**Route**	**Dosage**	**Dosing Interval**	**Comments**
Celecoxib	Oral	100–400 mg	Twice a day	• 400 mg initial dose recently FDA-approved for acute pain • Subsequent dosing should be 200 mg, twice a day • Contraindicated in patients with allergic reactions to sulfonamides • Can be taken with or without food
Parecoxib (currently unavailable in the United States)	Intravenous	20–40 mg	Twice a day	• Converted to valdecoxib, the active form • Valdecoxib reaches its T_{max} in about 30 minutes • 40 mg equivalent to 30 mg ketorolac • Contraindicated in patients with allergic reactions to sulfonamides • Oral valdecoxib was withdrawn from the U.S. market in April 2005

T_{max}, Time of maximum concentration.

COX-2 inhibitors have not been approved for use in children, but several published studies have demonstrated safe use and effective analgesia in pediatric surgery patients. Only oral preparations of COX-2 inhibitors are currently available in the United States.

Parecoxib, a prodrug converted *in vivo* to the active drug valdecoxib, is a new intravenous COX-2 selective NSAID undergoing late phase clinical trials in the United States. In patients in the early stages of recovery from general anesthesia or in patients not allowed oral intake, parecoxib is an attractive alternative to ketorolac for treating acute postoperative pain. Table 6-2 lists COX-2 inhibitors and adult acute-pain dosing guidelines. In patients at low risk for NSAID-induced side effects, lower-cost nonselective COX inhibitors can be utilized, such as ibuprofen, naproxen, and ketorolac (Table 6-3).

In September 2004, rofecoxib was voluntarily withdrawn from the market due to data showing an increased relative risk for cardiovascular events such as heart attack and stroke. These increased risks were observed after 18 months of continuous treatment in patients taking rofecoxib, as compared to patients taking placebo. Delays in approval of new COX-2 inhibitors and increased scrutiny on existing COX-2 inhibitors are likely. There is also evidence that the perioperative use of selective COX-2 inhibitors is associated with an increased incidence of vascular complications after coronary artery bypass surgery. In April 2005, valdecoxib was withdrawn from the market. Many questions remain unanswered. Is the short-term use of COX-2 inhibitors (using COX-2 drugs to treat acute pain) associated with increased risk of cardiovascular events for other surgeries?

Acetaminophen has significant analgesic properties and is well-tolerated in most patients without causing adverse effects on platelet function and gastric irritation. It is only available in oral and rectal administration forms

Table 6-3	Nonselective COX Inhibitors for Treating Acute Pain			
Drug	**Route**	**Dosage**	**Interval**	**Daily Maximum Dosage**
Ibuprofen	Oral	6–10 mg/kg	4 hours	• Up to 40 mg/kg/day, to a maximum of 2400 mg
Naproxen	Oral	5–6 mg/kg	12 hours	• Up to 24 mg/kg/day, to a maximum of 1000 mg
Ketorolac (for adults)	Oral, IV	10 mg po 15–30 mg/kg IV	6 hours	• 40 mg po • 120 mg IV • 5-day maximum duration of therapy; reduce dosing in patients over 65 years old
Ketorolac (for children ages 2–16)	IV	0.5 mg/kg, up to 15 mg maximum dose	6 hours	• Only single-dose approved • 2 mg/kg/day, up to maximum dose of 60 mg • Total dose of 60 mg/day is frequently used in hospitalized children

IV, Intravenous; po, by mouth.

in the United States. It is often combined with an opiate in a single oral tablet to simplify dosing. High acetaminophen doses can lead to hepatic dysfunction, however, and caution should be exercised in patients with concurrent alcohol use or hepatic disease. Most healthy adults should not ingest more than 4000 mg/day.

Oral acetaminophen dosing is delineated in Table 6-4. Neonates and infants have lower daily acetaminophen maximum doses of approximately 40 to 75 mg/kg/day. Single doses of 40 to 60 mg/kg acetaminophen administered rectally, after induction of general anesthesia, have been used successfully in young children. When used to treat acute pain, the ideal dose of acetaminophen is controversial, with a recent trend towards higher dosages, especially in children. Acetaminophen can be coadministered with another NSAID.

OTHER COANALGESICS AND NONPHARMACOLOGIC TECHNIQUES

Opiates, acetaminophen, nonsteroidal anti-inflammatory drugs, and local anesthetics are the most commonly prescribed perioperative analgesics. Other medications or coanalgesics that may contribute to improved pain control include ketamine, dextromethorphan, clonidine, dexmedetomidine, and gabapentin. Many of these drugs can be combined with local anesthetic regional techniques to enhance and prolong analgesia. Analgesics can also be applied topically, injected or instilled into wounds, or instilled into laparoscopic surgical fields using video assistance. Nonpharmacologic techniques, including physical measures (i.e., cold application and immobilization), transcutaneous electrical nerve stimulation, acupuncture, acupressure, hypnotic suggestion, and biofeedback, may help control pain with minimal side effects.

N-methyl-D-aspartate (NMDA) Antagonists

The N-methyl-D-aspartate (NMDA) receptor plays an important role in processing pain. Antagonizing the NMDA receptor may prevent induction and maintenance of central sensitization. The NMDA receptor may also mediate peripheral visceral and somatic sensitization.

Ketamine possesses NMDA-receptor-blocking properties when given intravenously, even after a single low dose of 0.1 to 0.2 mg/kg. At these reduced doses, ketamine is not usually associated with cardiovascular stimulation and unwanted psychological side effects. The S(+) isomer of ketamine possesses less psychic effects and is about four times as potent as the R(−) isomer and is undergoing clinical trials. Ketamine reduces opiate consumption, contributes to improved analgesia, may reduce postoperative nausea and vomiting, and may exert a preemptive analgesia effect. Use of ketamine as an analgesic in ambulatory patients is summarized in Table 6-5.

Dextromethorphan, available in oral and parental formulations, also antagonizes NMDA receptors, decreasing pain and reducing opiate consumption, without adverse effects on the respiratory or the cardiovascular systems. A preoperative dose and scheduled postoperative doses of dextromethorphan may play important roles in improving analgesia, especially after discharge from outpatient surgery. Further study is warranted.

α-2 Agonists

α-2 receptors play a role in modulating pain, and α-2 agonists reduce pain. Clonidine and dexmedetomidine stimulate presynaptic α-2 receptors and inhibit norepinephrine release from peripheral and central adrenergic nerves, decreasing peripheral vascular resistance and heart rate. Clonidine and dexmedetomidine provide good anxiolysis with minimal respiratory depression. Side effects include low blood pressure, bradycardia, dry mouth, and sedation. Using clonidine as an analgesic in ambulatory patients is delineated in Table 6-6. Dexmedetomidine, a more potent α-2 agonist than clonidine, has analgesic and anxiolytic properties. It decreased opiate consumption postoperatively when coadministered with intravenous morphine patient-controlled analgesia. In a recent study, when combined with lidocaine for intravenous regional anesthesia, dexmedetomidine shortened the onset of anesthesia, improved the quality of anesthesia, and prolonged postoperative analgesia.

Gabapentin

Gabapentin has been found to be useful in treating many chronic pain conditions. The most common side effects reported in patients taking gabapentin include dizziness and somnolence. Several recent studies have demonstrated

Table 6-4	Oral Acetaminophen Dosing Based on Body Weight				
<40 kg Dose	≥40 kg Dose	Interval (Hours)	Maximum Daily Dose <40 kg	Maximum Daily Dose ≥40 kg
10–15 mg/kg	650–1000 mg	4–6 hours	100 mg/kg/day	4000 mg/day

Table 6-5 Ketamine as an Analgesic in Outpatient Surgery Patients	
Ketamine Usage	**Comments**
Intravenous administration prior to incision	• Low doses may exert a preemptive analgesic effect • Adjunct for general anesthesia
Combined in infusion with propofol for intravenous sedation	• Eliminate opiate as a sedative adjunct during MAC or primary regional anesthetic cases • May substitute for (or augment analgesic effect of) opiates during sedation • Lower required dosage minimizes psychic effects
Caudal coanalgesic	• Prolongs duration of analgesia when compared to local anesthetic alone • (S+) ketamine combined with clonidine may provide extended analgesia in children
Intravenous regional anesthetic adjunct	• Delays onset of tourniquet discomfort • May contribute to postoperative analgesia
Intraarticular ketamine	• Improved analgesia when used alone in arthroscopic knee surgery • Adjunct analgesic in multimodal intraarticular instillation (bupivacaine + opiate + ketamine)

MAC, Monitored anesthesia care.

that a single preoperative dose of gabapentin reduced opiate consumption postoperatively after anterior cruciate ligament (ACL) and spinal surgeries, mastectomies, abdominal hysterectomies, and laparoscopic cholecystectomies. The ACL and spinal surgery, mastectomy, and laparoscopic cholecystectomy patients also exhibited decreased pain scores. Further controlled studies are necessary to define gabapentin's role in treating acute pain in ambulatory surgery patients, and the off-label use of gabapentin should be evidence-based. Somnolence may be a limiting dose-related issue after outpatient surgery.

Local Anesthetics

Local anesthetics can be applied topically to the eye and mucous membranes using drops, soaked sponges, or atomization. Application of a lidocaine (with or without prilocaine) topical cream mixture can be useful prior to vein puncture (or any needle introduction) or to superficial dermatologic procedures, and it can be used as a coanalgesic for decreasing pain after hemorrhoidectomies and pediatric circumcisions.

Local anesthetics can also be injected into the incision, and preincision preventive injection may work better than injecting the local anesthetic at the end of the procedure. Some surgeons inject a quick-onset short-acting local anesthetic prior to starting the procedure and follow up with a long-acting local anesthetic injection at wound closure. Wound instillation of bupivacaine prior to closure is an effective coanalgesic for inguinal herniorrhaphy in adults and is as effective as a single-shot caudal local anesthetic injection in pediatric inguinal hernia repair. Disposable infusion pumps can deliver local anesthetic into surgical wounds for 24 to 48 hours. Arthroscopic and laparoscopic portals can be injected with local anesthetic before incision and trocar introduction. Intraperitoneal video-guided bupivacaine instillation is useful as an analgesic adjunct for gynecologic laparoscopy and laparoscopic

Table 6-6 Clonidine as an Analgesic in Outpatient Surgery Patients	
Clonidine Usage	**Comments**
Preoperative oral adjunct to general anesthesia	• Decreases MAC and perioperative opiate requirements • May reduce PONV and shivering
Spinal and epidural adjunct	• Enhances block quality, increases block duration, and provides postoperative analgesia when combined with a local anesthetic in a multimodal neuraxial technique
Caudal adjunct	• Prolongs duration of analgesia when compared to local anesthetic alone • Combined with (S+) ketamine to provide extended analgesia
Peripheral nerve block adjunct	• Prolongs and enhances analgesia of short- and intermediate-duration local anesthetics
Intravenous regional anesthetic adjunct	• Delays onset of tourniquet discomfort • Analgesia persists for up to 6 hours after tourniquet deflation
Intraarticular adjunct for arthroscopy	• Prolongs duration and enhances quality of postoperative analgesia with intraarticular injection combined with bupivacaine and morphine

MAC, Minimum alveolar concentration of inhalation agent; PONV, postoperative nausea and vomiting.

cholecystectomy. Intraarticular injection of a local anesthetic alone or in combination with other analgesics (frequently opiates) improves pain control after knee and shoulder arthroscopic surgeries.

Nonpharmacologic Techniques

Cold application to surgery sites reduces pain and swelling, has been shown to be useful after extremity and oral-maxillofacial procedures, and may facilitate motion and physical therapy. Immobilization is helpful after shoulder surgery and is routinely employed after many types of outpatient orthopedic procedures. Transcutaneous electrical nerve stimulation (TENS), used as an analgesic therapy, is controversial. TENS is most effective after abdominal surgery, as demonstrated in some controlled trials, but the efficacy of TENS analgesia for procedures on other parts of the body is less supported in the literature, showing little or no improvement in analgesia. One study in the 1980s demonstrated that TENS was useful for analgesia and for improving muscle kinetics after arthroscopic knee surgery. Acupuncture or acupressure can be effective for acute pain management but is not frequently utilized in the United States. Cognitive interventions, such as hypnosis, biofeedback, and positive outcome suggestion, may help some patients, but well-controlled studies are needed to see if these nonpharmacologic interventions are beneficial.

REGIONAL ANESTHESIA AND ANALGESIC TECHNIQUES

Basic Issues

The use of regional anesthesia is growing in ambulatory surgery. Both surgeon and patient acceptance of regional techniques and expectation for availability of these techniques are also increasing. A majority of anesthesiologists would choose regional anesthesia for their own individual anesthetic requirements. Neuraxial techniques, peripheral nerve or plexus blockade, and intravenous regional anesthesia can be primary anesthetics in themselves or can be used in combination with general anesthesia. Biopsies, superficial procedures, and hernia repairs can be performed under local anesthesia or under surgical field block combined with intravenous sedation. In patients who wish to be asleep during their operations, a steady-state level of sedation can be readily achieved by using medication-infusion pumps. All patients should have, at a minimum, infiltration or instillation of a local anesthetic into the surgical wound as part of a multimodal perioperative analgesic plan.

Regional techniques are not for all patients and surgeons. The triad of patient acceptance, surgeon endorsement, and anesthesiologist willingness and ability to provide the technique must be present. Successful regional anesthesia with low complication rates is directly related to the performance frequency of the technique by the anesthesiologist. Success converts reluctant surgeons into advocates of regional anesthesia, and surgeon advocates willingly recommend regional anesthesia to their patients. Alert, comfortable patients without PONV will spread the word to friends and family.

Providing regional anesthesia and analgesic techniques can be a very demanding task in the rapid-turnover setting of outpatient surgery. Many anesthesiologists believe the advantages of regional anesthesia far outweigh the disadvantages. The time lost placing the block in the operating room can often be recouped at the completion of surgery, especially if general anesthesia is avoided, making for zero emergence time. A dedicated and independent anesthesia block team increases efficiency further, as the regional technique can be completed prior to entry into the operating room, utilizing no operating room time. Stage 1 recovery is frequently bypassed as many regional anesthesia patients are fast-tracked, alert and comfortable, to Stage 2 recovery. Analgesia is already established, leading to a reduction in opiate requirements, diminished nausea and vomiting, and a decreased length of stay at the ambulatory facility.

Indications and Contraindications to Regional Anesthesia

Regional anesthetic or analgesic techniques are indicated in most ambulatory surgery patients as part of a multimodal perioperative analgesic strategy. A primary regional anesthetic technique, coupled with a level of intraoperative sedation desired by the patient or with regional anesthesia in combination with general anesthesia, are highly recommended by the authors for most outpatient procedures and for almost any surgical site. Advantages of regional anesthesia are listed in Box 6-2. Contraindications to regional anesthesia in ambulatory patients are summarized in Box 6-3.

The American Society of Regional Anesthesia and Pain Medicine (ASRA) recently published an updated consensus statement on performing neuraxial anesthesia in patients receiving anticoagulants. The ASRA's evidence-based recommendations were designed to minimize risk of bleeding, neuraxial hematoma, and neurologic injury, thus encouraging safe, quality care. Bleeding risk is increased further when there is concurrent use of other medications that affect the clotting mechanisms. Educating surgeons regarding anticoagulation issues is critical so that medications that affect coagulation can be discontinued at the recommended time interval prior to surgery. The ASRA consensus statements regarding neuraxial anesthesia in the anticoagulated patient are summarized in Table 6-7.

Box 6-2 Advantages of Regional Anesthesia in Outpatients

Possible preemptive analgesic effect if nerve blockade exists before incision

Reduces surgical stress response

Preserves pulmonary function

May preserve cognitive function (?)

Allows monitoring the patient's mental status during the operation

Reduces aspiration risk

Avoids instrumentation of the airway

Provides postoperative analgesia

Decreases opiate requirements

Decreases postoperative nausea and vomiting

Bypasses Stage 1 recovery

Box 6-3 Contraindications to Regional Anesthesia in Outpatients

ABSOLUTE CONTRAINDICATIONS:

Patient or guardian refusal

Coagulation disorder or anticoagulant therapy

Active infection at the site of block placement

True local anesthetic allergy (very rare)

RELATIVE CONTRAINDICATIONS:

Preoperative unstable neurologic deficit

    Carefully document neurologic deficits prior to proceeding with regional anesthetic procedures.

Respiratory issues

    Interscalene brachial plexus blockade is contraindicated in patients requiring hemidiaphragm function to achieve effective minute ventilation.

    There is the potential for pneumothorax after supraclavicular brachial plexus block.

    High neuraxial block may be poorly tolerated in patients with chronic pulmonary diseases.

Cardiovascular issues

    Neuraxial blockade with resultant sympathectomy may not be tolerated well in patients with significant valvular heart disease or intravascular volume depletion.

Nonresponsive patients

    There is a long and safe record of performing regional anesthesia in anesthetized pediatric patients.

    Cognitively intact adults should have regional anesthesia performed while awake and properly sedated.

Epidural hematoma formation appears to be as likely during removal of an epidural catheter as during its insertion. Reports of epidural hematoma have occurred after outpatient surgery, and patients must be instructed to immediately report symptoms of localized back pain or leg pain associated with muscle weakness, sensory deficits, and bladder or bowel dysfunction. Early diagnosis and treatment are critical for the functional recovery of the patient, and magnetic resonance imaging of the spine is the diagnostic tool of choice.

The ASRA anticoagulation consensus statements can also be applied to peripheral and plexus nerve blockade, but these may be more conservative or restrictive than necessary. Of note, most case reports of major bleeding associated with peripheral nerve blocks occurred after lumbar sympathetic or psoas compartment blocks. Coagulation issues and regional anesthesia should be addressed on a case-by-case basis, analyzing the risk-to-benefit ratio for each patient.

PERIPHERAL NERVE AND NERVE PLEXUS BLOCKADE

Basic Issues

Peripheral nerve or nerve plexus block can be utilized for neck, trunk, and extremity surgeries. Single-shot peripheral block techniques are the most common, but there is increased utilization of continuous catheter techniques, even in outpatients, and the reader is referred to one of the many recently published regional anesthesia texts for detailed block descriptions. Placement is facilitated by thorough knowledge of the regional anesthesia block anatomy, including peripheral nerve location, nerve supply to the proposed surgical site, appropriate size and length of short-bevel insulated block needles, and nerve localization aids (i.e., peripheral nerve stimulators and ultrasound). Complications of peripheral nerve and nerve plexus blockade are not common, with the most common risk being a failed block. Most regional anesthesiologists would not repeat the same block if the first attempt failed. Risks associated with all peripheral regional anesthetics are listed in Table 6-8. Risks unique to a particular technique will be addressed within the individual nerve block presentation.

Today, most anesthesiologists performing peripheral nerve blockade use surface anatomy to determine the skin entry site and nerve stimulation of an insulated block needle of appropriate length to localize the desired peripheral nerves or nerve plexus. Depth markings on longer block needles are helpful. The black electrode (i.e., the negative electrode, or cathode) of the nerve stimulator is connected to the insulated needle and the red electrode (i.e., the positive electrode, or anode) is

Table 6-7   ASRA Consensus: Anticoagulation Medications and Neuraxial Anesthesia

Medication	Consensus Recommendations
NSAIDs	No contraindication
Clopidogrel	Discontinue before 7 days
Ticlodipine	Discontinue before 14 days
GP IIB/IIIa inhibitors	Discontinue before 8–48 hours • 4–8 hours for eptifibatide and tirofiban • 24–48 hours for abciximab
Subcutaneous heparin	No contraindication • Consider block placement at heparin nadir effect • Consider delaying administration until after block if technical difficulty is likely • Preblock platelet count when heparin therapy used >4 days • Remove catheter at nadir of SQ heparin effect
Intravenous heparin	Heparinize 1 hour after neuraxial technique • Remove catheter 2–4 hours after last heparin dose • Document acceptable PTT prior to catheter removal or, if heparin was stopped preoperatively, prior to block placement
Low molecular weight heparin (LMWH)	Preoperative use: • Delay neuraxial technique for at least 10–24 hours after the last LMWH (>24 hours for therapeutic doses of LMWH) Postoperative single daily prophylaxis dosing: • First LMWH 6–8 hours after needle or catheter placement • Second LMWH at least 24 hours after first dose • Remove catheter 10–12 hours after last LMWH dose • Hold next LMWH for at least 2 hours after catheter removal Postoperative twice-daily dosing: • Delay LMWH for 24 hours after surgery • Remove neuraxial catheter 2 hours before first LMWH dose
Warfarin	Discontinue preoperatively for 4–5 days • Document normal INR prior to block placement • After initiation (or restarting therapy), remove catheter when INR = 1.5
Thrombolytics	Contraindicated • No safety data
Herbal therapy	No evidence for mandatory discontinuation before neuraxial techniques • Garlic, gingko, and ginseng have the greatest impact on hemostasis • Consider potential anesthetic drug interactions

INR, International normalized ratio; PTT, partial thromboplastin time; SQ, subcutaneous.

placed on the skin away from the nerve. Initial (i.e., after skin entry) needle seeking intensities greater than 1.0 to 1.5 mA can cause discomfort to the patient and should be avoided. The desired motor response at a current output of 0.2 to 0.5 mA provides adequate localization of the nerve. Lower stimulating currents are unnecessary and indicate very close proximity to the nerve or, possibly, intraneuronal location of the block needle. Percutaneous nerve mapping (using a blunt probe or an alligator clip applied firmly to the skin at stimulating currents of 4 to 10 mA) prior to block needle insertion can help locate superficial nerves and determine the skin entry site. Mapping needle introducers (i.e., percutaneous electrode guidance [PEG]) allow transcutaneous localization of more superficial nerves (at 2 to 3 cm depth from the skin) and subsequent needle passage through the prepositioned introducer. Correlation with the PEG system is good when the stimulating current is ≤4 mA and the skin-to-nerve distance is ≤1 cm.

Ultrasound-assisted localization of neurovascular structures facilitates peripheral nerve and plexus blockade when compared to traditional localization techniques (i.e., blind and post-skin entry). Published reports of ultrasound guidance for regional anesthesia include brachial plexus (including interscalene, supraclavicular, infraclavicular, and axillary approaches), paravertebral, femoral, and popliteal blocks. Nerve and plexus components are identified as round to oval echoic structures in the transverse view. Color Doppler helps differentiate vascular hypoechoic structures; fat and bone are hyperechoic. The desired nerve location, the nerve depth (i.e., the distance from skin to nerve), the appropriate needle entry site, the subsequent needle path or direction, and the structures to avoid (e.g., vessels, lung, and bone) are

Table 6-8 Complications Applicable to All Peripheral and Plexus Nerve Blocks	
Complication	**Comments**

Failed block	• The most common complication
	• Move on to an alternative technique such as general anesthesia in a timely fashion
	• Skin anesthesia is often the last to set up
	  ○ Have the surgeon infiltrate incisions and portal sites
	  ○ Recommended for all surgeries as part of a perioperative multimodal analgesia strategy

Infection	• Very rare with single-shot techniques • Use an aseptic technique, including gloves
Hematoma	• Avoid multiple needle placements • Remember anatomy of vascular structures in proximity to the block needle path • Hold pressure for 5 minutes if there is unintentional vascular puncture of compressible vessels • See ASRA Anticoagulant Consensus Guidelines

Local anesthetic toxicity	• Calculate maximum dosage for each patient
	• Consider levobupivacaine or ropivacaine in blocks
	  ○ Performed at multiple levels or locations
	  ○ Performed with high total volume amounts
	  ○ Performed with more concentrated preparations of local anesthetic
	• Fractionate total dose into 3–5 mL volumes
	• Aspiration prior to each dose portion
	• Do not inject local anesthetic at rates faster than 20 mL/min
	• Avoid excessive injection pressure
	• Observe the patient for signs and symptoms of systemic uptake
	• In epinephrine-containing solutions, watch for ECG, HR, and BP changes

Nerve injury	• Do not inject local anesthetic if a paresthesia persists • Stop injection if it is painful • Avoid excessive injection pressure • Remove needle and verify patency • Withdraw the block needle when there is a twitch response at less than 0.2 mA; reacquire the twitch in the desired range of 0.2–0.5 mA • May represent intraneuronal needle-tip placement

BP, Blood pressure; ECG, electrocardiogram; HR, heart rate.

all determined before the needle is inserted. After needle entry, real-time guidance is used to direct the needle tip to the desired location. Ultrasound-guided needle positioning can be confirmed and fine-tuned with nerve stimulation of the insulated block needle (or, instead or additionally, by stimulating catheter).

Often the spread of the block solution is visible on the ultrasound screen, and circumferential spread around the nerve structures correlates with high block success rates. Increased block success rate, decreased block performance time, faster block onset, decreased vascular puncture rate (i.e., the block needle being steered away from blood vessels), avoidance of adjacent tissues (e.g., bone and lung), and improved patient comfort during the block (from fewer needle manipulations) may be associated with use of ultrasound. Larger-diameter block needles are used to insert catheters for continuous perineural local anesthetic infusions. Using ultrasound to avoid adjacent vascular structures with larger-diameter needles should decrease bleeding complications. Local anesthetic spread during catheter injection is visualized in real time. These potential advantages may lead to increased ultrasound utilization in regional anesthesia.

CLINICAL CAVEAT: DESIRED CHARACTERISTICS OF PERIPHERAL NERVE STIMULATORS

- Constant current output
- Accurate and easy-to-read current display
- Easy means to adjust current output
- A foot pedal control allows the person driving the needle to make the current adjustments
- Ability to adjust output by 0.01-mA increments between the 0.00 to 0.50 mA range
- A short pulse width of approximately 100 to 200 μs
- A stimulating frequency of 2 Hz
- More optimal localization than 1-Hz stimulation
- Disconnection and malfunction indicators

Portable ultrasound devices designed for vascular access are not the best choice for nerve block procedures. The maximum depth is often insufficient for deeper nerve localization, and nerve clarity on the display is suboptimal. It is hoped that the expense of higher-resolution portable ultrasound machines (with appropriate frequency probes) will not be an impediment to expanded (and, eventually, common) use of ultrasound. Early adopters of ultrasound imaging believe nerve blockade using the visually guided technique will result in easier and more rapid performance of safer single-shot and continuous peripheral nerve blocks at higher success rates, with fewer complications when compared to traditional methods.

Peripheral Nerve and Nerve Plexus Blockade—Neck Anesthesia

Many surgeries on the neck are performed on an outpatient basis. Preoperative injection of a parathyroid localization marker and the ability to measure blood parathyroid levels rapidly are prime examples how new technologies enable minimally invasive parathyroidectomy to be completed as an outpatient procedure under regional anesthesia. A cervical plexus block can be used for unilateral outpatient procedures including neck biopsies, minimally invasive parathyroidectomy, and thyroid surgery. Superficial cervical plexus block is safe and easy to perform and provides sensory analgesia to the skin of the neck and shoulder superior to the clavicle. Local anesthetic is injected subcutaneously along the posterior border of the sternocleidomastoid muscle, avoiding the external jugular vein. Cutaneous branches from the opposite side can be blocked by midline subcutaneous infiltration from the thyroid cartilage to the suprasternal notch, and this decreases medially directed skin-retractor discomfort. Deep cervical plexus block provides muscle relaxation and typically results in superficial cervical plexus blockade as well. Deep cervical plexus blockade has a higher rate of complications, including phrenic nerve block (which is common), recurrent laryngeal nerve block (i.e., the inability to immediately assess laryngeal function after thyroid or parathyroid surgery), hematoma, hypotension, local anesthetic toxicity (most likely secondary to intravascular injection in the vascular-rich neck), and spinal anesthesia (from injection of local anesthetic inside a dural sleeve). Local anesthetic supplementation by the surgeon is just as frequent, whether a deep cervical plexus block is or is not performed. Some anesthesiologists would rather have the surgeon inject local anesthetic into the deeper areas under direct vision rather than attempt a deep block in the neck.

Peripheral Nerve and Nerve Plexus Blockade—Upper Extremity Anesthesia

In choosing a regional technique for the upper extremities, considerations include the proposed surgical site, the estimated length of the operation, the use of a tourniquet, the positioning of the patient, any arm movement required to place the block, operative traction use (in shoulder arthroscopy), potential patient movement (in surgery using a microscope), the requirement of a neurologic assessment during surgery or shortly after the conclusion of the surgery, whether general anesthesia will be utilized in a combined technique, and the complications associated with the different regional approaches.

Anesthesia of the upper extremities can be achieved with a brachial plexus block performed at the root, trunk, division, cord, or distal branch portions of the plexus. The cervical paravertebral approach to the brachial plexus has been described recently, but it is not in common use at this time. Even in experienced hands, pneumothorax can occur with the supraclavicular approach to brachial plexus blockade. Since other techniques with fewer major side effects are available, the authors recommend avoiding supraclavicular brachial plexus block in the ambulatory setting (although further experience with ultrasound-guided techniques may change this opinion). At or beyond the axilla, the individual terminal nerve branches of the brachial plexus can be blocked.

Interscalene block is commonly employed in outpatient procedures, either as a primary regional technique or in combination with general anesthesia. Indications include shoulder arthroscopy, rotator cuff repair, shoulder stabilization, and upper arm procedures such as hemodialysis access and humerus surgery. Shoulder arthroscopy may not be amenable to a regional technique without supplemental sedation or general anesthesia because of positioning, claustrophobic draping over the patients face, and the use of upper-extremity traction. Shoulder surgery is a prime example of how the combination of regional and general anesthesia can result in favorable outcomes (e.g., reduced nausea and vomiting, prolonged postoperative analgesia, and improved patient satisfaction). Less bleeding and enhanced intra-articular imaging during the course of surgery due to better intraoperative hemodynamic control are advantages that have increased surgeon acceptance of this technique. Portal insertion for shoulder arthroscopy may occur outside the cutaneous distribution of interscalene block, and the surgeon should always infiltrate local anesthetic into the portal placement sites.

The interscalene approach to the brachial plexus block is performed with an awake or slightly sedated patient who is positioned supine with the head turned slightly to the opposite side and the ipsilateral arm extended at the body side, off the abdomen. The groove between the anterior and middle scalene muscles is palpated just lateral to the posterior belly of the sternocleidomastoid (SCM) muscle at the level of the cricoid cartilage. Often the groove is in proximity to the external jugular vein, about 1 cm lateral to the cleido portion of the SCM. Having the patient lift his or her turned head helps one locate the posterior portion of the SCM, and performing a large sniff tenses the scalene muscles. Some anesthesiologists perform the block more distally in the interscalene groove (lower than the cricoid cartilage), approximately 3 to 4 cm above the clavicle.

Percutaneous nerve localization (i.e., mapping) prior to needle placement can be helpful in patients with poorly defined surface anatomy. A 22-gauge 25 to 50 mm insulated block needle is introduced perpendicular to the skin into the interscalene groove. The interscalene approach is a shallow-depth block, and the needle, in most instances, should not be advanced greater than 25 mm. Twitches of the deltoid, pectoralis, biceps, triceps, forearm, or hand muscles at a current of 0.2 to 0.4 mA are indicative of adequate nerve proximity of the needle tip. Stimulation of the diaphragm indicates the needle is inserted too far anterior, and movement of the scapula or trapezius muscle indicates too-posterior needle placement. Seepage of local anesthetic onto neighboring nerves results in a 100% incidence of ipsilateral phrenic nerve block. Some patients also develop hoarseness, ipsilateral Horner syndrome, and nasal congestion. Preoperative educational warning and gentle reassurance is typically all that is required if these occur. The ulnar nerve (C8-T1) is frequently spared, making interscalene approach undesirable for hand surgery.

Infraclavicular approach to the brachial plexus blockade is gaining in popularity and has replaced the axillary approach for some anesthesiologists. For surgery at or below the elbow, the infraclavicular approach is safe and easy to perform, even with patient positioning restrictions, and usually provides arm tourniquet analgesia. Two approaches allow the practitioner some flexibility in placement. One technique is performed with the patient supine, head facing away from the side to be blocked, the arm abducted 90 degrees, and elbow flexed 90 degrees. This is similar to the positioning for an axillary block, and one can quickly change to the axillary approach if having difficulties.

The anesthesiologist stands opposite the side that is to be blocked. The needle insertion site is identified 3 cm below the midpoint from a line drawn between the medial head of the clavicle and the coracoid process. A 22-gauge 100-mm insulated needle with depth markings, its bevel facing downward, is directed at a 45-degree angle parallel to the line between the coracoid and medial clavicular head. (Some direct toward the pulse of the axillary artery just beyond the lateral pectoralis muscle border.) Pectoralis twitch occurs from direct muscle stimulation as the needle passes through this muscle layer. The initial stimulating current is reduced to below 1 mA after disappearance of the pectoralis twitch. Hand twitch is sought at a final reduced current of 0.2 to 0.3 mA. (A typical needle depth range is 5 to 8 cm and is just beyond cessation of the pectoralis

twitch.) Median nerve stimulation is preferred, but radial or ulnar nerve stimulation can be accepted as long as there is hand twitching. Axillary nerve stimulation causing deltoid twitch indicates the needle is placed too caudad. Musculocutaneous nerve stimulation causing biceps twitch indicates the needle is placed too cephalad. Both of these nerves may have exited the brachial sheath proximal to the coracoid process and are not acceptable stimulation endpoints. Latissimus-resembling twitch indicates local stimulation of the subscapularis muscle and too-deep insertion of the needle. This laterally directed approach (directed away from the chest cavity) has an extremely rare incidence of pneumothorax, and there is usually no effect on diaphragmatic respiratory function as the block solution remains below the clavicle. It is also well-suited for placement of a catheter for continuous infusion.

Another popular infraclavicular technique is the posterior directed coracoid technique. Advantages include a consistent, reliable, and palpable bony landmark (i.e., the coracoid process); the fact that the arm to be blocked can be in any position; avoidance of neurovascular structures in the neck; low risk of pneumothorax; and a reliable block of the musculocutaneous nerve. The patient is positioned supine with his or her arm to the side. The insulated needle is inserted 2 cm caudad and 2 cm medial to the coracoid process. The needle is advanced slowly and directly posterior until median nerve stimulation is obtained, as in the laterally directed approach previously described. Again, if no stimulation is found, the needle is withdrawn superficially and directed more caudad or cephalad, making sure not to direct either medially or laterally. Hematoma is possible secondary to inadvertent subclavian vessel puncture, but typically it is of little consequence when using a 22-gauge stimulating needle.

The axillary approach is probably the best known and simplest to perform brachial plexus block. Despite this, it is still an underutilized regional anesthetic technique for surgery on the elbow, forearm, and hand. The block itself is done with the patient supine, arm abducted 90 degrees and elbow flexed 90 degrees. The axillary artery is palpated high in the axilla, just lateral to the pectoralis major muscle. A vascular Doppler or percutaneous nerve mapping can help define the needle insertion location in patients whose axillary arteries are difficult to palpate. Many nerve localization techniques have been described, including the paresthesia-elicited technique, the transarterial technique (i.e., transvascular blood aspiration), creating an anesthetic barrier by perivascular fanwise infiltration above and below the artery, nerve-stimulator-guided techniques, and, recently, ultrasound-guided localization. Regardless of the technique, the musculocutaneous nerve is often spared with the axillary approach, but it can readily be blocked by local anesthetic infiltration in a fanwise manner into the coracobrachialis muscle just superior to the axillary artery. If an arm tourniquet is needed or the surgical field involves the median antebrachial cutaneous or the medial brachial cutaneous nerves, local anesthetic is infiltrated in the subcutaneous tissue inferior to the axillary artery and parallel to the axillary skin crease. This also blocks the intercostobrachial nerve.

A wrist block can be used for procedures on the hands and fingers since the terminal branches of the radial, median, and ulnar nerves are easily blocked in this area. Wrist block is generally adequate unless an arm tourniquet is required. The median nerve is blocked between the tendons of the flexor carpi radialis and the palmaris longus, where the wrist meets the hand. The ulnar nerve is blocked just above the ulnar styloid process under the tendon of the flexor carpi ulnaris. Radial nerve block at the wrist is essentially a field block since the radial nerve has already divided into multiple cutaneous branches. Paresthesias are not usually sought, nor is a nerve stimulator used. Local anesthetic volumes in the range of 5 to 8 mL are used for each nerve.

Peripheral Nerve and Nerve Plexus Blockade—Trunk Anesthesia

Paravertebral blocks can be performed at the thoracic and lumbar levels and are useful for outpatient procedures such as breast surgery and inguinal hernia repair. The local anesthetic is injected in the area in which the spinal nerves exit the intervertebral foramina, resulting in ipsilateral somatic and sympathetic nerve blockade, usually with no significant hemodynamic effects. Multiple levels are usually blocked, although some anesthesiologists perform a single injection with a larger volume of local anesthetic. Paravertebral catheters have also been used on outpatients to provide a continuous infusion of local anesthetic for up to 48 hours.

Intercostal or rib blocks are rarely performed in outpatient settings. There has been recent controversy as to whether women undergoing breast surgery should have surgery only as inpatients, so more nursing care can be provided, or as outpatients, so they can remain home with family. Regional anesthesia decreases PONV and prolongs postoperative pain relief, and therefore makes outpatient surgery a reasonable choice. Injecting a local anesthetic into the thoracic paravertebral spaces from T1 through T6 can block pain from partial or simple mastectomy or cosmetic breast surgery. Patients having herniorrhaphy can benefit from a thoraco-lumbar paravertebral block of T9 through L1. Complications of paravertebral block include epidural or spinal spread of the local anesthetic, hematoma, local anesthetic toxicity (to avoid, calculate the total dosage with multilevel blocks), nerve injury, pneumothorax (if the pleura is penetrated), paravertebral muscle pain (to avoid, use small 22-gauge needles), and infection. Never redirect the needle medially, as it may pass intraforaminal and cause spinal cord injury. Paravertebral block at the L2 level is avoided for

hernia repair because of potential quadriceps weakness and subsequent inability to ambulate.

Other blocks are helpful for inguinal hernia repair. Injecting local anesthetic 1 cm medially and 1 cm superiorly to the anterior superior iliac spine readily blocks the ilioinguinal and iliohypogastric nerves. The needle is directed posterior to a depth of 3 to 4 cm, and local anesthetic is injected as the needle is slowly withdrawn. A second pass of the needle is made inferiorly to a similar depth, and local anesthetic again is injected as the needle is removed. This block can be reinforced by blocking the genital branch of the genitofemoral nerve by injecting just below the inguinal ligament, just lateral to the pubic tubercle. These blocks can be used either prior to surgery as the primary anesthetic or as an adjunct to general anesthesia. They provide good postoperative pain relief.

Peripheral Nerve and Nerve Plexus Blockade—Lower Extremity Anesthesia

Patients having ambulatory surgery involving the lower extremity are candidates for peripheral nerve or nerve plexus blockade. Femoral nerve block is easy to perform with a single injection of bupivacaine, and it can provide up to 24 hours of knee analgesia after knee surgery. Complex knee procedures with a posterior pain component require a sciatic nerve block in addition to femoral blockade. Lumbar plexus or psoas compartment block can be done in lieu of femoral nerve block. Unlike a femoral nerve block, these reliably block the lateral femoral cutaneous and obturator nerves in addition to the femoral nerve. Popliteal block is useful for lower leg and foot procedures. Less extensive foot procedures can be performed with an ankle block.

The popularity of ultrasound-guided lower-extremity peripheral nerve block techniques is growing. These blocks can be used as a sole technique or in conjunction with general anesthesia. They should be considered as part of a multimodal perioperative analgesic strategy for lower extremity outpatient surgery.

Femoral nerve block is indicated for anterior thigh and anterior knee procedures. Although not often used for surgeries below the knee, a femoral nerve block at the level of the inguinal crease also blocks the saphenous branch of the femoral nerve, which continues below the knee to the medial leg, the medial ankle, and the dorsal-medial top of the foot. Femoral nerve block, combined with local anesthetic infiltration in the distribution of the genitofemoral nerve, has been used as a primary anesthetic for saphenous vein stripping. Femoral nerve block is performed with the patient supine, with both legs extended, and the head of the bed flat. The femoral artery is palpated at the inguinal or femoral skin crease below the inguinal ligament. A vascular Doppler can be used to identify the femoral artery in obese patients.

Landmarks should be marked with a marking pen, the skin prepped, and local anesthetic infiltrated subcutaneously in a lateral direction from the femoral artery, where subsequent block needle entry will occur. An insulated block needle is introduced just lateral to the femoral artery at the level of the skin crease and is directed cephalad, at about a 60-degree angle to the thigh. Quadriceps twitching at a current of 0.2 to 0.4 mA is the desired endpoint. Sartorius twitching (i.e., band-like contractions across to the medial thigh without patellar movement) is common and is not an acceptable endpoint as the femoral nerve branches to the sartorius may reside outside the femoral sheath, leading to incomplete block.

Lumbar plexus block is indicated for anterior knee, anterior thigh, and hip procedures, and when combined with sciatic nerve block, provides anesthesia for the entire lower extremity. The femoral, lateral femoral cutaneous, genitofemoral cutaneous, and obturator nerves are branches of the lumbar plexus. To place this block, the patient should be in the lateral decubitus position with a slight pelvic tilt forward and the operative leg up so that the quadriceps muscle is easily observed. A line is drawn midline over the lumbar spinous processes, and a second line is drawn from the iliac crest down and perpendicular to the spinous process line. A 21- to 22-gauge 100-mm insulated needle with depth markings is inserted 4 cm lateral to the intersection of the two landmark lines, perpendicular to the skin. Stimulation of the quadriceps muscle is sought at 0.5 to 1 mA and is generally encountered at a depth of 6 to 8 cm in patients of normal body habitus. Lower stimulating currents are avoided as quadriceps contraction at low currents may represent needle placement inside a dural sleeve, causing subsequent spread into the epidural or subarachnoid space. Risks of lumbar plexus block include hematoma, infection, vascular puncture (to prevent this, avoid deep insertions), local anesthetic toxicity (to prevent this, calculate the maximum dose for each patient), nerve injury, and hemodynamic effects (i.e., hypotension secondary to unilateral sympathetic block or epidural spread of local anesthetic). Complications are more frequent with lumbar plexus block than with femoral nerve blocks.

Sciatic nerve block is indicated for surgery on the knee (in conjunction with lumbar plexus block as a primary anesthetic of the lower extremity and for analgesia for posterior knee pain postoperatively), tibia, ankle, and foot. The saphenous branch of the femoral nerve provides cutaneous innervation of the medial surface of the lower leg. All other innervation below the knee is from the sciatic nerve and its branches. The sciatic nerve can be blocked at several levels and by using different methods. Block sites include the posterior transgluteal approach, the posterior and lateral popliteal approaches, and approaches at the terminal branches of the sciatic nerve in the ankle.

A posterior sciatic nerve block is performed with the patient in the lateral position with the operated leg up and placed on top of the dependent leg so twitches of the foot and toes are easily visible. The operative side knee is placed in front of the dependent knee and provides some forward tilting away from the true lateral position. A line is drawn between the posterior superior iliac spine on the side facing the greater trochanter and the posterior portion of the greater trochanter of the femur. A second line is drawn perpendicular and inferior to the midpoint of the first line. Needle entry occurs on this second line, 4 cm inferior to the trochanter-iliac spine line. After subcutaneous infiltration with local anesthetic, a 100-mm insulated block needle is inserted perpendicular to the skin at an initial current of 1 to 1.5 mA. The needle is advanced, causing local gluteal muscle twitches, which disappear as the needle is advanced deeper. With a slowly advancing needle, hamstring, calf, foot, or toe twitches are sought at a final current of 0.2 to 0.5 mA (typically at a depth of 50 to 80 mm). Twenty milliliters of plain local anesthetic are injected after negative aspirations, using divided doses. Epinephrine is avoided in proximal sciatic nerve blocks because of the variable blood supply and the potential for nerve stretching or compression (i.e., from tourniquet use or sitting postoperatively). Complications of transgluteal sciatic nerve block include hematoma, vascular puncture (to prevent this, avoid deep insertions), infection, local anesthetic toxicity (especially when combined with lumbar plexus block), and nerve injury.

Popliteal block of the sciatic nerve is performed at the level of the popliteal fossa and is indicated for ankle and foot surgery. Posterior and lateral approaches are used with a stimulating needle. Twitching of the toes or foot at 0.2 to 0.5 mA is an acceptable endpoint, with dorsiflexion and eversion indicating common peroneal nerve stimulation. Planter flexion and inversion indicates tibial nerve stimulation. A 35- to 45-mL injection of local anesthetic solution is given. Complications of popliteal block include hematoma, vascular puncture, local anesthetic toxicity, infection, nerve injury, and tissue pressure injury secondary to an insensate extremity.

For the posterior approach, the patient is placed prone, with feet extending beyond the bed so foot and toe movements are readily visible. The popliteal skin crease and biceps femoris and semitendinosus muscles are marked. A 50-mm insulated block needle is inserted at the midpoint of a line drawn between the two tendons, 7 cm above the popliteal crease. The initial current is set at 1 to 1.5 mA, and the needle is advanced until foot or toe movement is observed. At that point, the current is dropped into the 0.2- to 0.5-mA range. Occasionally, stimulation only occurs between 0.5 and 1 mA, and this is acceptable if the muscle response is clearly felt or visible. Calf muscle twitching is not acceptable because these nerve branches may be located outside the nerve sheath.

The lateral approach to popliteal block is performed with the patient in the supine position. The groove between the vastus lateralis and biceps femoris muscles is marked. The needle insertion point is in this groove, 8 cm above the popliteal skin crease (or 7 cm above the lateral femoral condyle). A 100-mm insulated needle with depth markings is inserted parallel to the floor and perpendicular to the long axis of the leg until the femur is contacted, and this depth is noted. After withdrawing the needle to the skin, the needle is redirected 30 degrees posterior until foot or toe twitches are obtained. This is typically 1 to 2 cm deeper than the femur contact depth, at a total depth of 5 to 7 cm. Stimulation currents are the same as for the posterior approach. The local anesthetic solution is injected in divided doses. If no motor response is elicited, the needle is withdrawn to the skin level and redirected 5 to 10 degrees posterior, repeating this maneuver a second time if necessary.

Ankle blocks are indicated for surgery of the toes and foot in cases in which a leg tourniquet is not required for longer than a few minutes. Local anesthetic solution without epinephrine and a 25-gauge 1.5-inch needle are used. The posterior tibial nerve is blocked in a fanlike manner just behind the medial malleolus. The deep peroneal nerve is blocked in a fanlike manner just lateral to the external hallicis longus at the level of the malleoli and lateral to the dorsalis pedis artery. The needle is introduced until bony contact occurs, is withdrawn 1 to 2 mm, and local anesthetic is injected. The superficial terminal branches of the saphenous, superficial peroneal, and sural nerves are each blocked with a subcutaneous infiltration of local anesthetic at the level of the tibial malleoli. The saphenous and superficial peroneal field blocks can often be performed from the deep peroneal skin entry site without removing the needle. Complications of ankle block are rare; however, care should be taken to avoid the saphenous vein.

REGIONAL ANESTHESIA FOR OPTHALMIC PROCEDURES

With health care reimbursements declining, all surgeries have to be done in an efficient manner in order to be sustainable for the outpatient surgery center. This is especially true for ophthalmologic surgery. Cataract surgery, particularly, has a narrow economic margin. Ophthalmologists often perform local or regional anesthesia for eye surgery, with sedation administered by a nurse or anesthesia provider. In order to be the most efficient, the outpatient center can be set up to facilitate case turnover so that the next patient's eye block is being performed while the prior case is proceeding. There is a multitude of options to anesthetize the eye. Local anesthetic instilled directly to the eye is the simplest,

whereas retrobulbar block involves the most risk. Branches of the facial nerve may also be blocked.

Retrobulbar block involves the injection of local anesthetic into the central cone behind the eye. Risks include globe penetration and retrobulbar hemorrhage. A peribulbar block is the injection of local anesthetic outside of the muscle cone of the eye; the local anesthetic gains access to the muscle cone and ciliary ganglion. Peribulbar block is associated with less risk at the price of slower onset and lesser efficacy (i.e., the need for repeat injection) when compared to retrobulbar block. Complications of eye blocks include oculocardiac reflex (causing bradycardia) and local anesthetic toxicity (from retinal artery injection). Intramuscular injection may lead to extraocular muscle damage. Globe perforation by the needle is possible, as are retrobulbar hemorrhage, brainstem anesthesia, and sedation complications (i.e., apnea, hypoventilation, hypoxemia, and airway obstruction).

INTRAVENOUS REGIONAL BLOCK

Intravenous regional anesthesia (IVRA) is a simple, reliable, and economically feasible anesthetic for short procedures on the hand, forearm, ankle, or foot. A 22-gauge intravenous catheter is placed in the operative limb, as close to the operative site as possible. The limb is exsanguinated (with elevation for 1 to 2 minutes followed by a tight esmarch elastic bandage wrapping), and a pneumatic tourniquet is inflated (to at least 300 mm Hg, or to 100 mm Hg above systolic pressures >200 mm Hg). After verification of tourniquet inflation integrity, local anesthetic is injected over 90 seconds into the previously placed 22-gauge intravenous catheter. Commonly, 0.5% lidocaine, 3 mg/kg, up to a maximum dose of 250 mg, is injected in a 50-mL (in the arm), or 70-mL (in the leg) total volume. Rapid injection may create high venous pressures and tourniquet leakage into the systemic circulation. Local anesthetic in the now-distended venous system diffuses retrograde and contacts nerve endings, producing anesthesia. If surgery is short, the tourniquet should remain inflated for at least 20 minutes to lessen the chance of local anesthetic toxicity after extremity washout. If less than 30 to 40 minutes have elapsed, the tourniquet is deflated for 10 seconds and then reinflated for 1 to 2 minutes prior to final tourniquet deflation. (Some anesthesiologists repeat this deflation/inflation cycle several times.) The tourniquet or tourniquets should be clearly labeled and operating room staff instructed that only the anesthesia provider is allowed to control the tourniquet. Unintentional tourniquet deflation must be avoided to prevent local anesthetic systemic toxicity.

Drawbacks of IVRA include tourniquet discomfort (avoided by limiting duration to 45 to 60 minutes), a 10-

to 15-minute onset time for surgical anesthesia, and rapid resolution of the anesthetic with lack of postoperative analgesia once the tourniquet is deflated.

Many anesthesiologists use a double-tourniquet system to gain some additional time when the patient complains of tourniquet pain. After exsanguination, with an Esmarch's bandage still in place, the distal tourniquet is inflated and followed by proximal tourniquet inflation. The distal tourniquet is then deflated, and injection of the local anesthetic solution is begun. If the patient complains of tourniquet pain, the distal tourniquet is inflated over the anesthetized area and then the proximal tourniquet is deflated.

A forearm tourniquet can be used for some procedures, depending on surgeon preferences. Advantages of a forearm tourniquet include a 50% dose reduction of local anesthetic and a delayed onset of tourniquet discomfort of a lesser degree. A sterile forearm cuff can be used as a rescue cuff for bothersome tourniquet discomfort from a double-cuff upper-arm setup.

Longer-acting local anesthetics have been used for IVRA, including ropivacaine and levobupivacaine. Results have shown slower onset times compared with lidocaine. Duration of postoperative analgesia was increased, but to a much lesser extent when compared

to the use of adjuncts such as ketorolac or clonidine added to lidocaine (see below).

Additives to lidocaine may aid in combating tourniquet pain and provide extended postoperative analgesia (Table 6-9). Ketorolac, clonidine, ketamine, neostigmine, meperidine, and magnesium sulfate have all been studied for use in IVRA, with variable success. The authors' standard cost-effective multimodal IVRA block mixture is 0.5% lidocaine plus 10 mg ketamine plus 15 mg ketorolac (unless there are platelet or bone-healing issues, which should be discussed with the surgeon ahead of time). Clonidine is relatively more expensive unless the standard vial is divided into unit doses and is used on multiple patients. If no IVRA adjuncts are employed, surgeons should be encouraged to infiltrate a longer-duration local anesthetic in the surgical field.

NEURAXIAL REGIONAL TECHNIQUES

Neuraxial regional anesthetic techniques (i.e., subarachnoid and epidural) are underutilized in ambulatory surgery despite allowing for more alert and comfortable patients in the postoperative period. A reduced incidence of PONV, when compared to patients recovering from

---

Table 6-9 Useful Pharmacologic Adjuncts Added to Lidocaine for IVRA

Drug and Dosage	Comments
Ketamine 0.1 mg/kg	• Enhances intraoperative analgesia • Less need for intraoperative opiate • Reduces tourniquet discomfort to a great degree
Clonidine 1–1.5 µg/kg (50–100 µg)	• Reduces tourniquet discomfort • Contributes to postoperative analgesia for up to 6 hours

Dexmedetomidine
  0.5 µg/kg
	• Single study demonstrated:
	  ○ Shortened sensory and motor block onset times
	  ○ Enhanced intraoperative analgesia
	  ○ Reduced tourniquet discomfort
	  ○ Contribution to postoperative analgesia for at least 6 hours

Ketorolac
  20 mg (for arm tourniquet)
  10 mg (for forearm tourniquet)
	• Reduces tourniquet discomfort
	• Contributes to postoperative analgesia for up to 12–16 hours
	• Concerns regarding platelet effect and bony osteogenesis should be discussed with the surgeon prior to using ketorolac as an adjunct

Atracurium 30 µg/kg	• Improves operating conditions when motor blockade is desired (e.g., for tendon repair or fracture reduction) • Delayed return of muscle strength after tourniquet deflation
Meperidine 1 mg/kg	• Intrinsic local anesthetic activity
Neostigmine 0.5 mg	• Improvement described when combined with prilocaine • No large-scale experience

Magnesium sulfate
  10 mL of 15% solution added to 50 mL
  of local anesthetic
	• Significant burning sensation can occur during injection
	• No large-scale experience

general anesthesia, is an additional benefit with these techniques. The ideal neuraxial technique would be easily and quickly performed, would have rapid onset with reasonable offset and street-readiness time, and would be associated with low risk and minimal side effects.

Lidocaine spinal anesthesia has the advantages of rapid onset with competitive recovery and discharge times when compared to general anesthesia for the same procedure. Unfortunately, the increased incidence of transient neurologic symptoms (TNS) with lidocaine spinal anesthesia has curtailed its use by many anesthesiologists.

Epidural anesthesia can be titrated using a catheter technique and has the advantage of more precisely matching anesthetic duration to the surgical duration. Compared to spinal anesthesia, epidural block placement time and the time to achieve surgical anesthesia are longer. The combined spinal–epidural (CSE) technique

takes advantage of the rapid onset of a dense and reliable spinal anesthetic, and the flexibility of extending anesthetic duration or intensifying blockade by additional dosing of the epidural catheter and use of CSE anesthesia for ambulatory surgery is increasing.

Caudal epidural injection of local anesthetic plus analgesic adjuncts can provide prolonged postoperative analgesia in pediatric outpatients. (See Chapter 10.)

Neuraxial Regional Techniques—Spinal Anesthesia

Spinal anesthesia can be used as the primary anesthetic for many outpatient surgeries that occur at or below the umbilicus. Most anesthesiologists can readily perform a successful spinal anesthetic in a timely fashion without increasing overall operating room time when compared to general anesthesia. Preparation for surgery can occur while the spinal is setting up, and emergence time is eliminated if general anesthesia is eliminated. When spinal anesthesia is the primary technique, surgeons should be reminded to inject incisions with a longer-duration local anesthetic as part of a multimodal postoperative analgesic strategy. Epidural catheter or CSE techniques are better suited for outpatient procedures lasting longer than 60 minutes. Peripheral nerve or nerve plexus blocks may be preferable for unilateral lower extremity procedures and have an additional advantage of providing prolonged postoperative analgesia, using either single-shot or continuous catheter infusion techniques.

The spinal anesthetic challenge is to best match the patient, surgeon, procedure, and estimated surgical duration with the optimal spinal local anesthetic and adjunct agents while considering the recovery profile and side effects of the selected spinal medication or medications. The goal of a timely recovery from spinal anesthesia must be matched with the anticipated length of the procedure. If surgical duration is longer than anticipated, supplemental local anesthetic infiltration by the surgeon and further intravenous sedation and analgesia may be required to finish the procedure. Conversion to general anesthesia may occur, and all patients should be informed of the potential need for general anesthesia preoperatively, regardless of the regional anesthetic technique. There is a low but universal incidence of failed blocks, even when placed by experienced and skillful anesthesia providers.

In current practice, lidocaine, bupivacaine, and procaine are the most commonly used local anesthetics for outpatient spinal anesthesia (Table 6-10). Hyperbaric solutions are preferred for surgeries at or above the inguinal ligament since spinal block density is less with isobaric solutions at dermatome levels above T12 through L1. Preservative-free 2-chloroprocaine has demonstrated

CLINICAL CAVEAT: TRANSIENT NEUROLOGIC SYMPTOMS (TNS) AND SPINAL LIDOCAINE

- Increased TNS risk in outpatients receiving spinal lidocaine
  - 16% to 40% reported incidence
  - TNS onset within 12 to 24 hours of surgery, lasting for 6 to 96 hours
    - Sensory or pain abnormalities in the anterior or posterior thighs +/− extension into legs +/− back pain
    - Discomfort typically mild to moderate, but it can be marked
    - No motor weakness
    - No neurologic abnormalities
  - Treatment of TNS consists of NSAIDs and oral opiates
    - Consider muscle relaxant and warm heat if muscle spasm present
    - Trigger point injections may also be helpful for muscle spasm
- TNS factors
  - Lithotomy position, obesity, and knee arthroscopy increase risk of TNS
  - Lidocaine dose, dilution, and baricity appear to have no effect on TNS incidence
- Does TNS represent low-grade lidocaine neurotoxicity?
  - Possible measures to minimize lidocaine neurotoxicity
    - Limit lidocaine dose to 50 to 60 mg maximum
    - Lidocaine concentration should not exceed 2.5%
    - Dilute commercial hyperbaric 5% lidocaine solution 1:1 with cerebral spinal fluid
    - Do not use epinephrine as an adjunct to prolong duration

promising short-acting and timely-offset properties without increased incidence of TNS in volunteers. Larger clinical trials utilizing 2-chloroprocaine are underway. Microcatheter spinal techniques are being reevaluated for efficacy and safety after being withdrawn from the market secondary to the association with caudal equina syndrome. Less neurotoxic local anesthetics, such as bupivacaine, can be titrated in small doses through the spinal microcatheter, allowing for surgical duration flexibility coupled with a low risk of postdural puncture headache. Fentanyl, epinephrine, and clonidine are the most common adjuncts coadministered with a local anesthetic for multimodal spinal anesthesia (Table 6-11). Water-soluble spinal opiates are not appropriate for ambulatory surgery secondary to risks of sedation, delayed respiratory depression, pruritus, and urinary retention. Complications of ambulatory spinal anesthesia are listed in Table 6-12.

Neuraxial Regional Techniques—Epidural and Combined Spinal–Epidural Anesthesia

Epidural anesthesia for outpatient surgery can be performed using either a single-shot or a continuous catheter technique. The block should be placed closest to the dermatome level of the procedure to provide intense neural blockade at the surgical site, utilizing the smallest effective local anesthetic dose. Abdominal surgeries below the umbilicus can be performed with lumbar epidural catheters using larger local anesthetic doses, but

---

Table 6-10   Spinal Local Anesthetics for Outpatient Surgery

Spinal Agent	Comments

Lidocaine	• Traditional ambulatory spinal anesthetic of choice
	• Quick onset, short duration, and rapid recovery
	• Associated with transient neurologic symptoms (TNS)
	• Controversy regarding its continued use
	• Consider using in supine patients not undergoing knee arthroscopy (to minimize TNS risk) for expected surgical durations < 60 minutes
	  ○ Desired block < T10
	    ■ 30–40 mg isobaric 2% lidocaine plus 10–20 µg fentanyl
	  ○ Desired block = T10
	    ■ 50–60 mg hyperbaric 2.5% lidocaine plus 10–20 µg fentanyl
	    ■ Dilute 5% lidocaine in D7.5W with an equal volume of aspirated CSF

Bupivacaine	• Lowest reported incidence of TNS (0–2%)
	• Conventional doses (10–15 mg) associated with prolonged block resolution and delayed discharge from outpatient unit
	  ○ Large standard deviations of length of blockade and recovery time when compared to lidocaine (i.e., poor recovery predictability)
	  ○ Consider continuous epidural anesthesia or CSE for expected surgical durations >60 minutes
	• Lower-than-traditional bupivacaine dose increases failure rate
	• Multimodal spinal anesthesia
	  ○ Low-dose bupivacaine (4–7.5 mg) plus 10–20 µg fentanyl
	  ○ Increases the success rate
	  ○ Maintains a favorable recovery profile and a competitive discharge time

Procaine	• Shortest-acting local anesthetic approved for spinal anesthesia • Time to home-readiness is longer when compared to lidocaine • Failure rate of approximately 1 in 7 • Fentanyl coadministration decreases failure rate • Increased incidence and severity of pruritus when compared to fentanyl plus lidocaine or bupivacaine • High incidence of postoperative nausea (17%) • TNS incidence of 1–6%
Mepivacaine	• No advantage over lidocaine
Ropivacaine	• No advantage at equipotent doses over the less-costly bupivacaine
Levo-bupivacaine	• No advantage over the less-costly bupivacaine
2-Chloroprocaine	• Encouraging (but small in number) studies show short duration, favorable recovery, and low TNS incidence

CSE, Combined spinal–epidural anesthesia.

Table 6-11	Spinal Anesthetic Multimodal Adjuncts for Outpatient Surgery

Spinal Adjunct	Comments
Fentanyl	• 10–25 µg prolongs and intensifies surgical anesthesia without increasing recovery time • Respiratory depression highly unlikely at these doses • Dose-related, but typically mild, pruritus in up to 50% of patients • Increases spinal success rate when coadministered with reduced doses of local anesthetic • Decreases lower-extremity tourniquet discomfort • Contributes to early postoperative analgesia
Epinephrine	• Prolongs sensory and motor block • Delays time to void and increases length of stay • Consider epidural analgesia if longer block duration is desired • Not recommended as spinal anesthetic adjunct for outpatient surgery
Clonidine	• 15–75 µg potentiates spinal local anesthetic and contributes to postoperative analgesia • Unacceptable rate of side effects (e.g., sedation and hypotension) • Lowest effective spinal anesthetic dose with minimized side effects not established • Not recommended as spinal anesthetic adjunct for outpatient surgery at this time
Neostigmine	• Potentiates spinal local anesthetic and contributes to postoperative analgesia • Unacceptable rate of nausea and vomiting • Not recommended as a spinal anesthetic adjunct for outpatient surgery • Not FDA-approved for subarachnoid use

time to bladder sensation recovery and patient discharge is typically prolonged.

Single-injection epidural techniques are best suited for surgeons performing procedures predictably lasting less than 1 to 1.5 hours. The epidural local anesthetic is chosen based on anticipated surgical duration to facilitate timely block offset and a favorable recovery profile. Preservative-free 3% 2-chloroprocaine provides surgical anesthesia for 45 to 60 minutes without prolonging ambulatory discharge times. Lidocaine at 1.5% to 2% provides 60 to 90 minutes of surgical anesthesia. Local anesthetic dosing through the epidural needle avoids epidural catheter placement and catheter malpositioning problems (i.e., intravascular, intrathecal, or one-sided block). One can also coadminister 1 µg/kg of fentanyl with the epidural local anesthetic to enhance analgesia. The preservative-free preparation of 2-chloroprocaine is associated with less muscular backache when compared to the ethylenediamine tetraacetic acid (EDTA) preparation. Longer-acting amide local anesthetics are usually avoided due to prolonged times to discharge.

Epidural catheter techniques allow the flexibility of further local anesthetic dosing to intensify the block or to prolong block duration; catheters are recommended for ambulatory procedures expected to last longer than 1 to 1.5 hours. CSE anesthesia, as popularized for obstetrical analgesia, is finding its way into ambulatory surgery centers. A pencil-tip small-gauge long spinal needle is placed through a prepositioned epidural needle. Local anesthetic with or without fentanyl is injected into the spinal fluid, followed by epidural catheter placement and subsequent local anesthetic supplementation through the catheter, as required. CSE has a more rapid onset and a higher success rate when compared to conventional epidural anesthesia.

Complications of epidural anesthesia are similar to those of spinal anesthesia. Hypotension is more gradual in onset with epidural anesthesia. The incidence of TNS is very low after epidural anesthesia. Post-dural puncture headache (PDPH) is less common with epidural anesthesia since the accidental dural puncture rate is less than 1% to 2% in experienced hands. An immediate-onset headache is often seen after unintentional dural puncture using an air loss of resistance technique, resulting in pneumoencephalitis. Unfortunately, depending on the age and gender of the patient and the level of puncture, a significant proportion of patients develop PDPH after unintentional dural puncture with large-diameter epidural needles. Epidural hematoma has occurred after outpatient epidural anesthesia. Risk of local anesthetic systemic toxicity and total

Table 6-12   Spinal Anesthetic Complications

Complication	Comments
Hypotension	• Secondary to arteriolar dilation and venous pooling from sympathetic blockade • High blockade produces loss of cardioaccelerator innervation and a decrease in cardiac output
Bradycardia	• High thoracic (T1–T2) sympathetic block of cardiac accelerators with unopposed action of the vagus nerve • Rare progression to asystole, especially in vagotonic patients • IV epinephrine indicated to restore circulation for severe bradycardia and asystole
Total spinal anesthesia	• Unusual with lower doses currently used for ambulatory patients • Avoid high doses of hyperbaric solutions, extreme patient movement, and the head-down position
Delayed discharge	• Use the lowest effective dose of local anesthetic • Use fentanyl as an adjunct • Avoid epinephrine adjunct

Urinary retention	• Avoid epinephrine adjunct
	• Voiding unnecessary prior to discharge with currently recommended outpatient spinal local anesthetic doses in low-risk patients with ultrasound scanned bladder volumes <400 mL
	• Some populations are at high risk for urinary retention after neuraxial anesthetic:
	  ○ Inguinal hernia, anal, and urologic procedures
	  ○ Age greater than 70
	  ○ Patient history of difficulty voiding

Post-dural puncture headache (PDPH)	• Incidence <1–3% using small-diameter 25- to 27-gauge noncutting pencil-point-tip needles (use these needles in high-risk patients, such as patients of age <30 years and females) • Headache occurs with upright posture and is clearly improved with supine posture • Associated symptoms include nausea, neck pain, diplopia, hearing loss, or tinnitus • Two-thirds of headaches resolve within 1 week • Epidural blood patch (10–20 mL blood) is indicated for bothersome headaches that limit patient function
Transient neurologic symptoms	• Relatively common after lidocaine spinal anesthesia • Low incidence with spinal bupivacaine • No cases of permanent neurologic damage reported
Backache	• Secondary to needle trauma or ligament stretching after muscle relaxation; may actually be transient neurologic symptoms
Neurologic injury	• Baseline neurologic exam is essential • Document presence, location, and duration or persistence of paresthesia if elicited (reported paresthesia incidences of 5–6%) • Stop spinal injection if the patient reports discomfort
Infection	• Extremely rare • Use sterile technique • Avoid if patient is bacteremic
Hematoma	• Extremely rare • Follow ASRA Consensus Guidelines (see Table 6-7)

spinal anesthesia is greater for the epidural technique since the total dose of local anesthetic is 5 to 10 times greater for epidural administration when compared to the spinal local anesthetic dose. Fractionated doses with observation periods for signs and symptoms of systemic uptake (in intravascular injection) or pronounced local anesthetic blockade (in subarachnoid injection) between doses must be utilized because of the large doses of local anesthetic used for surgical epidural anesthesia. Unilateral or incomplete patchy blocks occasionally occur, and it is best not to advance multiholed epidural catheters beyond 4 to 5 cm and the end-holed single-orifice catheters beyond 2 to 3 cm.

ACUTE PAIN MANAGEMENT IN THE OPIATE-DEPENDENT OUTPATIENT

Many patients who present for outpatient surgery may be opiate dependent or at least moderately tolerant to the therapeutic effects of opiate analgesics. Prolonged opiate therapy can lead to cellular and intracellular changes, including activation of N-methyl-D-aspartate receptors. Such changes may contribute to pharmacologic opiate tolerance, increased sensitivity to pain (manifested as apparent opiate tolerance), or both. Prolonged opiate treatment may also result in hormonal changes and may alter immune function. These effects may be exacerbated by dose escalation in some circumstances. Patients may also experience opiate-induced hyperalge-

sia (OIH), an increased sensitivity to pain. The immediate perioperative period is not the optimal time to attempt detoxification or rehabilitation management for any patient chronically using or abusing opiates. Methods for optimizing perioperative pain management for the patients chronically consuming opiates are complex. A suggested strategy (modified from two recent review articles) is listed in Box 6-4.

CONCLUSION

Appropriate use of regional anesthesia, combined with adequate postoperative analgesia, leads to successful outpatient surgery and highly satisfied patients.

Box 6-4   Acute Pain Management in Patients Chronically Consuming Opiates

PREOPERATIVE CONSIDERATIONS

Discuss the Following with Opiate-Dependent Patients:

- Precise opiate use
  - Identify chronic opiate-consuming patients with early recognition and high index of suspicion
  - Determine total dose, opiate type, route of injestion, etc.
- Potential for increased postoperative pain
  - All patients should be informed about the potential for aggravated pain and increased opiate requirements during the postoperative period
- Alternative analgesic techniques that complement opiates
  - Be sure to discuss appropriate regional techniques
- Effective management strategies after previous procedures
  - Also discuss ineffective strategies
    - Reluctance of care-givers to administer higher opiate doses
    - Incidents of inadequate analgesia
    - Relapse episodes
- Patient's fears and expectations related to pain management
  - Concerns related to the following:
    - Pain control
    - Anxiety
    - Risk of relapse
- Postoperative pain management plan
  - The patient and health care providers should formulate, at least in general terms, a perioperative pain management plan before surgery
  - Consider meeting with addiction specialists and pain specialists with regard to perioperative planning
  - Opiates remain an important component of postoperative pain therapy
  - An adequate opiate dose needs to be maintained to prevent opiate withdrawal

Initiation of Appropriate Preoperative Medications:

- Continue the preoperative opiate regimen on the day of surgery (i.e., oral, transdermal, intravenous)
  - Chronically opiate-consuming patients should receive their regular opiate dose on the day of surgery, especially if large doses of long-acting opiates are involved
  - Avoid withdrawal and the need to catch up with the patient's opiate requirement
- Consider administering 1000 mg of acetaminophen 1 to 2 hours before surgery
- Consider a COX-1 or COX-2 inhibitor
- Consider a single preoperative dose of gabapentin

(Continued)

Box 6-4   Acute Pain Management in Patients Chronically Consuming Opiates—Cont'd

INTRAOPERATIVE CONSIDERATIONS

Administration of Opiates to Meet the Following Requirements:

- Chronic pain
- Intraoperative surgical stimulation
- Anticipated postoperative pain
  - Long-acting opiates seem best suited for substituting the opiate dose taken chronically because relatively stable opiate plasma concentrations are produced
    - Often, the use of a continuous infusion of opiate is the best way to provide a steady serum concentration if the oral route is unavailable perioperatively
    - Although the use of short-acting opiates can be adequate for alleviating short-lasting stimulation caused by the surgical intervention, their sole use in opiate-dependent patients may result in very poorly controlled pain or even opiate withdrawal after surgery
  - One technique that may help gauge the adequacy of intraoperative opiate dosing is to reverse neuromuscular blockade and to allow patients to breath spontaneously at later stages of the general anesthetic
    - Patients with respiratory rates greater than 20 breaths/min and exhibiting slightly to markedly dilated pupils generally require additional opiate dosing
    - Intravenous boluses of morphine, fentanyl, or hydromorphone are titrated as needed to maintain a rate of 12–14 breaths/min and a slightly miotic pupil

Administration of Adjuvant Medications:

- Ketamine: 0.5 mg/kg IV bolus followed by 4 µg/kg/min infusion
- Ketorolac: 30 mg IV (if COX-1 or COX-2 inhibitor is not started preoperatively)
- Acetaminophen: 1000 mg orally if not started preoperatively

Institution of Appropriate Regional Technique:

- Continuous techniques (preferable)
  - Wound lavage or local infiltration with local anesthetic if another technique is not possible
- Despite a regional analgesic technique, opiate-dependent patients will still need their daily systemic opiate dose
  - Continuing daily systemic dose will prevent withdrawal
  - Daily systemic administration of at least half of the preoperative opiate dose is usually sufficient to prevent withdrawal when regional anesthetic techniques are used
  - Patient's chronic pain may not be improved by the surgical procedure

POSTOPERATIVE CONSIDERATIONS

- No predictions of opiate requirements can be made for individual patients
- Patients who use even modest opiate doses (i.e., <50 mg/day oral morphine equivalent) before surgery often require their baseline opiate dose plus 2 (or more) times the amount of opiates typically used for adequate pain control in opiate-naïve patients

Postoperative-Acute Phase:

- Titration of opiates, adjuvant medications, and regional techniques to patient comfort:
  - Expect postoperative opiate requirements to be up to 2 to 4 times the dose required in an opiate-naïve person
  - Remember that no individual's requirements can be predicted with confidence
  - Titrate opiates aggressively to achieve adequate pain control in the postoperative care unit
- Starting IV opiate patient-controlled anaglesia (PCA) (for inpatients):
  - If oral route is available, start with 1.5 times the preoperative oral opiate dose and use the IV opiate PCA for breakthrough pain
    - If oral route is unavailable, consider basal rate for PCA
  - Alternative approach
    - Sole use of intravenous opiates by PCA during the first 24 to 48 hours after surgery (the period during which opiate requirements are changing most rapidly)
    - After that period, the total dose delivered intravenously can be converted into a daily oral opiate dose sufficient for alleviating pain
  - The PCA device should be programmed to administer a patient-initiated dose of 3 to 5 mg morphine or 0.5 to 1 mg hydromorphone

(Continued)

Box 6-4 Acute Pain Management in Patients Chronically Consuming Opiates—Cont'd

- ○ Lockout interval should range from 6 to 10 min
- ○ A basal opiate infusion is often added to cover baseline requirements in patients who cannot take their daily dose of oral opiate
- • In patients undergoing a regional technique:
  - ○ Plan to administer at least half of the preoperative opiate requirement systemically
  - ○ Continue applicable regional techniques
  - ○ Consider using high-potency opiates such as fentanyl or sufentanil in place of morphine for epidural management (in inpatients)
- • Continue adjunct multimodal analgesics:
  - ○ Acetaminophen: 1000 mg every 6 hours, and/or
  - ○ NSAID or a COX-2 inhibitor, continued for several days (pay attention to renal function and risk of bleeding)
- • Ketamine (in inpatients)
  - ○ Continue ketamine if started in the operating room
  - ○ Consider instituting a ketamine infusion if pain proves refractory to other measures
- • Consider gabapentin
- • Consider α-2 agonists administered by oral, IV, or transdermal routes
- • Monitoring for oversedation and opiate withdrawal:
  - ○ Chronically opiate-consuming patients may be at higher risk for respiratory depression than opiate-naïve patients; they must be monitored appropriately with regular evaluation of sedation and oxygen saturation

Postoperative-Transition Phase:

- • Inpatients
  - ○ Chronically opiate-consuming patients require opiates for a prolonged period of time through the intravenous or epidural route when compared with opiate-naïve patients
  - ○ Monitoring of sedation should be maintained during this transition period
  - ○ Transition from regional and parenteral techniques to oral opiates or adjuvants:
    - ▪ Use the opiate requirements during the first 24 to 48 hours to determine daily oral opiate dose
    - ▪ Deliver half of the estimated oral requirement as a long-acting formulation to provide a steady baseline control of pain
    - ▪ During the early phases of the transition to oral opiates, time will be required for the serum levels of the long-acting opiates to approximate steady state; transition to oral medication should not be unduly delayed
    - ▪ Allow PRN use of a short-acting opiate every 3 hours in sufficient quantity to provide the remaining required opiate dose. This provides control of breakthrough pain
    - ▪ As the surgical pain subsides, cutting back on the breakthrough opiate medication is a simple way by which patients can reduce the total daily opiate dose
- • Both inpatients and outpatients
  - ○ Consider continuing acetaminophen and/or COX-1 (or COX-2?) inhibitors during the transition phase
  - ○ Plan to taper from postoperative opiate doses toward preoperative doses: discuss with patient or care provider
  - ○ Determine the need for specialty follow-up if regimen is particularly complex
  - ○ Discharging chronically opiate-consuming patients on the same opiate regimen they adhered to before surgery often results in inadequate pain control
  - ○ Develop a pain management plan before hospital discharge
  - ○ Provide adequate doses of opiate and nonopiate analgesics
  - ○ A slow tapering (over 2 to 4 weeks) from the oral dose on which the patient is stabilized at discharge is often a reasonable goal
  - ○ If surgery provides complete pain relief, opiates should be slowly tapered (no faster than 25% per day) rather than abruptly discontinued

Adapted from: Carroll I, Angst M, Clark J: Management of perioperative pain in patients chronically consuming opiates. Reg Anesth Pain Med. 29(6):576–591, 2004.
Mitra S, Sinatra RS: Perioperative management of acute pain in the opiate-dependent patient. Anesthesiology 101:212–227, 2004.

A shift towards multimodal analgesia reduces reliance on opiates and reduces opiate-related side effects. Newer developments in nerve localization will increase the popularity and utility of regional analgesia during outpatient surgery.

SUGGESTED READING

Apfelbaum JL, Chen C, Mehta SS, Gan TJ: Postoperative pain experience: results from a national survey suggest postoperative pain continues to be undermanaged. Anesth Analg 97:534–540, 2003.

Carroll IR, Angst MS, Clark JD: Management of perioperative pain in patients chronically consuming opiates. Reg Anesth Pain Med 29:576-591, 2004.

Chan, VWS: Nerve localization—seek but not so easy to find? Reg Anesth Pain Med 27:245-248, 2002.

Crews J: Multimodal pain management strategies for office-based and ambulatory procedures. JAMA 288:629-632, 2002.

Drasner K: Local anesthetic neurotoxicity: Clinical injury and strategies that may minimize risk. Reg Anesth Pain Med 27:576-580, 2002.

Evans H, Steel SM, Nielsen KC, et al: Peripheral nerve blocks and continuous catheter techniques. Anesthesiol Clin North America 23:141-162, 2005.

Gajraj NM, Joshi GP: Role of cyclooxygenase-2 inhibitors in postoperative pain management. Anesthesiol Clin North America 23:49-72, 2005.

Habib AS, Gan TJ: Role of analgesic adjuncts in postoperative pain management. Anesthesiol Clin North America 23:85-107, 2005.

Hadzic H, Vloka J: Peripheral Nerve Blocks: Principles and Practice. Philadelphia, McGraw-Hill Companies, 2004.

Horlocker T, Wedel D, Benzon H, et al: Regional anesthesia in the anticoagulated patient: defining the risks. Reg Anesth Pain Med 29(Suppl 1):1-11, 2004.

Joint Commission on Accreditation of Health Care Organizations: Pain: Current Understanding of Assessment, Management, and Treatments. Monograph—National Pharmaceutical Council, Inc. and JCAHO. http://www.jcaho.org/news+room+care +issues/pain_mono_npc.pdf

Mitra S, Sinatra RS: Perioperative management of acute pain in the opiate-dependent patient. Anesthesiology 101:212-227, 2004.

Perlas A, Chan V, Simons M: Brachial plexus examination and localization using ultrasound and electrical stimulation. Anesthesiology 99:429-435, 2003.

Pollack J: Transient neurologic symptoms: Etiology, risk factors, and management. Reg Anesth Pain Med 27:581-586, 2002.

Rathmell J, Neal J, Viscomi C: Regional Anesthesia: The Requisites in Anesthesiology. Philadelphia, Mosby, 2004.

Suresh S, Wheeler M: Practical pediatric regional anesthesia. Anesthesiol Clin North America 20:83-113, 2002.

White P: Changing role of COX-2 inhibitors in the perioperative period: Is parecoxib really the answer? Anesth Analg 100:1306-1308, 2005.

White P: The role of non-opiate analgesic techniques in the management of pain after ambulatory surgery. Anesth Analg 94:577-585, 2002.

Yoos JR, Kopacz D: Spinal 2-chloroprocaine for surgery: An initial 10-month experience. Anesth Analg 100:553-558, 2005.

CHAPTER 7

Postoperative Nausea and Vomiting

ASHRAF S. HABIB

TONG J. GAN

Postoperative nausea and vomiting (PONV) is a frequent and unpleasant side effect following surgery and anesthesia. The overall incidence of PONV has decreased from 60% from the time when ether and cyclopropane were used to approximately 30% nowadays. However, in certain high-risk patients this incidence may still approach 70%. Furthermore, it is estimated that approximately 0.2% of all patients may experience intractable PONV, resulting in delayed discharge from the recovery room, unplanned hospital admission following ambulatory surgery, or both, thereby increasing medical costs. The estimated cost of PONV to a busy ambulatory surgical unit ranges from $0.25 million to $1.5 million per year.

PONV is a major source of patient dissatisfaction with anesthetic care. In several studies, patients not only ranked the absence of PONV as being important, but also ranked it as more important than an earlier discharge from an ambulatory surgical unit. In one survey, patients were willing to pay up to $100, at their own expense, for completely effective antiemetic therapy after surgery.

In addition to the unpleasant experience and cost implications, PONV may rarely be associated with serious complications such as wound dehiscence, pulmonary aspiration of gastric contents, hematoma formation beneath skin flaps, dehydration, electrolyte disturbances, Mallory-Weiss tear, and esophageal rupture.

DEFINING EMETIC SYMPTOMS

Nausea is defined as a subjectively unpleasant sensation associated with awareness of the urge to vomit. Retching is defined as the labored, spasmodic, rhythmic contractions of the respiratory muscles, including the diaphragm, chest wall, and abdominal wall muscles, without the expulsion of gastric contents. Vomiting is the actual physical phenomenon of the forceful expulsion of gastric contents from the mouth and is brought about by the powerful sustained contraction of the abdominal muscles, the descent of the diaphragm, and the opening of the gastric cardia.

PHYSIOLOGY OF PONV

The complex act of vomiting involves coordination of the respiratory, gastrointestinal, and abdominal musculature. It is controlled by the vomiting center, which is located in the lateral reticular formation of the medulla oblongata in close proximity to the nucleus of the solitary tract in the brain stem, and has access to the motor pathways that are responsible for the visceral and somatic output involved in vomiting (Fig. 7-1).

The vomiting reflex has two main detectors of the need to vomit: the gastrointestinal tract (GIT) and the chemoreceptor trigger zone (CTZ) in the area postrema. The vagus is the major nerve involved in the detection of emetic stimuli from the GIT and has two types of afferent fibers involved in the emetic response: mechanoreceptors, which are located in the muscular wall of the gut and are activated by contraction and distension of the gut, and chemoreceptors, which are located in the mucosa of the upper gut and are sensitive to noxious chemicals. Stimulation of the vagal afferents leads to activation of the CTZ in the area postrema, a U-shaped structure which is a few millimeters long and is located on the dorsal surface of the medulla oblongata at the caudal end of the fourth ventricle. It is one of the circumventricular organs of the brain outside the blood-brain barrier and the cerebrospinal fluid barrier, and thus it can be activated by chemical stimuli received through the blood as well as through cerebrospinal fluid. Several other stimuli can affect the vomiting center, including afferents from the oropharynx, mediastinum, peritoneum, and genitalia, as well as afferents from the central nervous system (CNS) (i.e., the cerebral cortex, labyrinthine, visual, and vestibular apparatus).

Different types of receptors are involved in the transmission of impulses to the vomiting center. Cholinergic receptors are found in the vomiting center and the vestibular nuclei. The area postrema is rich in dopamine D_2, opioid, and serotonin $5HT_3$ receptors. The nucleus tractus solitarius is rich in enkephalins and in histaminic H_1, muscarinic cholinergic, and neurokinin-1 (NK1) receptors; the last of these is also found in the dorsal motor nucleus of the vagus nerve.

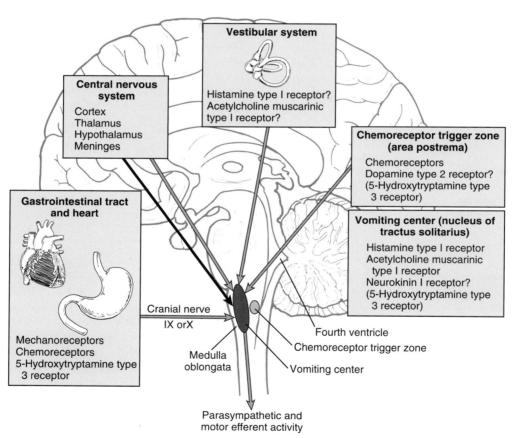

Figure 7-1 Vomiting centers and their input. Stimuli from the gastrointestinal tract, the vestibular system, the chemoreceptor trigger zone in the area postrema of the floor of the fourth ventricle and cortical centers in the brain can induce vomiting. (Adapted from Krakauer EL, Zhu AX, Bounds BC, et al: Case records of the Massachusetts General Hospital. Weekly clinicopathological exercises. Case 6-2005: A 58-year-old man with esophageal cancer and nausea, vomiting, and intractable hiccups. N Engl J Med 352(8):823, 2005.)

RISK STRATIFICATION

Universal PONV prophylaxis is not cost-effective and puts patients at unnecessary risk of drug-related adverse effects. The use of a risk-adapted prophylactic strategy allows targeting prophylaxis to those who will benefit most from it. Patient-, anesthesia-, and surgery-related risk factors have been identified.

Patient-related factors include female gender, a history of PONV or motion sickness, and nonsmoking status. Age has a nonlinear impact on PONV. Postoperative vomiting occurs infrequently in neonates and toddlers, but the incidence increases to 20% to 40% in school children, with little influence of gender before puberty. The incidence is highest in young adults and decreases continuously in the elderly. However, the impact of age is not as strong as the previously mentioned risk factors. It is believed that obesity and the stage of the menstrual cycle do not affect the incidence of PONV.

Anesthesia-related risk factors include the use of volatile agents, which cause PONV during the early postoperative period (within 0 to 2 hours); nitrous oxide, which increases the risk for postoperative vomiting (avoidance of nitrous oxide reduces the risk of PONV by 12%); opioids; and high doses of neostigmine (>2.5 mg) for the reversal of neuromuscular blockade.

There is controversy regarding a number of previously reported surgery-related risk factors. For example, some authors report that operations including breast surgery, laparoscopy, abdominal surgery, and ear, nose, and throat (ENT) surgery are associated with a high incidence of PONV.[1] Operations associated with a high incidence of postoperative vomiting in children include strabismus, adenotonsillectomy, hernia repair, orchidopexy, and penile surgery. However, Apfel et al.[2] did not find the type of surgery, except for hysterectomy and laparoscopic cholecystectomy, to be an independent risk factor for PONV in adults. They suggested that the high incidence of PONV after certain operations might be caused by the inclusion of high-risk patients. In addition, the duration of surgery might have an impact on PONV. It was reported that each 30-minute increase in duration increases PONV risk by about 60%. Routine decompression of the stomach with a nasogastric tube does not reduce the incidence of PONV. Some postoperative factors may also affect the occurrence of PONV. For instance, pain can be associated with nausea. Sudden changes in position and motion, including transportation in a stretcher, wheelchair, or car, may trigger vomiting.

A number of PONV risk scoring systems have been developed. Apfel et al.[3] described one simple score that has been validated in a study of 2722 patients in two centers (in Wurzburg, Germany, and Olulu, Finland). This simplified risk score consists of four predictors: female gender, a history of motion sickness or PONV, nonsmoking status, and the use of opioids for postoperative analgesia. If none, one, two, three, or four of these risk factors are present, the incidences of PONV are 10%, 21%, 39%, 61%, and 79%, respectively. A risk-dependent antiemetic strategy based on this score results in a significant reduction in the incidence of PONV.

STRATEGIES FOR THE PREVENTION AND TREATMENT OF PONV

Strategies available for the management of PONV are summarized in Box 7-1. A number of systematic reviews have been published on the relative efficacy of various interventions. In this context, the number of patients needed to treat statistic (NNT) indicates how many patients must receive the antiemetic intervention to prevent one particular PONV event in one patient who would have had this event had he or she received a placebo or no treatment. Thus, the NNT is a useful estimate of clinical relevance of treatment effect. The NNT of different antiemetics is described below when such data are available. The NNT of antiemetics that were studied in systematic reviews are summarized in Table 7-1.

Antiemetics

Serotonin-Receptor Antagonists
Serotonin plays an important role in nausea and vomiting. It stimulates vagal afferent neurons that activate the vomiting center or directly activate the CTZ. The $5HT_3$-receptor antagonists are a unique group of drugs in that they were developed specifically for the management of nausea and vomiting. Members of this group exert their effects by binding to the $5HT_3$ receptor in the CTZ and to vagal afferents in the gastrointestinal tract. Their favorable side-effects profile, their lack of sedation effects in particular, makes them particularly suitable for ambulatory surgery. They are, however, more expensive than the older antiemetics.

Ondansetron was the first member of this group to be marketed in the United States and was the most widely studied. The antivomiting efficacy of ondansetron is better than its antinausea efficacy. This may explain why it is more effective in prophylaxis of postoperative vomiting in children compared to prophylaxis of both nausea and vomiting in adults. It is most effective when given at the end of surgery. The recommended dose for prophylaxis is 4 to 8 mg intravenously (IV) in adults and 50 to 100 μg/kg in children. The NNT to prevent PONV is between 5 and 6. The reported side effects include headache (number needed to harm [NNH] = 36), dizziness, flushing, elevated liver enzymes (NNH = 31), and constipation (NNH = 23).

Box 7-1 Options Available for the Management of PONV

PHARMACOLOGIC TECHNIQUES

Monotherapy

Older-Generation Antiemetics

Phenothiazines: aliphatic (i.e., promethazine and chlorpromazine) and heterocyclic (i.e., perphenazine and prochlorperazine) antiemetics

Butyrophenones: droperidol and haloperidol

Benzamides: metoclopramide and domperidone

Anticholinergics: scopolamine

Antihistamines: ethanolamines (i.e., dimenhydrinate and diphenhydramine) and piperazines (i.e., cyclizine, hydroxyzine, and meclizine)

Newer-Generation Antiemetics

Serotonin $5HT_3$-receptor antagonists: ondansetron, granisetron, dolasetron, and tropisetron

NK1-receptor antagonists

Nontraditional Antiemetics:

Dexamethasone and propofol

Combination Therapy of Two or More of the Above Antiemetics

$5HT_3$-receptor antagonists + droperidol

$5HT_3$-receptor antagonists + dexamethasone

Droperidol + dexamethasone

NONPHARMACOLOGIC TECHNIQUES

Acupuncture, acupressure, laser stimulation of the P6 point, transcutaneous acupoint electrical stimulation, and hypnosis

ADDITIONAL MEASURES WITH POTENTIAL ANTIEMETIC EFFECTS

Ephedrine

Supplemental oxygen

Benzodiazepines

Adequate hydration

Good pain relief

α_2-adrenergic agonists

MULTIMODAL APPROACHES

From Habib AS, Gan TJ: Evidence-based management of postoperative nausea and vomiting: a review. Can J Anesth 51:326–341, 2004.

Dolasetron is structurally related to tropisetron and granisetron. The recommended intravenous dose for prophylaxis and treatment of PONV is 12.5 mg. The timing of administration of dolasetron appears to have little effect on its efficacy when administered for the prophylaxis of PONV. Dolasetron is rapidly converted into hydrodolasetron, which has a long half-life.

Tropisetron has been studied in Europe and has shown efficacy in the management of PONV. The recommended prophylactic dose is 2 to 5 mg. The NNT (95% confidence interval [CI]) for the prevention of nausea and vomiting at 24 hours postoperatively was 6.7 (4.8 to 11.1) and 5 (3.6 to 8.3), respectively.

Granisetron has also been used in the management of PONV in a dose of 0.35 to 3 mg. Although most studies have demonstrated efficacy at 1 mg for prophylaxis, a recent study suggested it may be effective at lower doses. For the treatment of established PONV, a dose of 0.1 mg was found to be effective.

Ramosetron is another $5HT_3$-receptor antagonist with general properties similar to those of ondansetron. It is used in the management of nausea and vomiting induced by cancer chemotherapy. It has also been shown to be effective for PONV prophylaxis in a dose of 0.3 mg given at the end of surgery.

Polanosetron, a serotonin antagonist with a longer half-life, is currently being evaluated in clinical trials for the management of PONV.

There is no evidence that there is any difference in efficacy among the various $5HT_3$-receptor antagonists when appropriate doses are used. Therefore, acquisition cost is the main factor that differentiates the $5HT_3$ compounds from one another.

Steroids

The exact mechanism of action of corticosteroids in preventing nausea and vomiting is unknown. It has been suggested that prostaglandin antagonism, release of endorphins, and tryptophan depletion may play a role. It is also possible that the anti-inflammatory or membrane-stabilizing effect of corticosteroids contributes to the antiemetic effect of these drugs. A study suggests that betamethasone has no effect on ipecac-induced vomiting, a serotonin-mediated pathway.[4]

Both dexamethasone and betamethasone decrease the incidence of PONV when administered as prophylaxis. Dexamethasone has, however, been more extensively evaluated. It has the advantages of being inexpensive, devoid of sedative-adverse effects, and long-acting. The recommended dose is 5 to 10 mg in adults and 150 µg/kg in children. More recently, smaller doses (2.5 to 5 mg) have been found to be effective. Dexamethasone appears to be most effective in preventing early PONV (0 to 2 hours postoperative) when administered prior to induction of anesthesia rather than at the end of surgery. There are no reports of dexamethasone-related adverse effects in the doses used for the management of PONV. The long duration of action of dexamethasone makes it particularly effective for the control of late PONV. The NNT (95% CI) for the prevention of early (0 to 6 hours postoperative) and late (0 to 24 hours postoperative) nausea with 8 mg dexamethasone was 5 (2.2 to −21) and 4.3 (2.3 to 26), respectively. For early and late vomiting, the NNT (95% CI) was 3.6 (2.3 to 8) and 4.3 (2.6 to 12), respectively.

Anticholinergic Drugs

The vestibular apparatus is rich in muscarinic receptors; hence, this class of drugs is very effective in the

Table 7-1   NNT (95% CI) of Antiemetics Studied in Systematic Reviews

	Early Nausea	Late Nausea	Early Vomiting	Late Vomiting
ANTICHOLINERGICS				
Transdermal scopolamine		5 (3.2-11.1)		5.9 (4.2-11.1)
ANTIHISTAMINES				
Dimenhydrinate	8 (3-20)	6 (3-33)	7 (4-50)	5 (3-8)
BUTEROPHENONES				
Droperidol 0.5-0.75 mg	4.8 (3.0-12)	11 (6.9-25)	10 (4.6-51)	3.4 (2.4-5.7)
Droperidol 1-1.25 mg	6.1 (4.5-9.4)	6.8 (5.2-9.7)	7.6 (5.8-11)	8.2 (5.6-15)
Droperidol 1.5-2.5 mg	5.9 (3.8-13)	5.8 (3.8-12)	6.9 (4.7-13)	7.1 (4.2-23)
Droperidol 5-20 µg/kg				7.3 (4.5-20)
Droperidol 50 µg/kg			7.4 (3.9-58)	4.4 (2.5-17)
Droperidol 75 µg/kg			4.2 (3.3-5.9)	3.8 (2.8-5.2)
Droperidol in morphine (PCA)		5.1 (3.1-15)		3.1 (2.3-4.8)
5HT$_3$-RECEPTOR ANTAGONISTS				
Ondansetron				
Ondansetron 1 mg	21 (9-∞)		9 (5.3-30)	15 (8-210)
Ondansetron 4 mg	5.6 (4-9)	4.6 (4-5.5)	5.5 (4.4-7.5)	6.4 (5.3-7.9)
Ondansetron 8 mg	11 (4.2-∞)	6.4 (4.6-10)	6.4 (4.7-10)	5.0 (4.0-6.7)
Ondansetron 100 µg/kg			5 (3.7-7.6)	2.7 (2-4.2)
Ondansetron 150 µg/kg			2.5 (1.9-3.6)	2.7 (1.7-7.6)
Ondansetron in morphine (PCA)		−67 (−5.8-∞)		5.1 (2.8-23)
Tropisetron				
Tropisetron 2-5 mg		6.7 (4.8-11.1)		5 (3.6-8.3)
BENZAMIDES				
Metoclopramide 10 mg	16 (7.5 to −210)	12 (6 to −1587)	9.1 (5.5-27)	10 (6-41)
PROPOFOL				
Propofol induction	9.3 (6.1-19.4)	50.1 (7.6-∞)	13.7 (8.1-45.4)	14.9 (6-∞)
Propofol maintenance	8 (6.4-10.8)	5.8 (4.2-9.4)	9.2 (7.6-11.7)	10.1 (6.2-28.8)
STEROIDS				
Dexamethasone 8 mg	5 (2.2 to −21)	4.3 (2.3-26)	3.6 (2.3-8)	4.3 (2.6-12)
OTHER INTERVENTIONS				
Omitting nitrous oxide	30 (13.5-∞)	36.9 (11.8-∞)	11.8 (8.5-19.4)	13.8 (8.8-31.6)
Omitting reversal of neuromuscular block	−636	14	417	23
Nonpharmacologic techniques (0-48 hours postoperative)	4 (3-6)		5 (4-8)	14 (6-∞)

PCA, Patient-controlled analgesia.

treatment of motion sickness. They block muscarinic cholinergic CNS-emetic receptors in the cerebral cortex and the pons. Atropine and scopolamine are tertiary amines that cross the blood-brain barrier and have efficacy against motion sickness and PONV. Scopolamine has the most potent antiemetic properties in this class of drugs, with an NNT of 3.8 for the prevention of PONV. The transdermal preparation should be applied the evening prior to surgery or 4 hours before the end of surgery. It has been documented to effectively reduce PONV in children receiving patient-controlled analgesia with morphine and

after strabismus surgery. Its limitations include a 2- to 4-hour onset of effect, its medical contraindications, and its age-related considerations. The NNH for the most commonly reported side effects was 5.6, 12.5, 50, and 100 for dry mouth, visual disturbances, dizziness, and agitation, respectively. These side effects may limit the use of scopolamine patches in ambulatory surgery.

Antihistamines
The antihistamines are inexpensive, older antiemetic drugs. They act by blocking acetylcholine receptors in

the vestibular apparatus and histamine H_1 receptors in the nucleus of the solitary tract. They are particularly effective in the management of motion sickness and PONV following middle ear surgery.

The antihistamines include the ethanolamines (i.e., dimenhydrinate and diphenhydramine) and the piperazines (i.e., cyclizine, hydroxyzine, and meclizine). The NNT (95% CI) to stay completely free from nausea with dimenhydrinate was 8 (3 to 20) during the first 6 hours postoperatively and 6 (3 to 33) for the period from 0 to 48 hours. For vomiting, the NNT (95% CI) was 7 (4 to 50) and 5 (3 to 8) for the early period and the 48-hour postoperative period, respectively. In the pediatric population, the effective dose is 0.5 mg/kg. The NNT (95% CI) for the prophylaxis of postoperative vomiting (POV) in children was 5 (3 to 9). Cyclizine (50 mg), IV or intramuscularly (IM), is used extensively for the prophylaxis and treatment of PONV in the United Kingdom. The parenteral formulation is not available in the United States. The major disadvantages of the antihistamines include sedation, dry mouth, blurred vision, urinary retention, and delayed recovery room discharge, which limit their use in the ambulatory setting.

Benzamides

Metoclopramide is the most commonly used antiemetic in this group. It is a prokinetic agent that blocks D_2 receptors in the gastrointestinal tract and, centrally, in the CTZ and the area postrema. It also increases lower esophageal sphincter tone and enhances gastric motility, which may prevent the delayed gastric emptying caused by opioids. In addition, metoclopramide has parasympathomimetic activity. At high concentrations, it has been shown to have a weak serotonin-receptor antagonistic effect.

The efficacy of the usual dose of 10 mg of metoclopramide in preventing PONV in adults is uncertain, with approximately 50% of studies showing it to be no more effective than placebo. However, a dose of 0.25 mg/kg has been shown to be effective in children, with an NNT of 6. In adults, a meta-analysis reported that there was no significant antinausea effect.[5] The NNT to prevent early (0 to 6 hours postoperative) and late (within 48 hours postoperative) vomiting was 9.1 and 10, respectively. Another systematic review comparing the efficacy of metoclopramide with droperidol and ondansetron also concluded that it is inferior to both drugs for the prophylaxis of PONV in adults and children.[6] A Quaynor and Raeder study, however, suggested that 20 mg may be an effective dose.[7] Side effects include sedation, restlessness, and extrapyramidal symptoms. Children seem more predisposed to these side effects than adults. Rapid intravenous administration may also be associated with cardiovascular side effects (i.e., hypotension, bradycardia, or tachycardia). However, the incidence of adverse events is relatively low in the doses used for the management of PONV.

Domperidone is a benzimidazole derivative, pharmacologically similar to metoclopramide, with a similar efficacy for the prevention of PONV. However, it appears to be more effective than metoclopramide for the treatment of active PONV and is associated with a lower incidence of extrapyramidal symptoms. It is only available as an oral or rectal preparation. The parenteral formulation was withdrawn following several reports of serious cardiac arrhythmias after intravenous administration.

Butyrophenones

The neuroleptic drugs haloperidol and droperidol have significant antiemetic effects. They are strong D_2-receptor antagonists that act at the CTZ and the area postrema.

Droperidol has been extensively used in anesthesia. At a dose of 1.25 mg, it is more cost-effective than ondansetron (4 mg) and is recommended as a first-line agent for PONV prophylaxis. The NNT to prevent early nausea is 5. For both early and late vomiting, the best effective dose is 1.5 to 2.5 mg (NNT = 7). In children, the recommended dose is 50 to 75 mcg/kg, with a NNT of 4. Even though its half-life is relatively short (3 hours), it has a long clinical duration of action (as long as 24 hours following administration), probably due to its strong binding affinity to the emetic receptors.

Droperidol is most effective when given at the end of surgery. It is also effective when given concomitantly with a patient-controlled analgesia system using morphine with an NNT (95% CI) for the prevention of nausea and vomiting of 5.1 (3.1 to 15) and 3.1 (2.3 to 4.8), respectively, the first 24 postoperative hours. Sedation and drowsiness are important side effects of droperidol and are dose-dependent. Low doses of droperidol (0.625 to 1.25 mg) are not associated with any increased sedation or prolongation of postanesthesia care unit (PACU) stay compared to ondansetron (4 mg). Extrapyramidal reactions, which are most likely to occur in children, are recognized side effects of droperidol, but these are rare in the doses used to treat PONV.

It has been estimated that less than 1% of children receiving droperidol for POV prophylaxis experience extrapyramidal symptoms, and up to 16% develop minor central nervous system side effects.

CURRENT CONTROVERSY: DROPERIDOL HAS AN FDA BLACK BOX WARNING

- Droperidol may be associated with Q-Tc segment prolongation and torsades de pointes.
- The incidence of arrhythmias with droperidol use is estimated to be very low and is dose-dependent.
- Although use of droperidol in the United States has dropped significantly, some experts question the evidence justifying the black box warning.

In December 2001, the Food and Drug Administration (FDA) issued a new black box warning, the most serious warning for an FDA-approved drug, on droperidol. The FDA noted that its use has been associated with Q-Tc segment prolongation and torsades de pointes, and, in some cases, it has resulted in fatal cardiac arrhythmias. The incidence of cardiac-adverse events following the administration of droperidol has been estimated to be 74 in 11 million. Since the black box warning, there has been a tenfold decrease in the use of droperidol in the United States. The need for a black box warning on droperidol has, however, been challenged by a number of experts in the field. Several small studies either have not shown a significant increase in Q-T interval with small-dose droperidol or have shown little difference in short-term droperidol-induced Q-T prolongation compared to that produced by $5HT_3$ antagonists.

Phenothiazines

The antiemetic effects of phenothiazines have been attributed to blockade of D_2 receptors in the CTZ. They also have moderate antihistaminergic and anticholinergic actions. The phenothiazines have an aliphatic or heterocyclic ring attached to the tenth position of a tricyclic nucleus. The aliphatic phenothiazines (i.e., prome-thazine and chlorpromazine) have less antiemetic potency and more sedative effects than the heterocyclic phenothiazines (i.e., perphenazine and prochlorperazine). Promethazine is an effective antiemetic with a long duration of action. In a dose of 12.5 to 25 mg given toward the end of surgery, it is effective for PONV management. Its use, however, is limited by sedation and prolonged recovery from anesthesia. Yet, a recent study did not show increased awakening time or increased duration of PACU stay when compared to ondansetron and placebo in patients undergoing middle ear surgery.

Similarly, chlorpromazine demonstrated efficacy in the prevention and treatment of PONV. Its many side effects, particularly sedation and hypotension, limit its use as an antiemetic.

The heterocyclic phenothiazines have similar antiemetic efficacy, but perphenazine causes more sedation. The recommended dose for prochlorperazine is 5 to 10 mg IM in adults. In children, the recommended dose for perphenazine is 70 μg/kg. These compounds have, however, a higher incidence of extrapyramidal side effects compared to the aliphatic phenothiazines. Severe dystonic reactions have followed the use of prochlorperazine, particularly in children and adolescents.

Other Interventions with Antiemetic Effect

Propofol

Propofol is an IV anesthetic agent with antiemetic properties. Total intravenous anesthesia (TIVA) with propofol is associated with a lower incidence of PONV when compared with inhalation agents. This technique is equally efficacious when compared to ondansetron (4 mg) in the prevention of PONV. The antiemetic effect of propofol is most pronounced in the early postoperative period. It is not useful for PONV prophylaxis if given only as a bolus for induction of anesthesia. Continuous subhypnotic propofol infusion and the use of patient-controlled antiemesis with propofol boluses have been effective in the treatment of PONV. The effective plasma concentration of propofol for the 50% reduction in nausea scores is 343 ng/mL. This is much lower than the range required for sedation (900 to 1300 ng/mL) and anesthesia (3000 to 10,000 ng/mL). The use of TIVA, however, is associated with an increase in drug cost compared to maintenance of anesthesia with a volatile agent.

The mechanism of the antiemetic action of propofol is not known. It is not due to the intralipid emulsion in the formulation. Propofol appears to have a direct antiemetic property. A recent study demonstrated that propofol infusion was associated with a reduction in the levels of serotonin and its metabolite, 5-hydroxyindoleacetic acid (5-HIAA), in the area postrema and in the cerebrospinal fluid (CSF).

Acupuncture-Type Techniques

In a pilot study evaluating the use of acupuncture for the prophylactic treatment of migraine headaches, migraine episodes were less severe and were accompanied by less nausea and vomiting. Subsequently, the use of acupuncture for the management of perioperative nausea and vomiting has been investigated in a number of studies. Acupuncture, acupressure, and transcutaneous acupoint electrical stimulation at the Neiguan (P6) acupoint have been studied for the prophylaxis of PONV. In a systematic review of randomized controlled trials investigating acupuncture techniques, a significant reduction in early PONV (0 to 6 hours postoperative) occurred in adults treated with acupuncture when compared with placebo. Antiemetics (i.e., metoclopramide, cyclizine, droperidol, and prochlorperazine) are comparable to acupuncture techniques in preventing early and late (0 to 48 hours postoperative) PONV in adults. The nonpharmacologic techniques are more effective for controlling nausea than for controlling vomiting. Recently, acupuncture for the prophylaxis of PONV in children has been shown to be effective.

The ReliefBand is a commercially available device that provides transcutaneous acupoint electrical stimulation at the P6 point. It has been compared to ondansetron for both the prophylaxis and the treatment of PONV in ambulatory patients. When used for prophylaxis, the combination of ondansetron and acupoint electrical stimulation is associated with a lower incidence of PONV, less need for rescue antiemetics, and improved quality of recovery and patient satisfaction when compared to ondansetron alone. When used as a rescue therapy for the treatment of PONV after laparoscopic cholecystectomy, the combination of ondansetron and the ReliefBand is significantly more effective as a rescue antiemetic than ondansetron alone.

Benzodiazepines

Benzodiazepines are effective for the prophylaxis of PONV. The successful use of midazolam in cases of persistent PONV and following the failure of other antiemetics has also been described. The suggested mechanism of the antiemetic effect of midazolam is a decrease dopamine input at the CTZ and a decrease in anxiety levels. It may also decrease adenosine reuptake, leading to reduced synthesis, release, and postsynaptic action of dopamine at the CTZ. Alternatively, midazolam may reduce serotonin release by binding to the γ-aminobutyric acid (GABA) benzodiazepine complex.

Ephedrine

Intramuscular ephedrine (0.5 mg/kg) is effective for PONV prophylaxis, especially in the early postoperative period (0 to 3 hours postoperative). It has also been suggested that ephedrine might have a specific antiemetic effect since there is no difference in postoperative blood pressure between the ephedrine- and the placebo-treated patients.

α_2-Adrenergic Agonists

α_2-adrenergic agonists significantly reduce the incidence of PONV in both children and adults. It has been suggested that the antiemetic effect of clonidine might be secondary to a reduction in the use of volatile agents and opioids or a reduction in sympathetic tone.

Supplemental Oxygen

In two studies by one group, oxygen supplementation (80%), either intraoperatively or both intraoperatively and for 2 hours postoperatively, was effective in achieving a significant reduction in the incidence of PONV when compared to patients receiving 30% oxygen during intestinal surgery.[8,9] The authors suggested that supplemental oxygen might reduce PONV by ameliorating subtle intestinal ischemia, thereby reducing release of serotonin and other emetogenic substances from a compromised bowel. Three other studies of patients undergoing gynecologic, breast, or thyroid surgery did not reproduce these findings.[10,11,12]

Hydration

In patients undergoing ambulatory surgery, the administration of a 20-mL/kg bolus of an isotonic solution preoperatively is associated with significantly less nausea on the first postoperative day when compared to patients who received a bolus of 2 mL/kg. The precise mechanism is not known, but it may be related to a better perfusion of the gastrointestinal tract, reducing the release of peripheral serotonin from the gut. A combination of colloid and crystalloid fluid resuscitation is associated with less PONV and less use of rescue antiemetics, compared with the administration of crystalloids alone, in patients undergoing major abdominal procedures. This may be related to the large volume of crystalloids infused, which results in bowel edema.

Other Modalities

Hypnosis is effective in reducing the incidence of PONV when compared with placebo in females undergoing breast surgery.[13] A study involving the use of treatment modality music and therapeutic suggestions has, however, failed to demonstrate a benefit in reducing nausea and vomiting in ambulatory patients.[14] Although some earlier reports suggested that ginger root might have a beneficial effect for PONV prophylaxis, this has not been confirmed in a recent meta-analysis.[15] Inhaled isopropyl alcohol vapor was also reported to be of benefit for the treatment of established PONV.[16,17,18] Further well-controlled studies will be required to establish the role, if any, of these treatment modalities.

Future Therapies

The NK1 antagonist class of drugs may act on the final common pathway from the emetic center. These compounds are known to inhibit the effects of substance P in the brainstem regions associated with emesis. Animal studies demonstrated broader-spectrum antiemetic activity of NK1-receptor antagonists when compared with the $5HT_3$-receptor antagonists. In humans, NK1-receptor antagonists are effective for the prophylaxis and treatment of PONV.

In one study of females undergoing gynecologic surgery, the NK1-receptor antagonist CP-122721 provided better prophylaxis against vomiting when compared with ondansetron.[19] The combination of both agents also significantly prolongs the time to administration of rescue antiemetics compared with either drug alone, and it is associated with a very low incidence of emesis (2%). Cost may, however, be an issue when considering routinely using these newer drugs for PONV.

Aprepitant is the only drug of this class approved in the United States for chemotherapy-induced nausea and vomiting. Aprepitant and another NK1 antagonist, GW679769, are currently being evaluated for PONV prophylaxis.

Combination Antiemetics and Multimodal Management of PONV

A number of factors have stimulated interest in using a combination of antiemetic agents for the management of PONV. First, there are at least four major receptor systems involved in the etiology of PONV: histamine H_1, cholinergic muscarinic, dopamine D_2, and serotonin $5HT_3$ receptors. Second, the etiology of PONV is multifactorial, and no single antiemetic agent is close to 100% effective in either treating or preventing PONV. On the contrary, the efficacy of currently available antiemetics is disappointing, with the best NNT reported being about 4 to 6. Finally, data from chemotherapy clearly demonstrate the superiority of the combination approach for the management of chemotherapy-induced emesis.

The most frequently studied combinations are a $5HT_3$-receptor antagonist with droperidol, dexamethasone, or metoclopramide. Overall, the combination with metoclopramide does not seem to confer any additional benefit, whereas the combination with droperidol or dexamethasone is significantly more effective than monotherapy.

There is little data directly comparing the efficacy of different antiemetic combinations. Recent data suggest that the combination of the $5HT_3$-receptor antagonists with droperidol or dexamethasone, as well as the combination of droperidol with dexamethasone, have similar efficacy for the prophylaxis of PONV.

In an attempt to further enhance the efficacy of antiemetic prophylaxis, Scuderi et al.[20] introduced the concept of the multimodal approach to the management of PONV in females undergoing outpatient laparoscopy. Their multimodal critical care algorithm consisted of total intravenous anesthesia with propofol and remifentanil, no nitrous oxide, no neuromuscular blockade, aggressive intravenous hydration (25 mL/kg), triple prophylactic antiemetics (ondansetron, 1 mg; droperidol, 0.625 mg; and dexamethasone, 10 mg), and ketorolac (30 mg). Control groups included standard balanced outpatient anesthetic with or without 4 mg of ondansetron prophylaxis. Multimodal management resulted in a 98% complete response rate (i.e., no PONV and no antiemetic rescue) in the PACU. No patient in this group vomited before discharge, compared with 7% of patients in the ondansetron group (p = 0.07) and 22% of patients in the placebo group (p = 0.0003). Subsequently, more studies confirmed the efficacy of a multimodal approach compared to single-agent antiemetic prophylaxis, especially in high-risk patients. More recently, a multimodal approach incorporating TIVA with propofol, a combination of ondansetron and droperidol, and omitting nitrous oxide was associated with a higher complete response rate and greater patient satisfaction in the PACU, compared with similar antiemetic prophylaxis with isoflurane and nitrous-oxide-based anesthetic.

In a large prospective study, Apfel et al.[2] evaluated three antiemetic interventions (ondansetron, 4 mg; droperidol, 1.25 mg; and dexamethasone, 4 mg) and three anesthetic interventions (TIVA with propofol, omitting nitrous oxide, and substituting remifentanil for fentanyl) for the prophylaxis of PONV. The authors employed a multifactorial design, allowing them to evaluate the effectiveness of each of the interventions plus all possible combinations of two or three interventions. The resulting data suggested that antiemetics with different mechanisms of action had additive rather than synergistic effects on the incidence of PONV. Each antiemetic reduced the risk of PONV by about 26%. When combinations of interventions were used, the benefit of each subsequent intervention was always less than that of the first intervention. They also reported that the efficacy of the interventions depended on the patient's baseline risk; the greatest absolute risk reduction from the antiemetic interventions was achieved in patients with high risk for PONV.

PROPHYLAXIS VERSUS TREATMENT OF ESTABLISHED PONV

Controversy exists regarding the optimal cost-effective approach to the management of PONV. Although some have questioned the use of any prophylactic antiemetics, others do support this practice. Proponents of prophylaxis argue that PONV is one of the patients' highest concerns and that it increases time to PACU discharge, unanticipated hospital admissions, and costs. Opponents of prophylaxis point out that many studies of PONV prophylaxis use surrogate end points of the incidence of PONV without providing data on the more important issues of unanticipated hospital admission rates, PACU discharge times, and patient satisfaction. Scuderi et al.[21] randomized 575 patients undergoing outpatient surgery to receive prophylaxis with ondansetron (4 mg) or placebo. Patients who developed PONV were assigned to receive ondansetron (1 mg IV) or placebo as rescue treatment. The authors reported that prophylaxis is effective in reducing PONV, but it only increased patient satisfaction from 93% to 97%, with no change in PACU discharge times or in the time necessary to resume normal activities. They stated that it would require prophylactic administration of ondansetron to 25 patients, at an additional cost of $400, to increase satisfaction in one patient who would not have been otherwise satisfied. However, in the high-risk population, patient satisfaction is improved by more than 10% with prophylaxis. Other workers have also confirmed that PONV prophylaxis improves patient satisfaction in the high-risk group.

The most cost-effective approach to the management of PONV will differ between an ambulatory center and an inpatient hospital setting. In this context, nursing labor costs are more likely to be directly related to the duration of PACU stay in an office-based setting and, to a lesser extent, in an ambulatory surgery unit, whereas prolonged PACU stay may not have a significant impact in nursing labor costs in an inpatient hospital setting unless nursing staff can be reduced. Since lower doses of ondansetron (1 mg) are effective for treatment of established PONV compared with the doses needed for prophylaxis, Tramer et al.[22] concluded that prophylaxis with ondansetron in all patients is less cost-effective than treatment with the same drug.

In patients at high risk for PONV, however, Hill et al.[23] reported that prophylactic antiemetic use is cost-effective and is associated with greater patient satisfaction compared with no prophylaxis. They reported that the cost associated with PONV in placebo patients was 100 times more compared with the cost of prophylaxis with a generic compound. Most of the costs were from nursing labor costs secondary to prolonged PACU stay as a result of persistent PONV. The cost of treating vomiting was three times more than the cost of treating nausea.

Similar results were reported in another study in which both droperidol and dolasetron were more cost-effective than no prophylaxis in high-risk patients.[24] In two separate cost-effectiveness analyses, droperidol was more cost-effective than ondansetron for PONV prophylaxis.[24,25] In another analysis, prophylaxis was only cost-effective if the incidence of PONV exceeded 33% with ondansetron and 13% with droperidol.[26] However, following the FDA black box warning on droperidol, many hospitals have removed this cost-effective agent from their formulary. More cost-effectiveness studies are therefore required.

Since the different $5HT_3$-receptor antagonists have comparable efficacy and safety profiles, acquisition cost is the main factor that differentiates the $5HT_3$ compounds from one another.

CURRENT CONTROVERSY: PROPHYLAXIS VERSUS TREATMENT OF PONV

- Controversy exists regarding the optimal cost-effective strategy for the management of PONV: give prophylaxis or wait and treat only established PONV?
- Opponents of prophylaxis argue that prophylaxis is not cost-effective, that treatment is more successful than prophylaxis, and that prophylaxis does not improve patient satisfaction.
- Studies have shown that prophylaxis is cost-effective and is associated with a greater degree of patient satisfaction in patients at high risk for PONV.

POSTDISCHARGE NAUSEA AND VOMITING

Although the prophylaxis and management of PONV occurring in the PACU has significantly improved, nausea and vomiting occurring following discharge from the PACU remain undertreated; nausea and vomiting occurring in the PACU may not accurately predict the incidence after discharge. Approximately 36% of patients who experience postdischarge nausea and vomiting do

not experience any nausea or vomiting prior to discharge. In an analysis of all studies evaluating patient-reported symptoms after outpatient surgery, the overall incidence of nausea and vomiting occurring following discharge from the hospital has been estimated to be 17% (ranging from 0% to 55%) and 8% (ranging from 0% to 16%), respectively.[27] This not only leads to a delay in resumption of daily activities, but also to distress to the patients who lack available treatment.

Most of the available antiemetics have short half-lives and may not be effective after discharge. In a meta-analysis, the NNT to prevent postdischarge nausea following ambulatory surgery was 12.9, 12.2, and 5.2 following the prophylactic administration of ondansetron (4 mg), dexamethasone, and a combination of two antiemetics, respectively.[28] For postdischarge vomiting, the NNT was 13.8 for ondansetron (4 mg) and 5 for combination treatment. In this analysis, droperidol was not effective for the prophylaxis against postdischarge nausea and vomiting. These results suggest that prophylaxis with a single agent should not be used routinely in low-risk ambulatory patients and that high-risk patients are best managed with a combination strategy.

CLINICAL CAVEAT: POSTDISCHARGE NAUSEA AND VOMITING

- Postdischarge nausea and vomiting is common after ambulatory surgery.
- Postdischarge nausea and vomiting is distressing to the patient and delays the resumption of daily activities.
- Prophylaxis using a combination of two or more antiemetics is significantly more effective in reducing the incidence of postdischarge symptoms compared to prophylaxis using a single agent.

RECOMMENDATIONS FOR PONV PROPHYLAXIS

A strategy based on the patient's PONV risk should be adopted. No prophylaxis is recommended for patients at low risk for PONV except if they are at risk for medical consequences from vomiting (e.g., patients with wired jaws). Since regional anesthesia is associated with an elevenfold reduction in the incidence of PONV compared to general anesthesia, a regional technique should be considered for patients at moderate to high risk for PONV. If this is not possible or is contraindicated and a general anesthetic is used, every effort should be made to keep the baseline risk of PONV low. The following strategies can help to keep the baseline risk of PONV low:
1. Avoid emetogenic agents including nitrous oxide, inhalational agents, etomidate, and ketamine.

2. Minimize the use of opioids. Adequate analgesia should, however, be ensured by using local anesthetics, nonsteroidal anti-inflammatory drugs (NSAIDs), and opioids, as required.

3. Consider the following:
   a. Using total intravenous anesthesia with propofol,
   b. Limiting the dose of neostigmine to a maximum of 2.5 mg in adults,
   c. Adequate hydration, especially with colloids, and
   d. Using anxiolytics, including benzodiazepines, nonpharmacologic techniques (e.g., acupuncture), and α_2-adrenergic agonists.

Finally, the use of a combination of antiemetics acting at different receptor sites should be considered. The addition of TIVA with propofol to a combination of antiemetics results in further improved prophylaxis. A suggested algorithm for the prophylaxis of PONV is shown in Figure 7-2.

CLINICAL CAVEAT: POSTOPERATIVE NAUSEA AND VOMITING PROPHYLAXIS

- Determine the PONV risk for every patient.
- Keep the baseline risk of PONV low.
- Use prophylactic antiemetics according to the patient's risk.
- Use a combination of antiemetics or a multimodal approach in patients with higher risk for PONV.

RECOMMENDATIONS FOR THE TREATMENT OF ESTABLISHED PONV

In contrast to the plethora of trials investigating different regimes for the prophylaxis of PONV, there is a paucity of data on the use of antiemetics for the

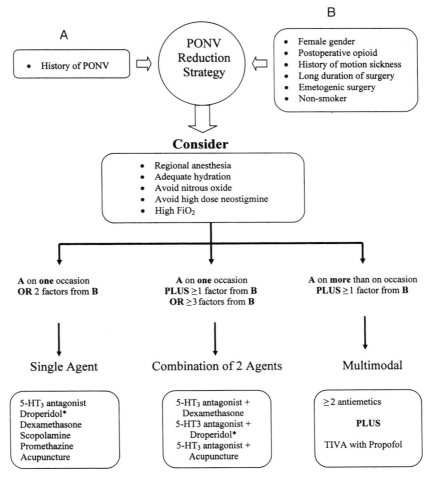

Figure 7-2   Algorithm for the prophylaxis of PONV. Emetogenic surgery is surgery with a high risk for PONV (e.g., intra-abdominal surgery, gynecologic surgery, breast surgery, strabismus surgery, and ENT surgery). (Adapted from Habib AS, Gan TJ: Evidence-based management of postoperative nausea and vomiting: A review. Can J Anesth 51:326–341, 2004.)

treatment of PONV in patients who failed prophylaxis or did not receive prophylaxis. The available evidence suggests that lower doses of antiemetics are effective for treatment compared to the doses required for prophylaxis. The serotonin-receptor antagonists are the most commonly studied agents in rescue trials. The following treatments are recommended for the treatment of established PONV: ondansetron (1 mg), dolasetron (12.5 mg), granisetron (0.1 mg), and tropisetron (0.5 mg). Similar to their use in PONV prophylaxis, the antivomiting efficacy of the $5HT_3$-receptor antagonists is better than their anti-nausea efficacy.

In patients who fail prophylaxis with one agent, it is unclear if an antiemetic acting at a different receptor would constitute a better agent for rescue. In one study, a repeat dose of ondansetron was not any better than placebo for the treatment of established PONV in patients who failed ondansetron prophylaxis. However, more studies are required on this issue.

When evaluating PONV following surgery, the role of factors other than anesthetics should be considered first. Contributing factors may include opiates, swallowing blood, or bowel obstruction. Appropriate rescue therapy must take these into account. Recommendations for the treatment of established PONV are summarized in Table 7-2.

SUMMARY

The etiology of PONV is multifactorial. Patient-, anesthesia-, and surgery-related risk factors have been identified. Universal PONV prophylaxis is not cost-effective. Identification of patients at high risk for PONV allows targeting prophylaxis to those who will benefit most from it. No prophylaxis is needed for patients at low risk for PONV. For patients at moderate risk for PONV, prophylaxis using a single antiemetic or a combination of two agents should be considered. Double- and triple-antiemetic

combinations should be considered for patients at high risk for PONV. Furthermore, a multimodal approach should be adopted incorporating steps to keep the baseline risk of PONV low. For the treatment of established PONV, smaller doses of antiemetics are required compared to those needed for prophylaxis. For patients who develop PONV despite prophylaxis, an antiemetic acting at a different receptor should be used for rescue.

REFERENCES

1. Sinclair DR, Chung F, Mezei G: Can postoperative nausea and vomiting be predicted? Anesthesiology 91:109–118, 1999.

2. Apfel CC, Kortilla K, Abdalla M, et al: A factorial trial of six interventions for the prevention of postoperative nausea and vomiting. N Eng J Med 350(24):2441–2451, 2004.

3. Apfel CC, Laara E, Koivuranta M, et al: A simplified risk score for predicting postoperative nausea and vomiting: Conclusions from cross-validations between two centers. Anesthesiology 91:693–700, 1999.

4. Axelsson P, Thorn SE, Wattwil M: Betamethasone does not prevent nausea and vomiting induced by ipecacuanha. Acta Anaesthesiol Scand 48(10):1283–1286, 2004.

5. Henzi I, Walder B, Tramer MR: Metoclopramide in the prevention of postoperative nausea and vomiting: A quantitative systemic review of randomized, placebo-controlled studies. Br J Anaesth 83:761–771, 1999.

6. Domino KB, Anderson EA, Polissar NL, Posner KL: Comparative efficacy and safety of ondansetron, droperidol, and metoclopramide for preventing postoperative nausea and vomiting: A meta-analysis. Anesth Analg 88:1370–1379, 1999.

7. Quaynor H, Raeder JC: Incidence and severity of postoperative nausea and vomiting are similar after metoclopramide 20 mg and onansetron 8 mg given by the end of laparoscopic cholecystectomies. Acta Anaesthesiol Scand 46:109–113, 2002.

8. Goll V, Akca O, Greif R, et al: Ondansetron is no more effective than supplemental intraoperative oxygen for

Table 7-2   PONV Treatment for Patients Who Failed Prophylaxis or Did Not Receive Prophylaxis

Initial Therapy	Rescue Treatment
No prophylaxis or dexamethasone	Low-dose $5HT_3$-receptor antagonist: ondansetron (1 mg), dolasetron (12.5 mg), or tropisetron (0.5 mg)
	Promethazine (6.25 mg) or droperidol (0.625 mg)
$5HT_3$-receptor antagonist plus a second agent	Antiemetic from a different class
Triple therapy: $5HT_3$-receptor antagonist plus two other agents when PONV occurs <6 hours postoperatively	Do not repeat initial therapy
	Use antiemetic from a different class
	Use propofol (20 mg) as needed in PACU (adults)
Triple therapy: $5HT_3$-receptor antagonist plus two other agents when PONV occurs >6 hours postoperatively	Repeat low-dose $5HT_3$-receptor antagonist and droperidol, but do NOT repeat dexamethasone or scopolamine
	Use an antiemetic from a different class

From Habib AS, Gan TJ: Evidence-based management of postoperative nausea and vomiting: A review. Can J Anesth 51:326–341, 2004.

prevention of postoperative nausea and vomiting. Anesth Analg 92:112-117, 2001.

9. Greif R, Laciny S, Rapf B, et al: Supplemental oxygen reduces the incidence of postoperative nausea and vomiting. Anesthesiology 91:1246-1252, 1999.

10. Purhonen S, Niskanen M, Wustefeld M, et al: Supplemental oxygen for prevention of nausea and vomiting after breast surgery. Br J Anaesth 91:284-287, 2003.

11. Joris JL, Poth NJ, Djamadar AM, et al: Supplemental oxygen does not reduce postoperative nausea and vomiting after thyroidectomy. Br J Anaesth 91:857-861, 2003.

12. Purhonen S, Turunen M, Ruohoaho UM, et al: Supplemental oxygen does not reduce the incidence of postoperative nausea and vomiting after ambulatory gynecologic laparoscopy. Anesth Analg 96:91-96, 2003.

13. Enqvist B, Bjorklund C, Engman M, Jakobsson J: Preoperative hypnosis reduces postoperative vomiting after surgery of the breasts. A prospective, randomized, and blinded study. Acta Anaesthesiol Scand 41:1028-1032, 1997.

14. Nilsson U, Rawal N, Enqvist B, Unosson M: Analgesia following music and therapeutic suggestions in the PACU in ambulatory surgery: A randomized controlled trial. Acta Anaesthesiol Scand 47:278-283, 2003.

15. Ernst E, Pittler MH: Efficacy of ginger for nausea and vomiting: A systemic review of randomized clinical trials. Br J Anaesth 84:367-371, 2000.

16. Smiler BG, Srock M: Isopropyl alcohol for transport-related nausea. Anesth Analg 87:1214, 1998.

17. Merritt BA, Okyere CP, Jasinski DM: Isopropyl alcohol inhalation: Alternative treatment of postoperative nausea and vomiting. Nursing Research 51:125-128, 2002.

18. Wang SM, Hofstadter MB, Kain ZN: An alternative method to alleviate postoperative nausea and vomiting in children. J Clin Anesth 11:231-234, 1999.

19. Gesztesi Z, Scuderi PE, White PF, et al: Substance P (Neurokinin-1) antagonist prevents postoperative vomiting after abdominal hysterectomy procedures. Anesthesiology 93:931-937, 2000.

20. Scuderi PE, James RL, Harris L, Mims GR 3rd: Multimodal antiemetic management prevents early postoperative vomiting after outpatient laparoscopy. Anesth Analg 91:1408-1414, 2000.

21. Scuderi PE, James RL, Harris L, Mims GR 3rd: Antiemetic prophylaxis does not improve outcomes after outpatient surgery when compared to symptomatic treatment. Anesthesiology 90:360-371, 1999.

22. Tramer MR, Phillips C, Reynolds DJ, et al: Cost-effectiveness of ondansetron for postoperative nausea and vomiting. Anaesthesia 54:226-234, 1999.

23. Hill RP, Lubarsky DA, Phillips-Bute B, et al: Cost-effectiveness of prophylactic antiemetic therapy with ondansetron, droperidol, or placebo. Anesthesiology 92:958-967, 2000.

24. Frighetto L, Loewen PS, Dolman J, Marra CA: Cost-effectiveness of prophylactic dolasetron or droperidol vs rescue therapy in the prevention of PONV in ambulatory gynecologic surgery. Can J Anaesth 46:536-543, 1999.

25. Tang J, Watcha MF, White PF: A comparison of costs and efficacy of ondansetron and droperidol as prophylactic antiemetic therapy for elective outpatient gynecologic procedures. Anesth Analg 83:304-343, 1996.

26. Watcha MF, Smith I. Cost-effectiveness analysis of antiemetic therapy for ambulatory surgery. J Clin Anesth 6:370-377, 1994.

27. Wu CL, Berenholtz SM, Pronovost PJ, Fleisher LA: Systematic review and analysis of postdischarge symptoms after outpatient surgery. Anesthesiology 96:994-1003, 2002.

28. Gupta AM, Wu CL, Elkassabany N, et al: Does the routine prophylactic use of antiemetics affect the incidence of postdischarge nausea and vomiting following ambulatory surgery? A systematic review of randomized controlled trials. Anesthesiology 99:488-495, 2003.

SUGGESTED READING

Carroll NV, Miederhoff P, Cox FM, Hirsch JD: Postoperative nausea and vomiting after discharge from outpatient surgery centers. Anesth Analg 80:903-909, 1995.

Gan TJ: Postoperative nausea and vomiting—can it be eliminated? JAMA 287:1233-1236, 2002.

Gan TJ, Meyer T, Apfel CC, et al: Consensus guidelines for managing postoperative nausea and vomiting. Anesth Analg 97:62-71, 2003.

Habib AS, Gan TJ: Combination antiemetics: what is the evidence? Int Anesthesiol Clin 41:119-144, 2003.

Habib AS, William DW, Eubanks S, et al: A randomized comparison of a multimodal management strategy versus combination antiemetics for the prevention of postoperative nausea and vomiting. Anesth Analg 99:77-81, 2004.

Kazemi-Kjellberg F, Henzi I, Tramer MR: Treatment of established postoperative nausea and vomiting: A quantitative systematic review. BMC Anesthesiol 1:2, 2001.

Kovac AL: Prevention and treatment of postoperative nausea and vomiting. Drugs 59:213-243, 2000.

Kovac AL, O'Connor TA, Pearman MH, et al: Efficacy of repeat intravenous dosing of ondansetron in controlling postoperative nausea and vomiting: a randomized, double-blind, placebo-controlled multicenter trial. J Clin Anesth 11:453-459, 1999.

Macario A, Weinger M, Carney S, Kim A: Which clinical anesthesia outcomes are important to avoid? The perspective of patients. Anesth Analg 89:652-658, 1999.

Watcha M, White PF: Postoperative nausea and vomiting: its etiology, treatment and prevention. Anesthesiology 77:162-184, 1992.

White PF, Watcha M: Postoperative nausea and vomiting: prophylaxis versus treatment. Anesth Analg 89(6):1337-1339, 1999.

Outpatient Anesthesia Complications

JOHN A. DILGER

HUGH M. SMITH

MICHAEL T. WALSH

Ambulatory surgical procedures have continued to increase over the last few decades in the United States. This dramatic increase has partly been a result of improved surgical techniques and the availability of better anesthetic agents with fewer side effects. Many procedures have moved from the traditional hospital into specific ambulatory surgery centers (ASCs) and office-based practices. The public perceives that these venues have a satisfactory safety record.

However, any ambulatory surgical center's quality and safety record is reflected in the center's morbidity and mortality rate. The complications that result from any procedure will, in many cases, have to be identified and managed outside the usual well-supported hospital setting. This puts considerable emphasis on communication between anesthesiologist and surgeon so that potential and actual problems may be identified and appropriately managed. Complications may also be responsible for patient transfers and admissions to the hospital. There are many causes of complications. There are surgical factors such as bleeding, anesthetic factors such as postoperative nausea and vomiting, and the patient's own medical conditions (e.g., uncontrolled diabetes mellitus) that may influence the likelihood of complications.

Perioperative complications may result despite optimal anesthetic and surgical care. There are many physiologic changes resulting from surgery, including a physiological stress response that causes release of inflammatory mediators. This stress response to surgery results from the activation of nociceptors and from an inflammatory response producing the release of cytokines, prostanoids, complement, and other tissue factors. The degree of the stress response relates to the severity of the surgical insult. By blocking the nociceptive input, the stress response may be decreased, but, except for prostaglandin inhibition, our ability to modulate the inflammatory response remains limited.

The inflammatory process may influence the development of complications. A stress response may lead to hyperglycemia, which, coupled with perioperative hypothermia or low wound perfusion, can lead to wound infections. Pain may lead to increased oxygen consumption, hypertension, tachycardia, or myocardial ischemia. Pain, along with the opioids given for pain control, disrupts rapid eye movement (REM) sleep, leading to daytime sleepiness and fatigue. Additionally, lack of REM sleep is associated with further increases in sympathetic tone. The resulting fluctuations in blood pressure and heart rate may result in myocardial ischemia. If anesthesiologists and surgeons are aware of and are committed to reducing the stress response from surgery, these complications may be mitigated, if not prevented.

So-called "minor" complications occur frequently after ambulatory surgery and may prolong the postoperative recovery. The duration of recovery is frequently viewed as an important outcome measure after outpatient surgery. Minor complications, although not a threat to life, may cause patients significant distress and serve to slow the normally rapid recovery in the outpatient setting. Minor complications create the need for extra treatments and prolonged recoveries in the postanesthesia care unit (PACU), thereby increasing costs. The delay in postoperative discharge is most frequently associated with the type of anesthesia and the type of surgical procedure. General anesthesia maintained with volatile agents is associated with twice as much postoperative nausea and vomiting (PONV) as a propofol-based intravenous technique. However, even general anesthesia maintained with propofol is associated with a higher incidence of PONV than is regional anesthesia. Orthopedic, urologic, and general surgical procedures may be more painful than other procedures and may cause prolonged recovery. Patient factors also affect the rapidity of recovery. Female patients are more likely to have PONV, and young patients are more at risk for PONV and severe pain. In contrast, elderly patients are less delayed by pain or PONV but are more at risk for cardiac complications. It is vital to appropriately manage patients who have preexisting conditions or who will have procedures associated with delayed recovery.

Unplanned hospital admission occurs when perioperative complications cannot be managed successfully in an ASC or office setting, and, therefore, much of the benefit of ambulatory surgery is lost. The incidence of unanticipated hospital admission ranges between 0.28% and 9.5%. Fortier et al.[1] reported that the causes of hospital admission could be placed into four categories. The most common reasons for hospital admission were surgical issues (38.1%) including pain, surgical complication, and bleeding. Anesthesia problems (25.1%) included PONV, somnolence, and sequelae of regional blocks. Social factors (19.5%) included a patient's or surgeon's request to admit or a lack of patient escort. General medical reasons accounted for 17.2% of admissions. Other factors increasing the likelihood of admission from an ASC include prolonged anesthesia, general anesthesia, painful surgery, and surgery ending late in the day.

Beyond these, an unplanned admission to a hospital because of recurring or new complications may occur even after the patient is discharged from the ambulatory setting. Twersky[2] in 1997 found that 1.3% of patients were readmitted to the hospital within 1 month for complications including bleeding, fever, infection, pain, wound disruption, and urinary retention. In a more recent study in 1999, Mezei[3] found a similar readmission rate of 1.1% and noted that transurethral biopsy tumor patients had the highest readmission rate (5.2%). There were no anesthesia-related causes for readmission in either study (Table 8-1).

Perioperative death after outpatient surgery is a rare event. The earliest study, in 1980 by Natof,[4] followed 13,433 patients for 2 weeks postoperatively and found no deaths. In 1999, Mezei[3] evaluated 17,638 cases for 30 days after surgery and found no mortality. Warner et al.,[5] in 1993, published a review of 38,598 outpatients and their 30-day postoperative recovery and found four deaths. Two of the deaths resulted from car accidents and two resulted from myocardial infarctions. In 2004, Fleisher et al.[6] evaluated the mortality rate in 564,267 patients and found a mortality rate for ambulatory surgery patients of 2.3/100,000 to 2.5/100,000 on the day of surgery, and the mortality at 7 days was between 25 and 50 out of 100,000.

The incidence of postoperative complications, with the exception of PONV and pain (discussed in greater detail within other chapters), is low. However, many complications can cause considerable morbidity in the perioperative period.

CARDIAC COMPLICATIONS

Myocardial Ischemia

Cardiovascular changes (e.g., bradycardia, tachycardia, blood pressure changes, and ischemia) are common intraoperative events during outpatient surgery. Significantly, perioperative cardiac complications are the leading cause of death in the perioperative period. Although rare, death usually occurs from myocardial infarction (MI), congestive heart failure, or a malignant arrhythmia.

A patient's perioperative risk will be greatly influenced by the preoperative presence of coronary artery disease, hypertension, or arrhythmias. Because of the increased incidence of these conditions in the elderly, cardiac events in this group are two times more common

Table 8-1	Unanticipated Hospital Admission After Ambulatory Surgery		
Surgical (38.1%)	**Anesthetic (25.1%)**	**Social (19.5%)**	**Medical (17.3%)**
Pain	PONV	Patient request	Patient comorbidity
Bleeding	Somnolence	Surgeon request	Unrelated medical
Other complication	Regional or other	No escort	

than in younger patients. Perioperative cardiac morbidity may be influenced by increased sympathetic tone, a hypercoagulable tendency after surgery, and tachycardia. Tachycardia in the presence of coronary stenosis impairs myocardial blood flow, resulting in subendocardial ischemia and myocardial dysfunction.

β-blocker drugs (and, recently, α-agonist drugs) play an important role in controlling heart rate. These drugs have clearly been shown to improve the long-term survival of patients after myocardial infarction. Myocardial infarctions typically occur silently within 24 to 48 hours of the day of surgery and are commonly of the non-Q-wave variety. In unselected patients more than 40 years old undergoing major noncardiac surgical procedures, the incidence of myocardial infarction is less than 2%. Higher-risk patients have an incidence of MI more than twice this rate. The mortality after perioperative MI is less than 10% to 15%, which is a lower incidence than earlier reports (50%). Estimates of the incidence of postoperative MI in outpatients are based on only a few studies. In the study by Warner et al.,[5] 14 MIs occurred out of 45,090 outpatient anesthetics. Fortier et al.[1] found 1 MI in 15,172 outpatients. Unfortunately, the largest study on outpatient complications, by Fleisher et al.[6] in 2004, did not examine the specific causes of morbidity.

Hypertension and Hypotension

Perioperative blood pressure changes may be caused by many different factors. Postoperative hypertension may result from poorly controlled existing primary hypertension, pain, anxiety, or bladder distention. The treatment for hypertension resulting from all but primary hypertension is straightforward: relieve the inciting factors. Importantly, the patient with poorly controlled primary hypertension may have wide fluctuations in blood pressure during induction and endotracheal intubation relating to volume deficits and baroreceptor dysfunction. There is considerable evidence that the uncontrolled hypertensive patient is at increased risk of myocardial ischemia from coronary artery disease, cerebral vascular disease, and heart failure. Therefore, if patients are treated with antihypertensive medications, they should usually take these medications preoperatively. Because of the risk of excessive intraoperative hypotension, some clinicians prefer that patients not take diuretics, angiotensin-converting enzyme-inhibiting or angiotensin-receptor-blocking drugs. Ideally, untreated hypertensive patients should be started preoperatively on medications. This can be done by the primary care provider or by the anesthesiologist acting as the perioperative physician.

Hypotension can occur postoperatively because of volume deficits, anemia, or vagal stimulation. Significant blood loss after ambulatory surgery is fortunately rare, but may increase in incidence when complicated procedures are performed. Large blood losses may result from the surgical technique itself, or they may be due to altered coagulation secondary to dilution or disseminated intravascular coagulation. Secondary effects of hypotension are a concern. However, it is controversial to link intraoperative hypotension and postoperative myocardial infarction. Indeed, Badner et al.[7] in 1998 failed to show an association. Furthermore, there was no clear association between postoperative hypotension and myocardial infarction. Despite this, a blood pressure within 20% of baseline is often a goal for at-risk patients during intraoperative and postoperative periods.

Tachycardia

Tachycardia may result from the same causes resulting in hypertension and hypotension, and the treatment is correcting these disorders. The risk of a perioperative MI in patients with coronary disease increases in proportion to the heart rate. Drugs that slow heart rate, such as β-blockers, may therefore be beneficial both in patients with cardiovascular risk factors and in those with documented coronary artery disease. Mangano et al.[8] showed that, when using atenolol for heart rate control, patients had better outcomes than did patients treated with placebo. Poldermans et al.[9] similarly found that administering bisoprolol to surgical patients lowered the rates for myocardial infarction compared to placebo-treated patents.

As yet, it is not proven that patients with known cardiac risk factors undergoing minor outpatient surgery benefit from β-blocker use. However, it does seem reasonable to treat patients with risk factors for coronary artery disease with β-blockers in order to control or prevent tachycardia in the perioperative period. It is unknown whether these patients should be continued on chronic β-blocker therapy after the surgical event. Involving the surgeon and the primary care physician in this decision is essential.

RESPIRATORY COMPLICATIONS

Respiratory events (e.g., apnea, bronchospasm, and laryngospasm) are the second most common intraoperative adverse event in ambulatory patients.

Hypoxia and Hypoventilation

The development of adverse pulmonary events in the PACU after general anesthesia was examined by Rose et al.[10] The study found an incidence of 1.3% for critical respiratory events, subdivided into 0.8% for hypoxia, 0.2% for hypoventilation, and 0.2% for airway obstruction. Associated factors included patient age greater than 60, male gender, obesity, and anesthetic factors (i.e., thiopental use compared to propofol and residual muscle relaxant effects).

The causes of perioperative hypoxia include low inspired oxygen concentration, hypoventilation, alveolar ventilation-perfusion mismatch, increased shunt, diffusion problems, and significant drops in cardiac output or hemoglobin. In the PACU, the most common causes of hypoxia are hypoventilation and ventilation-perfusion mismatching.

Hypoventilation may occur because of residual effects of anesthetics, opioids, or muscle relaxants given in the operating room; hypoventilation may result from airway obstruction. Patients with morbid obesity and obstructive sleep apnea (OSA) may be very sensitive to residual anesthetic effects, thereby causing significant airway obstruction and profound hypoxia. It may be important to use short-acting muscle relaxants and opioids so that they may be easily reversed either spontaneously or by specific antagonists. Ventilation-perfusion mismatching may occur after laparoscopic surgery or may result from hypoventilation or steep Trendelenburg positioning.

The pediatric patient may develop postintubation croup with hypoxemia, stridor, sternal retractions, barking cough, and hoarseness. In 1991, Litman[11] reported the incidence of croup after intubation to be 0.1%, and it occurred most commonly in patients between 7 months and 9 years of age. Patients were treated with humidified oxygen and did not require racemic epinephrine. All of the outpatients were discharged as planned.

Asthma

Asthma is a chronic disorder of the tracheobronchial tree, resulting from chronic inflammation of respiratory mucosa and intermittent constriction of bronchioles in response to antigens or nonantigenic stimuli such as cold or exercise. Perioperative bronchospasm is more common in patients with recent asthma exacerbations. If significant asthma symptoms exist, surgery should be delayed to avoid status asthmaticus and the inability to ventilate the lungs.

The cornerstone of the asthma patient's management is to continue metered-dose inhalers (i.e., β-agonists, steroids, or anticholinergics) and to consider use just prior to inducing anesthesia. Many practitioners prefer regional anesthesia for these patients, although the literature fails to show a significant advantage over general anesthesia in avoiding bronchospasm. At induction of general anesthesia, propofol has been shown to be superior to thiopental in reducing the incidence of bronchospasm after endotracheal intubation. Intravenous lidocaine may also be useful to reduce airway reactivity. Ketamine may have advantages in the emergency patient with asthma because of its bronchodilation effects,

although an increase in secretions and postoperative dysphoria may be problematic. Volatile anesthetic agents have bronchodilator effects and are often selected for the maintenance of general anesthesia. Sevoflurane is the least likely among inhaled agents to be irritating and is often chosen for the asthma patient undergoing ambulatory surgery.

Extubation of the asthmatic patient under general anesthesia ("deep" extubation) may decrease the risk of bronchospasm triggered by the endotracheal tube in a patient emerging from anesthesia. In the PACU, supplemental oxygen should be used because hypoxia may enhance airway reactivity. The overall incidence of a perioperative bronchospasm is 1.7%. Bronchospasm in the operating room or PACU may be treated with bronchodilator inhalers or nebulizers, subcutaneous or intravenous β-agonists, or systemic corticosteroids.

Pulmonary Aspiration

Pulmonary aspiration of gastric contents may produce mild to severe injury to the lung parenchyma and may result in chemical pneumonitis or pneumonia. The incidence of aspiration during elective surgery is quite low, occurring in 2.6/10,000 anesthetics, but during emergency surgery the incidence increases to 11/10,000 cases. The mortality from aspiration has been reported to be 0.14/10,000 and is increased in sicker patients. The incidence of aspiration is slightly more common in children and the elderly. There are factors that increase the risks of perioperative aspiration, including gastrointestinal obstruction, gastrointestinal reflux, emergency surgery, Trendelenburg's position, impaired laryngeal reflexes, and difficult airway management. The signs and symptoms of aspiration may include rales, wheezing, rhonchi, dyspnea, hypoxemia, and pulmonary infiltrates or edema. The magnitude of pulmonary injury depends on factors such as gastric volume, acidity, and particulate or fecal matter.

In patients at risk for aspiration, it is advised to pretreat with nonparticulate antacids to increase the gastric pH. A prokinetic agent such as metoclopramide may increase gastric emptying as well as increasing the lower esophageal sphincter tone. A rapid-sequence induction for general anesthesia is usually advised when the patient has preoperative risks for aspiration. The patient should be conscious before extubation to ensure the return of airway reflexes at the end of the surgery. The treatment for aspiration pneumonitis is individualized, so routine antibiotics and steroids are not recommended (Tables 8-2, 8-3).

An endotracheal tube has often been considered the best way to protect the airway from aspiration, but the use of laryngeal mask airways (LMAs) is increasing in ambulatory anesthesia. The laryngeal mask airway was

Table 8-2	Effect of Drugs on Lower Esophageal Sphincter Tone	
Decrease	**No Effect**	**Increase**
Anticholinergic drugs	Atracurium	Succinylcholine
Thiopental	Cimetidine	Ketamine
Propofol	Nitrous oxide (?)	Nitrous oxide (?)
Volatile anesthesia		Antacids
Opioids		Neostigmine
Metoclopramide		Metoprolol
Dopamine		
β-adrenergic agonists		
Tricyclic antidepressants		

Table 8-3	Factors Affecting the Risk of Aspiration	
Increased Risk of Aspiration	**Minimal Risk of Aspiration**	
Old age	Clear liquids ≥3 hours	
Obstetrics	Milk or light meal ≥6 hours	
Obesity	Cuffed tracheal tube	
Emergency surgery	LMA with spontaneous ventilation	
Lithotomy position	LMA with controlled ventilation	
Reflux or hiatal hernia	LMA with abdominal insufflation	
Difficult airway		

developed in the United Kingdom by Archie Brain as a compromise between endotracheal intubation and a facemask for airway management. Some consider the use of an LMA to be controversial because it cannot provide the same level of airway isolation and protection from aspiration as does a cuffed endotracheal tube. In a meta-analysis of studies recording the use of LMAs and aspiration, the incidence of aspiration was 3/12,901 anesthetics, and there were no cases involving children. In two of the three aspiration cases, there were risk factors for aspiration including one emergency anesthetic and one patient in Trendelenburg's position with abdominal insufflation.

The LMA has been shown to decrease the barrier pressure at the lower esophageal sphincter (LES) compared to the use of a facemask for anesthesia. There have been many studies evaluating the potential link between the LMA's change in LES barrier pressure and the subsequent risk of aspiration. Two studies were done comparing the LMA with a facemask for general anesthesia, using a pH probe inserted into the esophagus.[12,13] Both found that

significantly more patients in the LMA group had reflux at the LES probe than in the facemask group. However, in both reports, the LMA patients and the facemask patients had no pH differences found at the probe in the proximal esophagus. The cause of the pH drop at the LES in LMA-treated patients is unclear.

CASE STUDY: A SMALL AMOUNT OF BILE IS PRESENT IN THE LMA AFTER REMOVAL AT EMERGENCE

A 44-year-old female underwent a laparoscopic tubal ligation in Trendelenburg's position with controlled ventilation. The surgery was uneventful. The patient emerged and followed commands, and the LMA was removed, revealing bilious secretions on the tip. The patient is awake, alert, and in no respiratory distress.

CLINICAL NEED

The patient is stable and the surgeon asks whether to admit the patient for observation.

RESPONSE

The LMA was used in the procedure to facilitate airway control. There is evidence that an LMA may safely be used during laparoscopic surgery with controlled ventilation. The use of Trendelenburg's position may increase the risk of aspiration, although there are reports of series of patients with all three factors present without aspiration. There may be distal reflux or proximal reflux in the esophagus without gastric contents entering the oropharynx. To further confuse the issue, the presence of gastric fluid in the oropharynx does not mean clinically significant aspiration. The diagnosis of aspiration pneumonia may be made with a chest x-ray, but this may not be available at the freestanding ambulatory center or office-based practice. The x-ray will not immediately confirm the diagnosis, anyway.

In this patient, the vital signs are stable with normal oxygen saturations on room air. The exam reveals bilateral breath sounds without wheezing or rales. The patient is observed in the PACU for 2 hours and is unchanged on examination and saturation. This is consistent with recommendations by Warner et al.[14] in managing potential aspirations postoperatively. The patient had reflux during the procedure, but not a clinically significant aspiration, and the patient may be safely discharged.

CONCLUSION

A significant aspiration may be ruled out by observing the patient for 2 hours after the event or the extubation. If no symptoms of hypoxia, wheezing, or rales are present, the patient may be discharged home.

There has been concern that the LMA could allow aspiration during both spontaneous and controlled ventilation. Spontaneous ventilation causes subatmospheric intrathoracic pressure during inhalation. Under anesthesia, gastric contents may overcome the esophageal barrier pressure, causing reflux and aspiration. A study compared LMAs during spontaneous and controlled ventilation for laparoscopic gynecological procedures. Esophageal pH electrodes showed no significant difference in the incidence of reflux between the groups. In laparoscopic gynecologic patients in the head-down position, the LMA was compared to endotracheal intubation during controlled ventilation. There was no significant difference between the airway devices for reflux, and there were no cases of aspiration.

The results of these studies suggest that the low incidence of reflux in fasting patients is not influenced to a significant degree by the mode of ventilation, even in the presence of abdominal insufflation and Trendelenburg's position. Interestingly, the timing of the removal of the LMA after general anesthesia affects the incidence of reflux, but in a counterintuitive way. In patients who had the LMA removed during swallowing or struggling, the incidence of reflux was lower than when waiting for patients to open their mouth to command. A redesigned LMA, the LMA ProSeal, with an opening at the distal tip that allows a small esophageal suction catheter, has been introduced by the company. In addition to the distal tip, the device has increased seal pressure compared to the LMA classic. The device may be useful in the unexpected difficult airway when a full stomach is present. However, only the intubating LMA Fastrach can allow the blind direct introduction of an endotracheal tube to secure the airway.

Sleep Apnea

Obstructive sleep apnea (OSA) occurs because of episodic upper airway obstruction, although there may be a central-drive-to-breathe component as well. OSA causes daytime sleepiness and is present in 4% of males and in 2% of females in the middle age group. OSA is defined as the cessation of airflow for 10 seconds, resulting in hypoxemia, despite continued respiratory efforts, occurring five or more times per hour. OSA patients, while sleeping, relax their pharyngeal dilator muscles, causing airflow obstruction. This obstruction causes them to awaken, partially reestablishing tone in the muscles and reestablishing airflow. This cycle causes a lack of REM sleep, resulting in daytime somnolence. The severity of OSA is quantified using the "apnea index," which is the number of obstructions per hour (mild, 6 to 20; moderate, 21 to

50; and severe, >50). The risk factors for OSA are morbid obesity, a large neck circumference, severe tonsillar hypertrophy in children, and craniofacial abnormalities. Patients with OSA may have coexisting diseases including hypertension, coronary artery disease, and, in severe cases, pulmonary hypertension. The diagnosis is made with a sleep study using capnography, pulse oximetry, electroencephalogram (EEG), and chest-wall-movement detectors. The treatment for OSA is the application of a continuous positive airway pressure (CPAP) device, preventing the obstruction during REM sleep. OSA is often suspected because a spouse reports loud snoring, breathing cessation, and daytime sleepiness. If only due to the nationwide epidemic of obesity, increasing numbers of patients with diagnosed and undiagnosed OSA are presenting for surgery and anesthesia. Unfortunately, few patients have had a formal sleep study to confirm or refute the diagnosis.

CLINICAL CAVEAT: OBSTRUCTIVE SLEEP APNEA

- Diagnosed with a formal sleep study
- Presumptive diagnosis: large neck circumference, heavy snoring with breathing cessation, morning headaches, daytime somnolence
- Coexisting diseases: hypertension, hypoxia, pulmonary hypertension, congestive heart failure
- All general anesthetics and opioids worsen the obstruction
- Increased risk of obstruction after surgery lasts 1 week with major surgery
- Increased risk for difficult ventilation prior to intubation
- Regional analgesia is preferred
- Treatment is CPAP

All drugs causing central nervous system (CNS) depression will worsen OSA. Drugs including propofol, thiopental, opioids, benzodiazepines, volatile anesthetics, nitrous oxide, and neuromuscular blockers are implicated. These drugs may decrease the tone in the pharyngeal dilator muscles, allowing fat in the neck to cause complete obstruction by compressing the airway. Because of this, it may seem logical to manage OSA surgical patients with regional anesthesia and analgesia. The sole use of neuraxial or peripheral blockade would provide anesthesia and analgesia with no adverse effect on OSA. However, the concomitant use of sedatives and opioids during the block may increase OSA risk. The literature has failed to support the efficacy or safety of regional anesthesia compared to general anesthesia. If general anesthesia is selected for patients with OSA, airway access may not always be difficult, but if significant obesity or a thick neck is present, a difficult intubation may be encountered. For moderate to severely painful procedures of the upper or lower extremity, an ambulatory continuous nerve block may provide potent analgesia without sedation. Incisional pain in other locations may be treated by infusing a local anesthetic solution through small catheters placed in the wound and continuing the infusion through the painful portions of the recovery.

The postoperative care of OSA patients may be more difficult than the intraoperative management. From the available information, the type of anesthesia seems less important than the type of surgery in predicting outcomes with OSA. In total hip and knee patients, Gupta et al.[15] showed that patients with OSA had a longer hospital course with more complications, including requiring CPAP, intubation, or intensive care unit (ICU) admission.

The care of the recovering OSA outpatient will be even more challenging since the opportunity to monitor and treat episodes of obstruction is not present after discharge home. The care and discharge to home of the OSA patient will vary. Patients with OSA can be divided into three groups, and their PACU and discharge will vary accordingly. Some patients will have the diagnosis after a formal sleep study and are compliant with CPAP therapy. Other patients have a diagnosis of OSA and are not compliant with the use of CPAP. A third group has a presumptive diagnosis of OSA based on their symptoms of snoring, respiratory pauses, and daytime somnolence.

It has been common to perform ambulatory surgery on OSA patients with stable home CPAP treatment, although the safety of this practice has not been evaluated in prospective studies. The management of the OSA patient who has not been diagnosed or who is diagnosed but fails to follow the prescribed CPAP treatment is much more controversial. There is little written on how these groups should be managed as outpatients or if they are even appropriate candidates for ambulatory surgery.

There are general guidelines that may be suggested in the absence of evidence-based guidelines. Surgical procedures with OSA that involve little pain or that are for patients who use CPAP regularly may be done on an outpatient basis. All OSA patients must be observed postoperatively for an extended period until the anesthetic effects have dissipated. If patients require increasing doses of opioids for pain or if they continue to obstruct in the recovery phase, they should be admitted to a hospital for observation or CPAP therapy.

CURRENT CONTROVERSY: OUTPATIENT SURGERY IN PATIENTS WITH OBSTRUCTIVE SLEEP APNEA

- Postoperatively, the OSA is worsened for several days by residual anesthesia and opioid pain therapy followed by increased REM sleep
- CPAP is effective in eliminating the obstructive symptoms, but many are not compliant with treatment or are not formally diagnosed
- Outpatients using CPAP may be safely discharged from PACU once they are awake and alert
- Outpatients not treated with CPAP must be evaluated over several hours in the PACU prior to discharge to rule out significant obstruction and desaturation
- Patients with significant obstruction must be admitted for observation and monitored with pulse oximetry and capnography

---

Oropharyngeal Injury

A variety of injuries can occur during management of the airway. Dental injuries during airway instrumentation would seem common, but during laryngoscopy and endotracheal intubation, the incidence of injury is 1/4500 procedures. The development of a sore throat postoperatively is much more common, and it occurs in between 14% and 45% of procedures with endotracheal intubation and in 5.8% to 34% of procedure with LMA insertion. Risk factors for developing sore throat after endotracheal intubation include endotracheal tube size and pressure, female sex, age, surgery for gynecologic and thyroid procedures, intubation time, the use of nasogastric tubes, and the use of succinylcholine. The use of local anesthetics in the oropharynx increases the incidence of sore throat. Surprisingly, the ease of intubation has no effect on the incidence of sore throat. The soreness lasts, on average, 48 hours.

The use of endotracheal intubation with total intravenous anesthesia (TIVA) is associated with an even higher incidence of sore throat (50%). The incidence of sore throat with an LMA may vary considerably. If the LMA is inserted and fully inflated, the incidence of sore throat is 42%, but partial inflation reduces the incidence to 20%. By using a disposable soft-seal LMA, the incidence could be lowered further to 10%. This is comparable to conventional mask ventilation (8%). When a size 4 (versus a size 5) LMA is used in male patients, and when a size 3 (versus a size 4) LMA is used in female patients, there is a lower incidence of sore throat.

The treatment for sore throat is supportive, but if the discomfort is severe or is not resolved within 48 hours, an examination should be done looking for transmural pharyngeal or esophageal tears (Table 8-4).

Table 8-4	Factors Affecting the Risk of Postoperative Sore Throat	

Factors Increasing Risk	Factors Reducing Risk
Use of an endotracheal tube	Use of an LMA
Increased ETT size	Use of a size-4 LMA for males or a size-3 for females
High ETT cuff pressure	
Female gender	Use of a soft-seal LMA
Long duration of intubation	Partial inflation of the LMA cuff
Use of a nasogastric tube	Avoidance of local anesthetics in the oropharynx
Use of succinylcholine	
Gynecologic or thyroid surgery	
Combination of an ETT plus total intravenous anesthesia	

ETT, Endotracheal tube.

NEUROLOGIC COMPLICATIONS

Postoperative Delirium

Postoperative delirium is an acute change in the patient's baseline mental status that occurs after anesthesia. The symptoms can range from quiet confusion to frank violence and hysteria, which may cause injury to the patient and staff. Postoperative delirium is more common in both pediatric and elderly patients. However, usually only the elderly have a prolonged recovery.

Causes of delirium can include hypoxia and hypercarbia, so these must be immediately evaluated and corrected. Other causes include drugs having CNS anticholinergic effects, which result in patient confusion and agitation. Atropine is commonly implicated, although many other medications have central anticholinergic effects. Peripheral anticholinergic effects, which are not always present, include tachycardia, flushing, and anhidrosis. Intravenous physostigmine may improve the CNS abnormalities. Meperidine has a similar structure to atropine and may cause similar symptoms at higher doses. Benzodiazepines can cause postoperative confusion, particularly in the elderly. Because of its ability to cause hallucinations, ketamine may lead to postoperative delirium.

Surgical factors such as poorly controlled pain or bladder distention may cause agitation. Electrolyte and metabolic changes can cause mental status changes, so early evaluation of sodium, calcium, magnesium, and (especially) glucose levels are indicated. Patients with chronic alcohol consumption or substance abuse can develop delirium as a manifestation of withdrawal. After eliminating the more common causes, neurologic injury should be considered, and a thorough exam should be done with a possible neurologic consultation and CNS imaging.

An often-overlooked cause of early postoperative delirium and agitation is the patient with a history of posttraumatic stress disorder. Patients may or may not volunteer this problem during routine preoperative questioning.

Postoperative Cognitive Dysfunction

Postoperative cognitive dysfunction (POCD) is usually a complication of the elderly after general anesthesia for cardiac and other major surgeries. It may also occur with simpler surgeries normally done on an ambulatory basis. POCD may even occur with younger patients. POCDs are deficits in memory and cognition, which, in severe cases, include delirium. There are several theories as to the cause of POCD. One theory involves an imbalance of neurotransmitters in the presence of a decrease in physiologic reserve, as may occur in the elderly. Acetylcholine plays a role in activities of consciousness, and serotonin is important in mood, cognition, and sleep. Another possible etiology involves mediators of inflammation such as cytokines released during stress-affecting neurotransmitter function. Hormonal imbalances may also be involved. Cortisol elevation during stress may affect energy, cognition, and sleep. The diagnosis of POCD is made using perioperative neuropsychological testing (Table 8-5).

The incidence of POCD is higher for inpatient major surgery and is lower following outpatient surgery. Elderly patients have an incidence of POCD of 25.8% at 1 week and 9.9% at 3 months. A follow-up study by Canet et al.[16] found an incidence of POCD in the elderly after minor procedures of 6.8% at 1 week and 6.6% at 3 months. POCD incidence at 7 days after surgery is significantly lower in outpatients (3.5%) as compared to patients with short inpatient stays (9.8%).

Factors that may cause the increase in POCD with inpatients include sensory overload, sleep deprivation,

Table 8-5	Factors Affecting the Risk of Postoperative Cognitive Dysfunction	

Patient	Surgical	Postoperative
Age	Coronary artery bypass	Postoperative pain
Preexisting cognitive impairment	Length of procedure	Psychoactive medications
Alcoholism	Abdominal aortic aneurysm operation	Electrolyte abnormalities
	Hip fractures	Respiratory complications

immobility, and the absence of the familiar home environment. When major and minor surgery studies are compared, the major surgery patients had a significantly higher rate of POCD at 1 week and a higher rate at 3 months, thus reaffirming major surgery as a primary risk factor. The other significant risk factors that have been identified are advanced age, preexisting cognitive impairment, and the severity of any coexisting illness.

In a 2002 study of surgical patients, Johnson et al.[17] reported that, in patients between 40 and 60 years old, the POCD rate was 19.6% at 1 week and the 3-month incidence was 6.2%. This illustrates that POCD is not completely confined to the elderly. It has been suggested that regional anesthesia decreases the risk of developing POCD, but in a 2004 meta-analysis, Wu et al.[18] found no difference in the incidence of POCD when regional and general anesthesia were compared.

Most of the patients developing POCD see a resolution of symptoms by a week, but patients with persistent symptoms of POCD will have ramifications in quality of life as well as social and financial implications for the patient and family. Although major surgery is the primary cause, ambulatory surgery and anesthesia may also cause POCD.

Perioperative Headache

The development of a perioperative headache may be quite distressing to all because it is not directly related to the procedure or anesthesia and may prolong the PACU time. One of the most reliable predictors of perioperative headaches is a patient history of prior headaches. In 2003, Gill[19] found that caffeine withdrawal, the duration of fluid deprivation, and starvation were not significant factors in causing headaches. In an earlier study, Nikolajsen[20] found prior headaches to be a significant factor but also found that caffeine withdrawal (from consumption >400 mg/day) was a significant factor in headache development. In patients with high caffeine intake, prophylactic treatment with IV caffeine significantly decreased the incidence of postoperative headache. Further study is needed to define the specific causes of perioperative headache.

Regional Anesthesia

Postdural Puncture Headache

In addition to the aforementioned causes of headache, postdural puncture headache (PDPH) may follow spinal or epidural anesthesia. PDPH continues to occur despite advances in equipment and patient selection. Spinal needles in 25-gauge size with a pencil-point tip will cause PDPH in less than 1% of patients, including those in high-risk groups. Conversely, the incidence of headache is much greater when an accidental dural puncture occurs

with an epidural needle. When a PDPH occurs with a small pencil-point needle, the treatment may be conservative if the patient's symptoms are mild. With an epidural puncture, the symptoms may be more severe and more persistent. In this case, aggressive therapy is warranted. An epidural blood patch is the treatment of choice for PDPH when conservative measures (i.e., bed rest, hydration, and IV caffeine) fail. Epidural blood patching should be done when symptoms are not resolved and are debilitating. If left untreated, PDPH may impact the patient's quality of life and may actually cause further complications such as a subdural hematoma.

Of course, PDPH is a clinical diagnosis without a specific test, but the classic history of positional fronto-occipital headache pain following a neuraxial procedure is very reliable. Other causes of severe headache in the postoperative period must be considered and ruled out.

Transient Neurologic Syndrome

Occurring after spinal anesthesia, transient neurologic syndrome (TNS) is manifested by back pain that may radiate into the buttocks or legs. The back pain may be severe, lasting 3 or 4 days, and, at times, it may be worse than the surgical pain. TNS is most common with spinal lidocaine (33%), followed closely by mepivacaine (30%), and it is least common with bupivacaine (1%). Factors such as early ambulation, knee arthroscopy, and the lithotomy position increase the incidence of TNS. TNS does not appear to be a neurotoxic injury, such as occurs in cauda equina syndrome after lidocaine spinal anesthesia. The mechanism of TNS is not clear, and further study is needed.

Efforts to decrease TNS risk for lidocaine have included reducing the dose, changing baricity, and decreasing lidocaine concentration and volume. No alterations have been clearly effective. There is no equivalent lidocaine replacement with regard to efficacy and duration, but low-dose bupivacaine combined with fentanyl has been used with success in the outpatient setting. Additionally, intraspinal 2-chloroprocaine is being studied. Although TNS causes no serious injury, it does delay the patient's recovery and compromises early satisfaction with surgery.

Peripheral Nerve Injury After Regional Anesthesia

The use of regional anesthesia for ambulatory patients is ideal in that it avoids highly emetogenic drugs used for general anesthesia and postoperative analgesia. However, for several reasons, not all patients or surgeons are fully accepting of regional anesthesia. One reason is that nerve injuries may occur with the use of regional anesthesia. The incidence of a severe nerve injury because of a peripheral nerve block is very low. Interestingly, the most common nerve injury, one to the ulnar nerve at the elbow, actually occurs during general anesthesia. Most of the injuries to the ulnar nerve under general anesthesia have no identifiable cause.

The etiology of a nerve injury may relate to patient or surgical issues, or it may involve the actual regional technique. Patient issues would include preexisting neurologic diseases (e.g., diabetes mellitus) and surgical factors including positioning, trauma to or retraction of a nerve during the procedure, tourniquet ischemia, or a tight cast or dressing. Regional anesthesia may injure a nerve by needle trauma, injection of a local anesthetic into the nerve (causing an ischemic injury), or local-anesthetic neurotoxicity. Short-bevel or conventional needles may be used to elicit a paresthesia, whereas newer techniques use nerve electrolocation, ultrasound image location, or both. No technique appears to be associated with a lower rate of nerve injury.

A nerve injury would be suspected if a persistent paresthesia was present. Other less-common symptoms include a sensory or motor deficit. If a neurologic deficit is present, the patient should be referred for a neurological exam. This may include electromyography to ascertain the extent of the injury or the presence of a preexisting condition. The evaluation will help localize the injury so the etiology of the nerve injury is clarified and any possible treatment may occur immediately.

In the past, it was traditional to let all peripheral nerve blocks dissipate prior to discharge so that nerve injuries could be diagnosed. This practice has changed, and patients are now discharged with a single injection or a continuous nerve block (with a portable local anesthetic pump) immediately after surgery. This change has occurred for two reasons. Historically, in the early postoperative period, few nerve injuries were diagnosed, and recovery from the block was prolonged. The second reason is that regional anesthesia, using long-lasting local anesthetics, may be used for intentionally prolonged analgesia. This obviates the need for opioids and reduces the risk of PONV.

MISCELLANEOUS COMPLICATIONS

Urinary Retention

Anesthesia, surgery, and patient factors (i.e., prior urinary retention or benign prostatic hypertrophy) may cause postoperative urinary retention in outpatients. General anesthesia may cause bladder atony by interfering with the autonomic control of the bladder, and neuraxial anesthesia may interfere with the micturition reflex, resulting in detrusor muscle blockade. Surgeries, such as inguinal, gynecologic, pelvic, rectal, and urologic surgeries, are associated with a high risk of postoperative urine retention. Patients having procedures associated with a low risk for urinary retention may be

discharged prior to voiding, but patients in high-risk categories should be observed until the bladder is emptied because the urinary retention rate is 5% and, after discharge, recurs in 25% of affected patients. The use of peripheral blocks does not have the same effect on urinary function as general and neuraxial anesthesia in high-risk procedures. The incidence of urinary retention after inguinal herniorrhaphy with peripheral nerve blocks is 0.37%, which is significantly lower than the incidence with general (3.0%) or neuraxial (2.4%) techniques (Table 8-6).

Oral Intake

Oral intake prior to discharge affects discharge time, but opposite to the direction expected. In a study by Jin,[21] adult patients with postoperative oral fluid intake took significantly longer to ambulate and to achieve postanesthetic discharge criteria, and they had stay times in the ambulatory unit longer than their nondrinking counterparts. However, there was no difference in the incidence of PONV between the groups. In 989 pediatric patients (from ages 1 month to 18 years), mandatory oral fluid intake was associated with more PONV and a longer stay in the ambulatory unit than in the patients who had optional oral fluid intake; there were no readmissions for PONV or dehydration in either one of the study groups.

Postoperative Myalgias

Succinylcholine, which is a depolarizing muscle relaxant, is ideal for ambulatory surgery with its rapid, predictable onset and low cost and its record for spontaneous and rapid full recovery. Succinylcholine is associated with myalgias occurring up to 50% of the time. The myalgias are typically located in the neck, shoulder, and abdominal muscles and last 2 to 3 days postoperatively. Postsuccinylcholine myalgias are more common in females, but they are less common in the pediatric and geriatric populations and in the patient doing muscle training.

Table 8-6 Factors Affecting Risks of Postoperative Urinary Retention

Patient	High-Risk Surgery	Anesthetic
Age	Gynecologic	General anesthesia
Prior history of urinary retention	Urologic	Neuraxial anesthesia
Benign prostatic hypertrophy	Pelvic	Decreased incidence of urinary retention from peripheral nerve blocks
	Rectal	
	Inguinal	

Early ambulation after surgery increases the incidence and severity of the pain after succinylcholine. The intensity of the pain does not correlate with changes in the potassium or creatine phosphokinase (CPK) levels after succinylcholine. The mechanism of the pain is thought to result from fasciculations that cause muscle contraction without muscle shortening. This results in muscle bundle injury, which leads to myalgias.

The most common technique for the prevention of myalgias is pretreatment with a nondepolarizing muscle relaxant prior to succinylcholine. Lidocaine pretreatment has been shown to be effective in reducing postsuccinylcholine myalgias. Lidocaine pretreatment caused a lower rise in serum plasma potassium and a drop in calcium levels. This effect may result from lidocaine's cell-membrane-stabilizing properties, which prevent ionic exchange across the cell membrane and thereby decrease the myalgias. A superior pretreatment strategy appears to be the combination of nondepolarizing drugs and lidocaine; this combination is more effective than either drug alone in preventing postoperative myalgias.

The best way to prevent postsuccinylcholine myalgia is to avoid the use of succinylcholine. Alternatives include regional anesthesia, performing general anesthesia without muscle relaxants, or using nondepolarizing muscle relaxants. The patient requiring a rapid sequence induction for severe reflux may be a good candidate for succinylcholine; however, even in this setting, rocuronium may be a suitable option.

Corneal Abrasion

The incidence of corneal abrasion was once reported to be as high as 44%, but, currently, the rate is much lower because of our understanding of the mechanisms and prevention. A corneal abrasion can be very painful for the patient and, although very uncommon, can cause permanent loss of vision. The symptoms of corneal abrasion include pain, a foreign body sensation, loss of visual acuity, photophobia, and tearing. Because corneal reflexes are reduced or abolished during or after sedation and general anesthesia, eye injuries can occur. In addition, in the operating suite, a chemical injury is possible from prep solutions or from gastric secretions contaminating the surface of the eye. During general anesthesia, the eyes should be protected with tape, adhesive patches, padding, or a combination thereof as soon as is practical after the patient loses consciousness. In the case of prep solution contamination, the surface of the eye should be generously irrigated with preservative-free saline.

The diagnosis of corneal abrasion is made using fluorescein dye and a slit lamp. Treatment may consist of a local anesthetic solution, an antibiotic ointment, and patching for 24 hours. When a serious eye injury occurs, immediate ophthalmologic consultation should be obtained. Minor corneal abrasions may be examined by the anesthesiologist, who can make a decision on the need for referral. The majority of injuries heal spontaneously without intervention. Usually, with the proper perioperative measures, including protecting the patient from their own probing hands during emergence, corneal abrasions may be avoided.

Postoperative Hyponatremia

There are several risk factors for postoperative hyponatremia. These include preoperative hyponatremia, the use of low-sodium IV solutions, the absorption of low-sodium irrigation solutions, an excessive

---

CASE STUDY: A PATIENT HAS MASSETER SPASM WITH SUCCINYLCHOLINE AFTER INDUCTION OF ANESTHESIA

A 15-year-old male patient with severe reflux underwent an inguinal hernia repair under general anesthesia. After the induction, the patient had a mild masseter spasm and was subsequently intubated without problem.

CLINICAL NEED

The patient is recovered from anesthesia and is being observed for malignant hyperthermia (MH).

RESPONSE

MH is a rare autosomal-dominant trait that predisposes individuals exposed to triggering agents (i.e., succinylcholine and volatile anesthetics) to a hypermetabolic reaction affecting skeletal muscle, leading to hyperthermia and massive rhabdomyolysis. The incidence of MH reactions during anesthesia is estimated at from 1/15,000 in children to 1/50,000 in adults. One of the risk factors for the development of MH is masseter spasm. Early diagnosis is key, and dantrolene is the treatment.

Masseter spasm and the patient's age were risk factors for the development of MH in this case. This patient developed a mild masseter spasm during the procedure. The rest of the anesthetic and procedure were uneventful. The patient should be observed for 12 hours and monitored for the development of temperature elevation, increasing pulse rate, abnormality of acid and base status, myoglobinuria, or dark-colored urine. In the absence of these symptoms, the patient may be discharged after this period of observation. In the case of severe masseter spasm, the patient should not be discharged as an outpatient; he instead should be admitted to the hospital for observation.

increase in antidiuretic hormone (ADH) levels due to surgical stress, and female gender. It has also been seen with excessive oral intake of low-sodium liquids due to overzealous patient or caregiver recovery efforts. Patients may progress to develop symptoms including nausea, headaches, seizures, or other hyponatremic encephalopathy in extreme cases. Management includes following electrolyte levels and careful correction, as needed, with isotonic or hypertonic saline.

SUMMARY

The high quality of ambulatory anesthesia and surgical care has dramatically reduced morbidity and mortality. This chapter has identified the most frequent perioperative problems, including PONV and pain, which cause patients significant distress. Anesthesiologists have made great strides with perioperative prevention and management of these potential problems. This has resulted in more rapid recovery, sometimes bypassing the PACU altogether. Furthermore, the use of techniques such as continuous home regional analgesia will advance the perioperative treatment of pain. In the future, we must look closely at issues that include postoperative functional status, the impact of anesthesia and surgery on patients' quality of life, and satisfaction with the management of their care. We have clearly cut the perioperative cost of surgery by doing more procedures on an outpatient basis. We must aim for better recovery strategies and fewer complications so that patients may resume their daily activities sooner. In this way, we can avoid simply transferring management of perioperative complications into the home environment.

REFERENCES

1. Fortier J, Chung F, Su J: Unanticipated admission after ambulatory surgery: A prospective study. Can J Anaesth 45:612-619, 1998.

2. Twersky R, Fishman D, Homel P: What happens after discharge? Return hospital visits following ambulatory surgery Anesth Analg 84:319-324, 1997.

3. Mezei G, Chung F: Return hospital visits and hospital readmissions after ambulatory surgery. Ann Surg 250:721-727, 1999.

4. Natof HE: Complications associated with ambulatory surgery. JAMA 244:1116-1118, 1980.

5. Warner MA, Shields SE, Chute CG: Major morbidity and mortality within 1 month of ambulatory surgery and anesthesia. JAMA 270:1437-1441, 1993.

6. Fleisher LA, Pasternak LR, Herbert R: Inpatient hospital admission and death after outpatient surgery in elderly patients: Importance of patient and system characteristics and location of care. Arch Surg 139:67-72, 2004.

7. Badner NH, Knill RL, Brown JE: Myocardial infarction after noncardiac surgery. Anesthesiology 88:572-578, 1998.

8. Mangano DT, Layug EL, Wallace A: Effect of atenolol on mortality and cardiovascular morbidity after noncardiac surgery. Multicenter Study of Perioperative Ischemia Research Group. N Engl J Med 335:1713-1720, 1996.

9. Poldermans D, Boersma E, Bax JJ: The effect of bisoprolol on perioperative mortality and myocardial infarction in high-risk patients undergoing vascular surgery. N Engl J Med 341:1789-1794, 1999.

10. Rose DK, Cohen MM, Wigglesworth DF, DeBoer DP: Critical respiratory events in the postanesthesia care unit. Anesthesiology 81:410-418, 1994.

11. Litman RS Keon TP: Postintubation croup in childern. Anesthesiology 75(6):1122-1123, 1991.

12. Owens TM, Robertson P, Twomey C: The incidence of gastroesophageal reflux with the laryngeal mask: A comparison with the face mask using esophageal lumen pH electrodes. Anesth Analg 80:980-984, 1995.

13. Roux M, Drolet P, Girard M: Effect of the laryngeal mask airway on oesophageal pH: Influence of the volume and pressure inside the cuff. Br J Anaesth 82: 566-569, 1999.

14. Warner MA, Warner ME, Weber JG: Clinical significance of pulmonary aspiration during the perioperative period. Anesthesiology 78:56-62, 1993.

15. Gupta RM, Parvizi J, Hanssen AD: Postoperative complications in patients with obstructive sleep apnea syndrome undergoing hip or knee replacement: A case-control study. Mayo Clin Proc 76:897-905, 2001.

16. Canet J, Raeder J, Rasmussen LS: Cognitive dysfunction after minor surgery in the elderly. Acta Anaesthesiol Scand 47:1204-1210, 2003.

17. Johnson T, Monk T, Rasmussen LS, et al: Postoperative cognitive dysfunction in middle-aged patients. Anesthesiology 96:1351-1357, 2002.

18. Wu CL, Hsu W, Richman JM, Raja SN: Postoperative cognitive function as an outcome of regional anesthesia and analgesia. Reg Anesth Pain Med 29:257-268, 2004.

19. Gill PS, Guest C, Rabey PG, Buggy DJ: Perioperative headache and day case surgery. Eur J Anaesthesiol 20:401-403, 2003.

20. Nikolajsen L, Larsen KM, Kierkegaard O: Effects of previous frequency of headache, duration of fasting and caffeine abstinence on perioperative headache. Br J Anaesth 72:295-297, 1994.

21. Jin F, Norris A, Chung F, Ganeshram T: Should adult patients drink fluids before discharge from ambulatory surgery? Anesth Analg 87:306-311, 1998.

SUGGESTED READING

Brimacombe JR, Berry A: The incidence of aspiration associated with the laryngeal mask airway: A meta-analysis of published literature. J Clin Anesth 7:297–305, 1995.

Held PH, Yusuf S: Effects of beta-blockers and calcium channel blockers in acute myocardial infarction. Eur Heart J 14 (Suppl F):18–25, 1993.

Ho BY, Skinner HJ, Mahajan RP: Gastro-oesophageal reflux during day case gynaecological laparoscopy under positive pressure ventilation: Laryngeal mask vs. tracheal intubation. Anaesthesia 53:921–924, 1998.

Landesberg G: The pathophysiology of perioperative myocardial infarction: facts and perspectives. J Cardiothorac Vasc Anesth 17:90–100, 2003.

Moller JT, Cluitmans P, Rasmussen LS, et al: Long-term postoperative dysfunction in the elderly: ISPOCD 1 study. Lancet 351:857–861, 1998.

Skinner HJ, Ho BY, Mahajan RP: Gastro-oesophageal reflux with the laryngeal mask during day-case gynaecological laparoscopy. Br J Anaesth 80:675–676, 1998.

Van Zundert AA, Fonck K, Al-Shaikh B, Mortier E: Comparison of the LMA-classic with the new disposable soft seal laryngeal mask in spontaneously breathing adult patients. Anesthesiology 99:1066–1071, 2003.

Hospital-based anesthesiologists tend to focus primarily on initial patient recovery in the postanesthetic recovery unit (PACU). The ambulatory anesthesiologist, in contrast, must plan for, observe, and personally deal with recovery issues that include both initial and extended recovery from anesthesia. In fact, ambulatory anesthesiologists must consider concerns that extend beyond the time of facility discharge.

There are many aspects of outpatient care that are important to the efficient and economical management of an ambulatory surgery center (ASC) or office-based surgery practice. However, it has been asserted that the recovery phase determines more than 35% of total perioperative costs. Although the tendency has been to separate medical care costs from an episode of care into individual cost centers, the total cost of care must be the ultimate concern. Intraoperative techniques that prevent or treat pain and postoperative nausea and vomiting (PONV) may be relatively expensive. However, the cost of treating complications and side effects during the recovery phase may far exceed preventative expenses. When developing perioperative care strategies, it is important to remember that rapid and efficient recovery and discharge of satisfied patients and families should be a prime goal.

Recovery from ambulatory anesthesia and surgery has traditionally been thought of as taking place in three distinct stages. In the Phase 1 recovery process, patients return to consciousness and achieve stabilization of basic physiologic functions, including self-maintenance of a patent airway, and maintain acceptable and stable pulmonary and cardiovascular function. This typically occurs in a PACU room adjacent to the operating room suites. In the second stage of recovery, patients develop greater return of mental capacity and acquire the ability to take care of many of their own basic needs. This often occurs in a separate Phase 2 area that may be shared with the preoperative preparation area. In Phase 3 of recovery, patients return to their preoperative state and activity level, usually in their own homes (Box 9-1).

In the past, recovery from surgery and anesthesia was often determined by a minimum fixed time requirement. For example, it was usual to have a minimum PACU time

---

Box 9-1   Three Phases of Recovery

Phase 1 recovery: The patient undergoes return of basic physiologic functions.
Phase 2 recovery: The patient reacquires the abilities needed for activities of daily living and becomes capable of safely returning home.
Phase 3 recovery: The patient returns to baseline function and can resume normal activities.

of 30 minutes. Today, the modern principle is that recovery should be guided by patient-specific achievement of minimum criteria. This criteria-based recovery practice allows flexibility in advancing patients through all stages of recovery.

In addition, standardization of perioperative care can guide and improve the prophylaxis and treatment of common postoperative complications and side effects. Agreement about clinical care pathways by both physicians and nursing staff can improve the efficiency and safety of the ambulatory facility. The ambulatory surgery environment does not lend itself well to unnecessary variation in provider practices. An active quality-improvement program is essential to direct clinical practice for ambulatory facilities.

PHASE 1 RECOVERY

Monitoring

Immediately after emergence from anesthesia, patients are transported to the Phase 1 PACU. A typical Phase 1 recovery room is essentially a mini–intensive care unit (ICU) and usually has a patient-to-nurse ratio of 2:1. The capability for physiologic monitoring in a PACU is similar to that of the operating room. Upon arrival, patients immediately have oxygen saturation, respirations, pulse, blood pressure, and temperature recorded. The level of consciousness and extent of any block, if regional anesthetic was used, is determined. A recovery score is obtained initially and every 10 to 15 minutes subsequently. Continuous pulse oximetry monitoring is often maintained until discharge from the Phase 1 PACU. Any supplemental oxygen is weaned, as tolerated, to maintain an oxygen saturation of 92% or greater or, if patient baseline was lower than this, at preoperative levels. Unacceptable degrees of pain and nausea are identified and treated. Regional blocks for analgesia, such as femoral nerve blocks following anterior cruciate ligament (ACL) reconstruction, may be performed. Upon the attainment of satisfactory discharge criteria, the patient can be transferred to a Phase 2 recovery area.

PACU Aldrete Score

The evolution of modern-day discharge criteria for the Phase 1 PACU began in 1970 with Dr. Aldrete's[1] discharge criteria, also known as the postanesthesia recovery score or "Aldrete score." These discharge criteria, or a modification of them, are the most widely used criteria for discharge of patients from Phase 1 recovery rooms in both the inpatient and outpatient surgical settings. Oxygen saturation has replaced the antiquated use of skin color as a criterion. A score of 8 to 10 is considered adequate to discharge a patient safely from the PACU, with no score of zero allowed in any category (Table 9-1).

FAST TRACKING

Fast tracking is the process of bypassing the Phase 1 recovery room and transferring the patient to Phase 2 recovery directly from the operating room. This practice was common in the past for procedures performed with only local anesthesia or light sedation, but recently has been advocated after general anesthesia for selected patients and procedures. Apfelbaum et al.[2] showed that significant cost-savings, without compromising patient outcomes, could occur with fast tracking. Minimally invasive surgical techniques, multimodal analgesia, level-of-consciousness monitoring, and shorter-acting anesthetics have all contributed to fast tracking becoming an option for more patients. Fast tracking has even been reported to be possible with selected geriatric patients and school-age children.

There is some evidence that bypassing Phase 1 recovery can shorten time to discharge. This, however, requires nursing staff acceptance of patients coming directly from the operating room. Unfortunately, this may

Table 9-1	A Modified Postanesthesia PACU Aldrete Score

ACTIVITY	SCORE
Able to move four extremities voluntarily or on command	2
Able to move two extremities voluntarily or on command	1
Unable to move extremities voluntarily or on command	0
RESPIRATION	
Able to breathe deeply and cough freely	2
Dyspnea or limited breathing	1
Apnea	0
CIRCULATION	
BP ± 20% of preanesthetic level	2
BP ± 20–49% of preanesthetic level	1
BP ± 50% of preanesthetic level	0
CONSCIOUSNESS	
Fully awake	2
Arousable on calling	1
Not responding	0
O$_2$ SATURATION	
Able to maintain O$_2$ saturation >92% on room air	2
Needs O$_2$ inhalation to maintain O$_2$ saturation >90%	1
O$_2$ saturation <90% even with O$_2$ supplement	0
TOTAL SCORE	**10**

BP, Blood pressure.
From Aldrete, JA: The post-anesthesia score revisited. J Clin Anesth 7:89–91, 1995.

be a significant issue limiting the expansion of fast tracking in many facilities.

Physical space arrangements and flexibility-in-care plans can serve to facilitate fast tracking. If the Phase 1 and Phase 2 areas are located on a continuous floor plan rather than as separate rooms, it is more likely that nursing ratios can be flexible. In this situation, patients can float to the required level of care, and the geographic location is not the determinant for the level of care. Another modification is to admit the fast-tracked patients into the PACU and to discharge them home directly from the PACU. Using this scheme for significant numbers of patients has limited utility since the bed space available in a PACU is often considerably less than in a Phase 2 area.

Fast Tracking Criteria

A commonly used system for fast tracking is White's and Song's[3] scoring method. Except for the added criteria of pain and nausea/vomiting, this system is similar to the modified Aldrete PACU discharge approach. Because the fast-tracked patient enters an area in which the nurse-to-patient ratio is lower than that of the PACU, care is less intense; therefore, patients should be relatively awake and comfortable if fast-tracked (Table 9-2, Box 9-2).

Fast Tracking Impact

There are several advantages and potential drawbacks to fast tracking. Advantages include possible facilitation of a faster discharge home, eliminating unnecessary stays in the expensive PACU area, a more rapid return to a more comfortable surrounding, decreased monitoring requirements and paperwork, and overall reduced health care costs.

The ability of fast tracking to decrease costs is promoted as a reason to adopt this strategy. The recovery care for Phase 2 patients is less labor-intense than that of Phase 1 patients. The American Society of Postanesthesia Nurses (ASPAN) staffing guideline recommends a routine Phase 1 nurse-to-patient ratio of 1:2, and they seek a 1:3 ratio for Phase 2. If fast tracking is adopted consistently for a significant number of patients, PACU personnel costs may be decreased. Even if a smaller number of patients bypass the PACU, the recovery room could be closed earlier at the end of the clinical day if the last patients are fast-tracked.

Disadvantages to fast tracking include a possible loss of facility revenue from recovery room stay, an increased need for cross-training of nursing personnel, increased work for nursing staff in the Phase 2 recovery area, and, possibly, an increased risk of postoperative complications. No data exist to support an increased risk for complications with fast tracking, but, as with any change in

Table 9-2	White and Song's Scoring System: Criteria for Fast Tracking After Outpatient Anesthesia

A minimal score of 12 (with no score <1 in any individual category) is required for a patient to be fast tracked (i.e., to bypass the postanesthesia care unit) after general anesthesia.

LEVEL OF CONSCIOUSNESS	SCORE
Awake and oriented	2
Arousable with minimal stimulation	1
Responsive only to tactile stimulation	0

PHYSICAL ACTIVITY	
Able to move all extremities on command	2
Some weakness in movement of extremities	1
Unable to voluntarily move extremities	0

HEMODYNAMIC STABILITY	
Blood pressure <15% of baseline MAP value	2
Blood pressure 15–30% of baseline MAP value	1
Blood pressure >30% below baseline MAP value	0

RESPIRATORY STABILITY	
Able to breathe deeply	2
Tachypnea with good cough	1
Dyspneic with weak cough	0

OXYGEN SATURATION STATUS	
Maintains value >90% on room air	2
Requires supplemental oxygen (nasal prongs)	1
Saturation <90% with supplemental oxygen	0

POSTOPERATIVE PAIN ASSESSMENT	
No or mild discomfort	2
Moderate to severe pain controlled with IV analgesics	1
Persistent severe pain	0

POSTOPERATIVE EMETIC SYMPTOMS	
No or mild nausea with no active vomiting	2
Transient vomiting or retching	1
Persistent moderate to severe nausea and vomiting	0

TOTAL SCORE	14

MAP, Mean arterial pressure.
From White PF, Song D: New criteria for fast-tracking after outpatient anesthesia: A comparison with the modified Aldrete's scoring system. Anesth Analg 88:1069–1072, 1999.

Box 9-2	Simplified Fast Tracking Criteria

Patient meets discharge criteria from Phase 1 recovery.
Patient does not need immediate treatment for nausea, pain, or shivering.

clinical practice, advocates of this system in a facility may need to justify the recovery change and to support claims of safety by sharing quality data with all facility personnel.

PHASE 2 RECOVERY

Upon arrival to the second stage of recovery, patients should encounter surroundings designed to help them progress toward discharge. Accommodations are generally available for limited numbers of friends or family. Patients often are transitioned from a flat gurney into a reclining chair that can be adjusted, eventually, to a sitting position. Typically, clear liquids and limited amounts of carbohydrates are provided. If solids are offered, they should be free of fat and protein to allow easy digestion while the body deals with pain, residual anesthetic agents, and opioids. A restroom should be situated nearby for easy access. Pain and nausea are treated as needed. When the patient tolerates even minimal oral intake, oral, rather than intravenous, analgesic medications may be administered. Monitoring includes checking the patient's basic vital signs approximately every 30 to 60 minutes. At intervals, nursing staff should assess the patient's recovery by means of the facility's discharge scoring system, used in a fashion similar to the PACU discharge system.

Written and verbal information must be provided to the patient and family, and this should include advice on postoperative follow-up and instructions about what action to take if complications occur. A responsible person who will take the patient home and stay with him or her overnight should also be given the instructions for later care of the patient to reinforce the patient's memory. Written instructions are a practical, as well as a legal, necessity. After receiving sedative-hypnotic and amnesic medication, patients are not likely to retain many details of even simple verbal instructions. Preprinted instructions for various common anesthetic and surgical procedures should be developed to standardize and comprehensively address postdischarge care. Depending on the facility's patient population, foreign language versions may be necessary. The instructions should contain an area for additional written provider comments concerning specific issues for each patient.

Modified Postanesthesia Recovery Discharge Systems

Standard recovery scoring systems have been developed for facility discharge of ambulatory surgical patients. Examples of these include the Modified Postanesthesia Recovery Score for Ambulatory Patients developed by Aldrete[1] and the Modified Postanesthesia Discharge Scoring System (PADSS) developed by

Chung.[4] Patients are considered fit for discharge when they achieve at least a score of 18 out of 20 by the Aldrete system or 9 out of 10 by the PADSS.

Scoring systems for discharge from an outpatient facility have common themes of requiring appropriate and stable vital signs, return of adequate mental capability and ambulation, control of nausea and pain, and the presence of minimal bleeding at incision sites. However, facilities may want to modify the published scoring criteria to deemphasize drinking, eating, and urination for most patients (Tables 9-3, 9-4).

Oral Intake and Urination Recovery Requirements

As opposed to the earlier days of ambulatory anesthesia, modified scoring systems in present practice do not place as much emphasis on minimum predischarge oral intake or on waiting until urination occurs. Clinical experience and multiple studies have shown that, except in selected situations, requiring all patients to drink and urinate prolongs discharge time without decreasing the risk of postdischarge problems. Requiring patients to drink or eat may actually increase the risk of nausea and vomiting, thus further delaying discharge.

Although often considered a minor risk, urinary retention can have serious consequences. Care should be taken to ensure that patients do not develop urinary retention and that the urinary bladder does not become overdistended before or after discharge. If the adult bladder contains significantly more than 600 mL for more than 4 hours, short- or long-term derangements in bladder function may result. Excessive bladder wall stretch can lead to bladder wall ischemia and long-term urinary dysfunction.

CLINICAL CAVEAT: CHANGING DISCHARGE REQUIREMENTS

Recent information indicates that requiring all patients to drink fluids, eat food, and urinate before discharge unnecessarily prolongs recovery and may actually increase unwanted effects.

Although all patients should usually be asked to urinate before surgery, not all should be required to do so before discharge. Patients can be divided into those who are at low risk and those at high risk for postoperative bladder retention. Patients at high risk for retention include those who have had inguinal hernia, penile, rectal, urologic, or other pelvic surgery. Also at high risk are those patients with a history of urinary retention or those who had a preoperative urinary catheter, those requiring

Table 9-3 Modified Postanesthesia Recovery (PAR) Score for Ambulatory Patients	
ACTIVITY	**SCORE**
Able to move four extremities voluntarily or on command	2
Able to move two extremities voluntarily or on command	1
Unable to move extremities voluntarily or on command	0
RESPIRATION	
Able to breathe deeply and cough freely	2
Dyspnea, limited breathing, or tachypnea	1
Apneic or on mechanical ventilation	0
CIRCULATION	
BP ± 20% of preanesthetic level	2
BP ± 20–49% of preanesthetic level	1
BP ± 50% of preanesthetic level	0
CONSCIOUSNESS	
Fully awake	2
Arousable on calling	1
Not responding	0
O$_2$ SATURATION	
Able to maintain O$_2$ saturation >92% on room air	2
Needs O$_2$ inhalation to maintain O$_2$ saturation >90%	1
O$_2$ saturation <90% even with O$_2$ supplement	0
DRESSING	
Dry and clean	2
Wet but stationary or marked	1
Growing area of wetness	0
PAIN	
Pain-free	2
Mild pain handled by oral medication	1
Severe pain requiring parenteral medication	0
AMBULATION	
Able to stand up and walk straight*	2
Vertigo when erect	1
Dizziness when supine	0
FASTING OR FEEDING	
Able to drink fluids	2
Nauseated	1
Nausea and vomiting	0
URINE OUTPUT	
Has voided	2
Unable to void but comfortable	1
Unable to void and uncomfortable	0
TOTAL SCORE	**20**

BP, Blood pressure.
*May be substituted by Romberg's test or picking up 12 clips in one hand.
From Aldrete, JA: The post-anesthesia score revisited. J Clin Anesth 7:89–91, 1995.

Table 9-4 Modified Postanesthesia Discharge Scoring System (PADSS)	
VITAL SIGNS	**SCORE**
Vital signs stable and consistent with age and preoperative values.	
BP and pulse within 20% of preoperative value	2
BP and pulse within 20–40% of preoperative value	1
BP and pulse >40% of preoperative value	0
ACTIVITY LEVEL	
Patient must be able to ambulate at preoperative level.	
Steady gait, no dizziness	2
Requires assistance	1
Unable to ambulate	0
NAUSEA AND VOMITING	
Minimal, successfully treated with oral medication	2
Moderate, successfully treated with intramuscular medication	1
Severe, continues after repeated treatment	0
SURGICAL BLEEDING	
Postoperative bleeding consistent with expected blood loss.	
Minimal	2
Moderate	1
Severe	0
PAIN ACCEPTABILITY	
The level of pain should be acceptable to the patient.	
Yes	2
No	0
TOTAL SCORE	**10**
Patients with a score of 9 are considered fit for discharge home.	

BP, Blood pressure.
Modified from Marshall S, Chung F: Assessment of home readiness: Discharge criteria and postdischarge complications. Curr Opin Anaesthesiology 10:445–450, 1997.

raxial anesthesia may have a distended bladder, making initiation of micturition difficult for some patients. Patients at low risk for urinary retention can be discharged without urination. Those at high risk must urinate before discharge. If high-risk patients cannot urinate but are otherwise ready for discharge, the patient's bladder may be catheterized. Alternatively, small, portable ultrasound devices are increasingly being used in ambulatory facilities. These can accurately determine bladder volume, assisting in therapy decisions. All patients should be instructed to call or to return to medical care if they are unable to urinate within 6 to 8 hours after discharge or if they have a painfully distended bladder.

Postoperative Escort and Recovery Attendant

An almost universal requirement for discharge from ambulatory surgical facilities is that a responsible person should accompany the patient to the location where the

large amounts of opioids, patients with any neurologic disease affecting the micturition reflex, or those who have received spinal or epidural anesthesia with long-acting local anesthetic agents. Patients who have received large amounts of intravenous fluids under general or neu-

patient plans to stay for the first postoperative night. The ASA Ambulatory Anesthesia guidelines specifically state: "Patients who receive other than unsupplemented local anesthesia must be discharged with a responsible adult." However, the definitions of "responsible" and "adult" vary among centers, and there is usually no way, other than the patient's own promise, to assure that the patient actually has an escort after leaving the facility.

Most facilities have a policy that a patient who has received sedative-hypnotics or opioids (for an opioid-naïve patient) should not operate a motor vehicle or bicycle after leaving the surgery facility. In addition to the residual effects of medications, the effect of pain or limitations from the surgical procedure may make vehicle operation difficult. An escorted patient may travel home after surgery on public transportation after minor procedures, but patients should not, as a rule, leave the surgical facility alone.

Another common surgical facility requirement is that postoperative patients should have a capable, responsible attendant stay with them overnight. A "responsible attendant" can be defined as a person who has the physical and mental ability to assist the patient and to summon help should the patient be unable to do so. The minimum age of this attendant could range from 16 to 18 years, depending on facility policy. If the presence of this person is required by facility policy and is actually not available, surgery should be cancelled or arrangements made to admit the patient for observation to a suitable overnight health care facility.

Clearly, there is no way to confirm that an attendant will actually remain with the patient once the patient arrives at home. Patients who have no method of summoning emergency services (e.g., land phone line or cell phone) should not usually be allowed to recover at home. A difficult situation arises postoperatively when the patient or escort actually informs caregivers that there will not be a previously promised overnight attendant. It may be more difficult for some facilities to arrange admission to another health care facility at a late hour. Another problem is the postoperative patient who has promised to provide a discharge escort but then insists on leaving without one. Some states may place a legal obligation on caregivers to inform local authorities if it is suspected that the patient intends to operate a motor vehicle after receiving sedatives or anesthetics. Even if there is no legal obligation, many maintain that there is an ethical obligation to protect the public.

Each facility should develop policies and procedures to address these escort and attendant issues. Policies should be written to anticipate difficult management situations. It should be remembered that a strictly set policy must actually be enforced. All patients and surgeons should understand the facility's policies before arriving for the procedure.

> ### CLINICAL CONTROVERSY: ESCORT AND ATTENDANT POLICIES
>
> If patients do not have an escort from the facility or have an attendant to assist them at home, what policies do the ambulatory facility have in place and how strict are they? Does the facility policy allow providers to make exceptions, and is this safe for patient care?

The Ambulatory Anesthesia guidelines (2003) from the American Society of Anesthesiologists (ASA) state, "A licensed physician should be in attendance in the facility or, in the case of overnight care, immediately available by telephone, at all times during patient treatment and recovery and until the patients are medically discharged." Also written is, "Qualified personnel and equipment should be on hand to manage emergencies. There should be established policies and procedures to respond to emergencies and unanticipated patient transfer to an acute care facility." The guidelines further stipulate, "Discharge of the patient is a physician responsibility."

Factors Affecting Discharge Time

In 1998, Pavlin et al.[5] studied factors affecting discharge time in adult outpatients. Anesthetic technique was the most important determinant of discharge time. The second most important factor was the Phase 2 nurse. Some nurses were, and some were not, quite skilled at facilitating discharge. Systems factors were the primary cause of Phase 2 delays (41%). The most common cause (53%) of systems-related delay in discharge from Phase 2 recovery was awaiting a responsible person to arrive and take the patient home.

Other causes of medical discharge delay include true side effects or complications of anesthesia and surgery. Pain, sedation, and nausea and vomiting were the three most common medical causes of delays. Other medical or surgical factors, such as unsteady gait, dizziness, bleeding, or cardiopulmonary problems, may all increase the time in the ASC or office and, ultimately, cause unanticipated transfer to an acute care facility.

Regional Anesthesia and Analgesia

The use of regional anesthesia for outpatient surgery deserves special emphasis in discussions about recovery. Patients who have peripheral or plexus nerve blocks for appropriate surgery are more comfortable and have less PONV, sedation, and bladder dysfunction than matched patients having general anesthesia. As a result, patients with nonneuraxial blocks can bypass the PACU and may be discharged home faster. When long-lasting local anesthetics are used, patients remain more comfortable and have fewer opioid-related side effects for extended periods. In fact, the growing use of continuous peripheral nerve or plexus catheter techniques may extend comfort several days out from surgery and reduce home recovery adverse opioid side effects. Of course, patients must be made aware of any special care necessary to prevent accidental injury to an insensate limb. An anesthesiologist should be on call to respond to analgesic-infusion-related questions or problems.

Epidural and subarachnoid blocks may be performed for outpatient surgery. Before patients are allowed to ambulate, motor and sensory block must have regressed to where there is normal perianal (i.e., S4 through S5) sensation, plantar flexion of the foot, and proprioception of the great toe. The use of long-acting neuraxial local anesthetics has been associated with delayed recovery, slow ambulation, and higher incidences of urinary retention. These patients should urinate before discharge. Mulroy et al.[6] have shown that patients who have neuraxial anesthetics with short-duration local anesthetics without epinephrine may be discharged without requiring urination. These patients should be instructed to return only if they cannot urinate after approximately 4 to 6 hours. Delayed urination has not been associated with local anesthetics used for pediatric caudal analgesia.

SPECIFIC SITUATIONS

Premature Infants

Infants who have a history of premature birth (i.e., gestational age less than 37 weeks) must be monitored postoperatively for longer periods before discharge home. Although there may be no postconceptual age at which a premature infant is totally without risk for postoperative apnea, experts have recommended infants at postconceptual age 60 weeks as being at lower risk. If the infant is younger than this, depending on the nature of the anesthesia and surgery, up to 12 hours of apnea-free recovery may be required before discharge home. If post-premature infants have hemoglobin levels of less than 10 gm/dL, a continuing history of apnea, or significant health issues such as bronchopulmonary dysplasia, admission may be advised even if they are of more than 60 weeks postconceptual age.

Malignant Hyperthermia History

Patients with a personal or family history of possible malignant hyperthermia may have ambulatory surgery and anesthesia performed safely. Local anesthesia, regional blocks, or nontriggering general anesthesia are acceptable options. These patients can be discharged after uneventful recovery following these types of anesthesia. Depending on the history and the type of surgery and anesthesia, 3 to 6 hours of observation may be appropriate. Specific discharge instructions and patient follow-up should be considered.

Obstructive Sleep Apnea

Patients with obstructive sleep apnea (OSA) are often dilemmas for recovery plans. The decision to discharge these patients depends on factors such as the severity of OSA, the extent of the surgical procedure, the predicted need for postoperative opioid analgesics, the presence of coexisting obesity and other medical conditions, and the ability to use continuous positive airway pressure (CPAP) devices at home. In most instances, OSA patients having airway surgery should be admitted because of airway risk after surgery and the common contraindication to the use of CPAP devices after airway surgery. If patients are chronically using CPAP at home, they must agree to diligently use the device at home. OSA patients with severe OSA, with a body mass index (BMI) greater than 40, or requiring large amounts of opioids should be admitted for observation. Patients with mild OSA, with a BMI between 30 and 40, and requiring only a modest amount of opioid analgesia are in a medical gray area: judgment may be used to determine appropriateness for discharge home. Preoperative assessment and risk stratification is essential to avoid patient and provider aggravation and delays or cancellations on the day of the procedure. The ASA has released practice guidelines for the perioperative management of patients with OSA.[7]

PHASE 3 RECOVERY

The third stage of recovery takes a variable length of time, depending on a multitude of factors including surgery, anesthetic technique, and the age and condition of the patient. Outpatient surgery implies that the patient adequately recovers and travels home to begin resuming normal activities. This may be true for relatively minor procedures and for relatively young and healthy patients. However, for many patients, especially those who have had extensive procedures, the full recovery period can take weeks. Studies have reported extended periods of recovery and loss of work time after outpatient surgery.

Patients are routinely advised not to drive or make any important decisions for at least 12 to 24 hours after having received general anesthesia or sedative-hypnotics. If patients are taking opioids for postoperative pain control, they are advised not to drive or operate dangerous machinery while under the influence of these medications.

Some centers and offices utilize extended recovery care, either on-site or at freestanding recovery centers. Suitable trained personnel and adequate resources should be available at these locations to care for postoperative patients. More outpatient centers are also arranging home health care assistance, especially when extensive procedures are performed. Anesthesiologists should assure themselves that patients are discharged to a safe environment.

The home stage of recovery may be associated with significant risks and burdens on patients and families. The postoperative period can be a stressful time for both patients and caregivers. It has been said that, in some ways, the cost savings of outpatient surgery have taken place at the cost of the time and effort of the people who care for the patient at home. Increased attention and research is needed to reduce risk and to make this final recovery stage easier for patients and caregivers.

CLINICAL CONTROVERSY: PHASE 3 RECOVERY

Ambulatory surgical providers and facilities have a responsibility to consider the burden placed on patients and families when the ambulatory pathway is selected. What resources should the ambulatory surgery center provide to assist with Phase 3 recovery?

REFERENCES

1. Aldrete JA: The post-anesthesia score revisited. J Clin Anesth 7:89–91, 1995.

2. Apfelbaum JL, Walawander CA, Grasela TH: Eliminating intensive postoperative care in same-day surgery patients using short-acting anesthetics. Anesthesiology 97(1): 66–74, 2002.

3. White PF, Song D: New criteria for fast-tracking after outpatient anesthesia: A comparison with the modified Aldrete's scoring system. Anesth Analg 88:1069–1072, 1999.

4. Chung F: Discharge criteria: A new trend. Can J Anaesth 42:1056–1058, 1995.

5. Pavlin DJ, Rapp SE, Polissar NL, et al: Factors affecting discharge time in adult outpatients. Anesth Analg 87: 816–826, 1998.

6. Mulroy MF, Salinas FV, Larkin KL, et al: Ambulatory surgery patients may be discharged before voiding after short-acting spinal and epidural anesthesia. Anesthesiology 97: 315–319, 2002.

7. American Society of Anesthesiologists: Practice Guidelines for Perioperative Management of Patients with Obstructive Sleep Apnea. 2005. Available at http://www.asahq.org/publicationsAndServices/sleepapnea103105.pdf

SUGGESTED READING

Benumof JL: Obstructive sleep apnea in the adult obese patient: Implications for airway management. J Clin Anesth 13:144–156, 2001.

Chung F, Mezei G: Factors contributing to a prolonged stay after ambulatory surgery. Anesth Analg 89:1352–1359, 1999.

Chung F: Recovery pattern and home-readiness after ambulatory surgery. Anesth Analg 80:896–902, 1995.

Cote CJ, Zaslavsky A, Downes JJ, et al: Postoperative apnea in former preterm infants after inguinal herniorrhaphy. A combined analysis. Anesthesiology 82:809–822, 1995.

Fengling J, Norris A, Chung F, Ganeshram T: Should adult patients drink fluids before discharge from ambulatory surgery? Anesth Analg 87:306–311, 1998.

Fortier J, Chung F, Su J: Unanticipated admission of ambulatory surgical patients. Can J Anaesth 45:612–619, 1998.

Hogue SL, Reese PR, Colopy M, et al: Assessing a tool to measure patient functional ability after outpatient surgery. Anesth Analg 91:97–106, 2000.

Keita H, Diouf E, Tubach F, et al: Predictive factors of early postoperative urinary retention in the postanesthesia care unit. Anesth Analg 101:592–596, 2005.

Marshall SI, Chung F: Discharge criteria and complications after ambulatory surgery. Anesth Analg 88:508–517, 1999.

Mattila K, Toivonen J, Janhunen L, et al: Postdischarge symptoms after ambulatory surgery: First-week incidence, intensity, and risk factors. Anesth Analg 101:1643–1650, 2005.

Pavlin DJ, Pavlin EG, Fitzgibbon DR, et al: Management of bladder function after outpatient surgery. Anesthesiology 91:42–50, 1999.

Pavlin DJ, Rapp SE, Polissar NL, et al: Factors affecting discharge time in adult outpatients. Anesth Analg 87: 816–826, 1998.

Shirakami G, Teratani Y, Namba T, et al: Delayed discharge and acceptability of ambulatory surgery in adult outpatients receiving general anesthesia. J Anesth 19:93–101, 2005.

Silverstein JH, Apfelbaum JL, Barlow JC, et al: Task force on postanesthetic care: practice guidelines for postanesthetic care. Anesthesiology 96:742–752, 2002.

Twersky R, Fishman D, Homel P: What happens after discharge? Return hospital visits following ambulatory surgery. Anesth Analg 84:319–324, 1997.

Twersky RS, Abiona M, Thorne AC, et al: Admissions following ambulatory surgery: Outcomes in seven urban hospitals. Ambulatory Surgery 3:141–146, 1995.

Wu CL, Berenholtz SM, Pronovost PJ, Fleisher LA: Systematic review and analysis of postdischarge symptoms after outpatient surgery. Anesthesiology. 96:994–1003, 2002.

APPENDIX: SUMMARY OF THE AMERICAN SOCIETY OF ANESTHESIOLOGISTS' PRACTICE GUIDELINES FOR POSTANESTHETIC CARE

Full document accessible at http://www.asahq.org/publicationsAndServices/postanes.pdf. Reprinted from Silverstein JH, Apfelbaum JL, Barlow JC, et al: Task force on postanesthetic care: practice guidelines for postanesthetic care. Anesthesiology 2002; 96:742-752.

General Principles

1. Medical supervision of recovery and discharge is the responsibility of the supervising practitioner.
2. The recovery area should be equipped with appropriate monitoring and resuscitation equipment.
3. Patients should be monitored until appropriate discharge criteria are satisfied.
4. Level of consciousness, vital signs, and oxygenation (when indicated) should be recorded at regular intervals.
5. A nurse or other individual trained to monitor patients and recognize complications should be in attendance until discharge criteria are fulfilled.
6. An individual capable of managing complications should be immediately available until discharge criteria are fulfilled.

Summary of Recommendations for Discharge

Requiring that Patients Pass Urine Prior to Discharge

The requirement for passing urine prior to discharge should not be part of a discharge protocol. The requirement for passing urine prior to discharge may only be necessary for selected patients.

Requiring that Patients Drink Clear Fluids Without Vomiting Prior to Discharge

The requirement of drinking clear fluids should not be part of a discharge protocol. The requirement of drinking clear fluids may only be necessary for selected patients.

Requiring that Patients Have a Responsible Individual Accompany Them Home

As part of a discharge protocol, patients should routinely be required to have a responsible individual accompany them home.

Requiring a Minimum Mandatory Stay in Recovery

Patients should be observed until they are no longer at increased risk for cardiorespiratory depression. A mandatory minimum stay should not be required. Discharge criteria should be designed to minimize the risk of central nervous system and cardiorespiratory depression following discharge.

Guidelines for Discharge

1. Patients should be alert and oriented. Patients whose mental status was initially abnormal should have returned to their baseline.
2. Vital signs should be stable and within acceptable limits.
3. Discharge should take place after patients have met specified criteria. Use of scoring systems may assist in documentation of fitness for discharge.
4. Outpatients should be discharged to a responsible adult who will accompany them home and be able to report any postprocedure complications.
5. Outpatients should be provided with written instructions regarding postprocedure diet, medications, activities, and a phone number to be called in case of emergency.

CHAPTER 1

Pediatric Ambulatory Anesthesia

JOAN BENCA

PEDIATRIC PATIENT SELECTION

Healthy infants and children are well-suited to ambulatory surgery. Advantages include less separation from parents, fewer disruptions in daily routines, less expensive care, and, possibly, a lower risk of infection. The main disadvantages of ambulatory surgery include less preoperative time to assess children, the unsuitability of some children or families to an outpatient experience, and the logistical difficulty of managing complications.

Patient selection is an important consideration when scheduling a child for an ambulatory surgical procedure. A freestanding ambulatory surgery center (ASC) will have more stringent patient selection criteria than an ambulatory facility that is located within a full-service hospital. There are also nonmedical considerations, including the distance the patient lives from the ambulatory surgery facility and an emergency room, the ability of the family to take care of the child after surgery, and the number of preoperative visits required to complete appropriate preoperative consultations and laboratory tests. All of these factors need to be considered when selecting patients for ambulatory surgery because, for a few families, an inpatient evaluation and surgery may actually be less financially and emotionally costly, as well as being safer for the child, than an ambulatory procedure.

Medical criteria for selecting which patients and which procedures are appropriate for ambulatory surgery vary from facility to facility. Currently, there are no evidence-based guidelines for pediatric selection. A minimum age for patients having ambulatory surgery has not been established. At 1 month of age, even healthy term infants might require postoperative observation. It is probably reasonable to schedule healthy term infants who have made the transition from an uneventful early neonatal period (i.e., ductus arteriosus has closed, pulmonary vascular resistance has decreased, and physiological jaundice has resolved) for ambulatory procedures that are short in duration, have minimal blood loss, and have only minor physiologic changes. The minimum age for ambulatory surgery and anesthesia should be made on a case-by-case basis in consultation with the anesthesiologist, surgeon, and pediatrician. A postconceptual age of 42 weeks is the youngest age reported in reviews of pediatric ambulatory anesthesia in which infants have been cared for as outpatients. Because of ready access to inpatient facilities, a hospital-based ambulatory surgery center may consider 42 to 44 weeks postconceptual age for a healthy term infant as a reasonable age limit.

CLINICAL CONTROVERSY

What is the lower limit of age that is acceptable for ambulatory surgery in term infants? There is little data to make recommendations.

Former premature infants must be evaluated carefully. Apnea after an anesthetic has been reported as late as 60 weeks postconceptual age. Also, infants who were born prematurely may have other residual problems, such as anemia, bronchopulmonary dysplasia, or gastroesophageal reflux, that make them poor candidates for ambulatory surgery at a freestanding facility. It is reasonable to schedule all infants as early-morning cases in the ambulatory surgery setting so that there can be a longer observation period after surgery and anesthesia.

Studies in former preterm infants after anesthesia report varying incidences of central apnea, and some include brief self-correcting apneic episodes that seem to have little clinical significance. It is difficult to compare the studies because the study groups are not homogeneous. Some series include children with other significant medical problems undergoing major invasive procedures. It is clear from the data that former premature infants are at risk for apneic episodes in the postoperative period. Infants with residual lung disease and a history of apnea are in the highest risk group. Former premature infants younger than 46 weeks postconceptual age are at greatest risk for postoperative apnea. The most conservative recommendation for postoperative admission monitoring is 60 weeks, from the study by Kurth et al.[1] The recommendation from Liu et al[2] and Welborn et al[3] is 44 to 46 weeks.

A general guideline regarding the age at which former premature infants without significant residual lung disease may have ambulatory anesthesia varies among centers from 50 to 60 weeks postconceptual age. Any former premature infant with symptomatic bronchopulmonary dysplasia appears to be at higher risk for postanesthetic apnea. Some states have legislated a minimum age at which an infant may have general anesthesia at a freestanding surgery center, and this may be as high as 6 months of age. The duration of monitoring after an anesthetic is also controversial. Monitoring for 12 hours after anesthesia is one minimum recommended observation period.

CLINICAL CAVEAT

Former premature infants who are also anemic (i.e., hematocrit less than 30 gm/dL) are at significantly increased risk for postoperative apnea, as are those former premature infants who have bronchopulmonary dysplasia or a history of previous central apnea.

CLINICAL CONTROVERSY

At what postconceptual age can a former premature infant be safely anesthetized in the ambulatory setting? Various authors report postgestational ages ranging from 44 to 60 weeks.

Other general categories of patient problems that a freestanding pediatric ambulatory surgery center must consider are latex-allergic patients, patients with Down syndrome or other craniofacial syndromes, juvenile-onset diabetic patients, patients who have uncorrected or surgically corrected congenital heart disease, and pediatric patients who have had solid-organ or bone marrow transplants. Patients in each of these categories may or may not be appropriate for the ambulatory setting depending on patient history, staffing level at the ambulatory surgery facility, and availability of laboratory testing.

Children with uncorrected or corrected congenital heart disease may be candidates for ambulatory surgery. The patient must be stable and have had a preoperative evaluation by a cardiologist. A child with a small atrial septal defect (ASD) or ventricular septal defect (VSD) may be a candidate for ambulatory surgery. Children who have had complete repair of more complex congenital heart disease may or may not be candidates depending on their risk for arrhythmias or congestive heart failure and the presence of significant residual shunting or pulmonary hypertension. A child with stable heart disease needing ear tube insertion may be acceptable. A complete discussion of all types of congenital heart disease and anesthesia is outside the scope of this chapter. More information is available in standard texts and at the following useful Web site: http://www.med.yale.edu/intmed/cardio/chd/.

Children with a personal or family history of malignant hyperthermia may have ambulatory procedures under anesthesia. A 10-year review of malignant-hyperthermia-susceptible children found no incidents of malignant hyperthermia using a nontriggering anesthetic technique. Both MHAUS (Malignant Hyperthermia Association of the United States) and SAMBA (Society for Ambulatory Anesthesia) consider malignant-hyperthermia-susceptible patients to be candidates for nontriggering anesthetics as outpatients. MHAUS recommends an observation period of 3 to 5 hours after an uneventful anesthetic and that families should be provided with an emergency contact in case problems arise after leaving the surgery center. The latest information is available from MHAUS and at their Web site, http://www.mhaus.org.

PREOPERATIVE EVALUATION

In general, only American Society of Anesthesiologists (ASA) physical status (PS) I and II children are routine candidates for ambulatory surgery, especially at freestanding centers. However, an ASA PS III child who has well-compensated, stable disease may be a candidate for a minor outpatient procedure. Adequate medical records from the primary care physician and prior consultation with the anesthesiologist are mandatory to plan a safe surgical experience.

A history of significant central or obstructive sleep apnea ordinarily limits a patient to a hospital-based ambulatory surgery center because the need for overnight monitoring is not predictable with currently available tests. Preoperative sleep studies may be useful as a predictor of postoperative apnea, but it is not clear if these should always be recommended for children. It is also not clear which children with a history of sleep apnea need a preoperative electrocardiogram (ECG) or echocardiogram to rule out pulmonary hypertension. Likewise, suspected difficult airway access or a history of difficult airway access might be a contraindication to care at a freestanding ambulatory surgery center, depending on facility resources and personnel experience.

Children with asthma require careful preoperative evaluation. A history of hospitalization for asthma, recent oral steroid use to control asthma symptoms, recent exacerbation of asthma symptoms, or abnormal room-air oxyhemoglobin saturation would make care at a freestanding ambulatory surgery center much less advisable. All children with asthma should continue their medications on the day of surgery. A thorough assessment of the patient, including chest auscultation, is mandatory on the day of surgery, and peak flows may be checked against baseline values.

Obesity is increasingly a problem in children. Morbidly obese children should not be scheduled at a freestanding surgery center without prior evaluation and approval by an anesthesiologist. Medical problems associated with obesity in children include obstructive sleep apnea, gastroesophageal reflux, hypertension, pulmonary hypertension, dyslipidemia, insulin resistance, and obesity-hypoventilation syndrome.

Children with seizure disorders are often not candidates for ambulatory surgery unless the seizures are well-controlled. Children with neurological problems, mucopolysaccharidosis, sickle cell disease, myopathy, severe cerebral palsy, or metabolic disorders are probably not good candidates for most freestanding and office-based ambulatory surgery facilities (Box 10-1).

Preoperative Assessment

Some centers utilize preoperative screening clinics, telephone consultations, or direct visits with an anesthesiologist for preoperative evaluation. Obtaining a history and physical exam (H&P) from the child's primary doctor or the surgical team is usually standard practice, although, in a few centers, the anesthesiologist may perform the H&P. It is preferable to have all preoperative evaluations completed prior to the patient's arrival on the day of surgery in order to minimize waiting times, patient and parental anxiety, and operative delays. Children with stable chronic diseases, heart murmur, or congenital heart disease usually need updated consulta-

Box 10-1   General Contraindications to Ambulatory Surgery at a Freestanding Facility

ASA III or IV patients with poorly controlled systemic disease (e.g., brittle insulin-dependent diabetics, symptomatic asthmatics, patients with uncorrected or partially corrected congenital heart disease with oxygen requirements or requiring multiple medications, and children with myopathy or debilitating neurologic disease)

Morbidly obese children with respiratory or cardiac problems

Former premature infants less than 60 weeks postconceptual age

Children with an unstable or inappropriate home environment that is unable to meet the needs of the child after surgery

Children with a known difficult airway

Children under age 2 to 3 years for tonsillectomy and adenoidectomy, children with severe obstructive sleep apnea, and children with Down syndrome undergoing tonsillectomy

tions with a subspecialty physician prior to the day of surgery. It is not efficient to obtain these consultations on the day of surgery.

Children who have an upper respiratory infection (URI) should be carefully evaluated on the day of surgery. Signs of lower respiratory infection (LRI), including fever, abnormal chest examination by auscultation, productive cough, and abnormal room-air oxygen saturation, are reasons to delay elective anesthesia. Children with mild upper respiratory infections are usually reasonable candidates for low-intensity surgery. Children with current and recent URIs are at slightly increased risk for respiratory complications, including breath-holding, laryngospasm, bronchospasm, severe cough, oxyhemoglobin desaturation, and postintubation croup, but can have elective surgery without significant increase in adverse outcomes. Every child with a URI should be evaluated on an individual basis and the parents should be informed of the risks. Children who require otolaryngology procedures often have frequent URIs. It can be difficult to schedule these children when they are completely free of signs and symptoms of mild respiratory illness (Table 10-1, Fig. 10-1).

It is of importance that children who live in households with exposure to cigarette smoke are also at increased risk for perioperative laryngospasm, wheezing, bronchospasm, stridor, breath-holding, coughing, and oxyhemoglobin desaturation. A recent URI may additionally increase the risk of these complications for these patients.

Table 10-1   Signs and Symptoms of Respiratory Tract Infection in Children with URI or LRI

	Mild URI	Severe URI	LRI	Allergic Rhinitis
History	No fever	Malaise, Fever	Severe cough	Atopy
			Sputum production	Seasonal history
	Minimal cough	Purulent coryza	± Fever	Sneezing
	Clear runny nose	Sneezing		
	Sneezing	Cough		
General exam	Nontoxic clear runny nose	Toxic-appearing	± Toxic	Allergic shiners
			± Fever	
			± Irritable	
Pulmonary exam	Clear lungs	± Clear lungs	Rales	Normal
	± Upper airway congestion	Upper airway congestion	Rhonchi	
			Abnormal SpO_2	
	Normal SpO_2	± Abnormal SpO_2		

LRI, Lower respiratory infection; URI, upper respiratory infection; ±, may be present or absent.
Adapted from Easley RB, Maxwell LG: Evidenced-Based Practice of Anesthesiology. Philadelphia, WB Saunders, 2004.

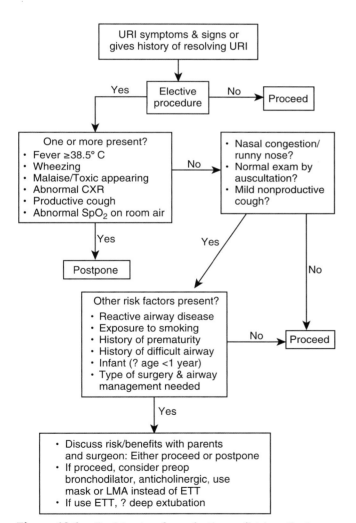

Figure 10-1 Decision tree for evaluating pediatric patients with preoperative respiratory symptoms.

A decreased incidence of respiratory tract complications has been reported with the use of a laryngeal mask airway, as opposed to an endotracheal tube, in children with recent URIs or in those who are exposed to cigarette smoke.

CLINICAL CAVEAT

Children with current and recent upper respiratory infection are at increased risk for respiratory complications including breath holding, laryngospasm, bronchospasm, severe cough, oxyhemoglobin desaturation, and postintubation croup, but some may have minor elective surgery.

CLINICAL CAVEAT

Children who live in households with smokers are at increased risk for respiratory complications.

CLINICAL CAVEAT

In children with a URI, there are fewer respiratory tract complications when a laryngeal mask airway is used instead of an endotracheal tube.

Murmurs in children are common and can be a diagnostic dilemma. However, it is reassuring if the child has no worrisome cardiac symptoms or signs and is growing normally and the murmur has typical innocent characteristics. Innocent heart murmurs have characteristics of being early- to midsystolic, softer than grade III/VI, low- to medium-pitch, musical, and not harsh in quality. Pathological-sounding murmurs should be evaluated prior to surgery by a cardiologist. Many anesthesiologists will proceed without cardiology evaluation if a child with an innocent-sounding murmur has a good activity history, has a normal oxyhemoglobin saturation on room air, does not have finger clubbing, has no history or other physical findings consistent with congenital or acquired heart disease, and has a normal ECG.

If there is any doubt, an ECG, chest x-ray (CXR), echocardiogram, and cardiology consultation should be obtained. Auscultatory findings alone may have low specificity, especially in infants. Therefore, all infants with murmurs, all children with signs or symptoms of cardiac disease, and those with murmurs that have pathological features should be referred for evaluation before elective surgery. If the murmur appears benign and the decision is made to proceed without a consultation or an echocardiogram, meticulous removal of air from intervenous (IV) lines and administration of bacterial endocarditis prophylaxis (according to American Heart Association [AHA] current guidelines) are in order. It may be prudent to obtain a cardiology evaluation after surgery (Table 10-2, Fig. 10-2).

Children with Down syndrome need careful preoperative evaluation for possible heart disease, atlantoaxial instability, a potential difficult airway or small trachea, and obstructive sleep apnea. There is a 10% to 20% incidence of atlantoaxial instability in these patients. Flexion of the neck is more hazardous than slight extension. Obtaining routine preoperative cervical spine films is controversial because it is not predictive of outcome in the absence of signs or symptoms of spinal cord compression. Many centers no longer routinely obtain cervical spine radiographs. Normal cervical spine films in flexion and extension do not guarantee the absence of

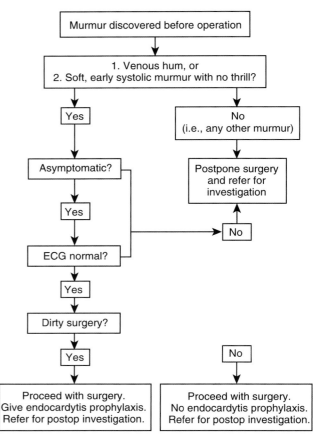

Figure 10-2　Decision tree for management of a preoperative murmur in children. (Adapted from McEwan AI, Birch M, Bingham R: The preoperative management of the child with a heart murmur. Paediatr Anaesth 5:151–156, 1995.)

atlantoaxial instability. Physical examination demonstrating gait disturbance, hyperreflexia, or new incontinence is concerning. It is reasonable to avoid extremes of cervical positioning in all children with Down syndrome, regardless of whether or not the patient has had cervical spine films.

Table 10-2	Characteristics of Pediatric Cardiac Murmurs

Innocent	Pathological
• Asymptomatic	• Symptomatic
• Lack of cardiac hypertrophy	• Associated with cardiac hypertrophy
• Soft	
• Early systolic only	• Holosystolic or late systolic
• Lack of thrill	
• Absent with position changes	• Diastolic
• Venous hum characteristics: best heard just above the right clavicle and sound radiates into neck	• Presence of thrill
• Continuous murmur characteristic: hum can be obliterated by brief digital pressure on the ipsilateral internal jugular vein or if child turns head	

CLINICAL CONTROVERSY

Should all children with Down syndrome undergo preoperative flexion and extension neck films, or are positioning precautions sufficient?

Preoperative Laboratory Tests

Routine laboratory tests are no longer required by most ambulatory surgery centers for preoperative preparation of most children. There are no evidence-based guidelines for acceptable preoperative hematocrit levels in children. Most centers routinely check a hematocrit for former premature infants under the age of 6 months, for children with hemoglobinopathies, for children with particular chronic diseases, and for patients undergoing procedures that might incur significant blood loss. Premature infants less than 6 months of age scheduled for elective surgery should be referred to their primary care doctor if the preoperative hemoglobin is less than 10 gm/dL. Routine coagulation screening is not necessary unless a child has a history of excessive bleeding, easy bruising, or a family history of bleeding disorder.

Preoperative pregnancy testing for girls after the age of menarche is not routine at all centers and is controversial. The opportunity for a confidential interview with adolescents is not always readily available prior to ambulatory surgery. The incidence of positive preoperative pregnancy tests in adolescents is reported to be as high as 0.5% to 1.2% in some urban centers. Other authors found that a careful history was as accurate as pregnancy testing. At the very least, it is important to question all female patients after menarche about menstrual history and the possibility of pregnancy. Each ASC should develop its own policy.

Many states now require testing for sickle cell and other hemoglobinopathies for newborns. These states have a central lab database of results, accessible by clinicians after patient consent. Hemoglobin electrophoresis should be obtained in all children under 1 year of age or in symptomatic children over age 1 to determine the presence of sickle cell or other hemoglobinopathies. Some clinicians require, at a minimum, a rapid slide test for sickle hemoglobin in all patients of African descent. It should be noted that although African descent is a risk factor for sickle hemoglobin, other ethnic groups might also have sickle cell disease (Box 10-2).

CLINICAL CONTROVERSY

Should preoperative pregnancy testing be mandatory for all girls after the age of menarche?

CLINICAL CONTROVERSY

Should preoperative hemoglobin electrophoresis be mandatory prior to elective surgery for all children at risk for sickle cell disease or only for those under 1 year of age?

Preoperative Eating and Drinking Guidelines

Increasing utilization of outpatient surgery has been one of the stimulants to making nothing-by-mouth (NPO)

Box 10-2	**Preoperative Laboratory Test Recommendations**

Hemoglobin: former premature infants less than 6 months of age
Hemoglobin electrophoresis: children under 1 year of age in ethnic groups at risk for sickle cell disease
Pregnancy testing: controversial
Glucose: diabetic patients
Coagulation profile: patient with a history of bleeding or a family history of bleeding

---

guidelines more liberal. It is more difficult for parents to withhold food and liquids for long periods at home than it is in the hospital setting. In children, prolonged preoperative fasting can result in irritability, hypotension from dehydration, and hypoglycemia. Preoperative instructions should include offering the child clear liquids 2 or 3 hours prior to the scheduled surgery time. Gastric volume does not decrease with a clear liquid fast of longer than 2 hours. Fasting time for breast milk is controversial. Some practitioners consider breast milk almost equivalent to clear liquids. Others are concerned about delayed gastric emptying after breast milk because the fat content of breast milk may vary with maternal diet. Most sources, including the ASA guidelines, recommend a 4-hour fast for breast milk for all infants. It is not known if breast-feeding for older children should have different NPO recommendations (Table 10-3).

PREMEDICATION AND PARENTAL PRESENCE AT INDUCTION

In the ambulatory surgery setting, a child's preoperative anxiety is addressed through premedication, behavioral intervention, or parental presence at induction. Preoperative visits to the surgical center, videotapes, and printed material are utilized at many centers, and it is not clear which method is most helpful or whether any of these methods influence patient anxiety in the perioperative period. The optimal technique to allay anxiety in

Table 10-3	**Minimum NPO Fasting Times (in hours)**		
Age (in months)	Breast Milk	Milk and Solids	Clear Liquids
0–6	4	6	2
6–24	4	6	2
>24	?	6–8	2

the pediatric patient may vary with the situation. The length of the procedure, patient and family characteristics, the personality of the anesthesiologist, and the age of the child may affect the technique used to allay a child's anxiety. Some studies suggest that premedication is more helpful than parental presence. However, most parents prefer to accompany their children if offered the opportunity.

Parental presence at induction of their child's anesthetic has become increasingly popular over the last 20 years. Parental presence policy is often determined by the medical center's overall philosophy regarding parental involvement. Not all parents are appropriate candidates for this technique. There are no evidence-based guidelines for the upper and lower age limits at which parental presence is helpful. It is probably most helpful for children in the 1 to 6 year age range. Some anesthesiologists offer parental presence at induction as soon as the child exhibits stranger anxiety (at approximately 6 to 8 months). Others feel more comfortable with premedication and delaying parental presence until the child is closer to 1 year of age. Many anesthesiologists will ask older children whether they would like their parents to accompany them. Parents often feel that accompanying their child to the operating room improves their and their child's surgical experience. There are studies to suggest that, compared with parental presence alone, premedication with midazolam improves children's postoperative behavior in the 2 weeks after surgery.

Two appendices at the end of this chapter show samples of surgicenter policy and information for parents on parental presence at induction.

CLINICAL CONTROVERSY

Which do parents, children, and providers prefer: premedication of pediatric patients with an anxiolytic, parental presence at induction, or both?

Not all children require premedication prior to all anesthetics, but there is no good way to identify all those who would benefit from premedication. Drugs used to reduce preoperative anxiety include midazolam by the oral (0.3 to 0.5 mg/kg), intranasal (0.2 to 0.3 mg/kg), intramuscular (0.08 to 0.3 mg/kg), or rectal route (0.4 to 1 mg/kg). The maximum dose by the oral route is 10 to 20 mg. Midazolam given orally has an onset time of 10 to 15 minutes and a duration of 1 to 2 hours. Oral midazolam is probably the most commonly used premedication in children for anxiolysis. It has a fast onset, a reasonably short duration of action, and consistent and predictable effects with minimal cardiac or ventilatory depression. Midazolam also provides anterograde amnesia in children. Side effects, including

paradoxical agitation, are rare, but do occur. The main drawback of midazolam premedication is that it has a very bitter taste. Most children do not like intranasal administration of midazolam because of bitterness and coughing, and rectal administration is not well tolerated above age 3. Midazolam premedication given orally 30 to 45 minutes prior to induction of anesthesia has been reported not to delay recovery time even after procedures of less than 30 minutes in duration.

Less commonly used premedication includes 5 to 6 mg/kg of oral or 2 to 3 mg/kg of intramuscular ketamine. Intramuscular ketamine and intramuscular midazolam are good backup plans for children who refuse oral agents and who are difficult to control. Intramuscular ketamine is usually combined with glycopyrrolate (0.01 mg/kg) as an antisialagogue. The addition of midazolam decreases the incidence of hallucinations. Within 2 to 4 minutes of intramuscular ketamine, most children will accept a facemask for induction. Ketamine provides excellent amnesia and analgesia. The main disadvantages of ketamine are salivation, hallucinations, and delirium. The incidence of delirium or hallucinations when intramuscular ketamine is followed by an inhalation anesthetic is low. With availability of local anesthetic creams prior to intravenous placement, some children may prefer to have an intravenous catheter placed for premedication and induction of anesthesia.

ANESTHESIA FOR AMBULATORY SURGICAL PROCEDURES

The most common method for induction of anesthesia used for children in the United States is an inhalation anesthetic. There are two options for well-tolerated potent inhalation agents for induction: halothane and sevoflurane. Some practitioners also administer 70% nitrous oxide and 30% oxygen for 30 seconds until the child is relaxed, prior to beginning halothane or sevoflurane, in order to increase patient acceptance. A number of authors have studied immediate use of 8% sevoflurane and have reported good patient acceptance and no adverse cardiovascular or respiratory events. It is not clear that sevoflurane has a better safety record than halothane for all practitioners, but the learning curve for halothane is significantly longer than that for sevoflurane. When sevoflurane goes off patent, there may be low, or no, availability of halothane.

CLINICAL CONTROVERSY

Which is the preferred potent inhalation agent: halothane or sevoflurane?

Box 10-3 Common Ambulatory Otolaryngology Procedures

Myringotomy and ear tube placement
Adenoidectomy
Tonsillectomy
Frenulectomy
Microlaryngoscopy
Functional endoscopic sinus surgery
Bronchoscopy
Nasal fracture reduction
Branchial cleft cyst excision

Anesthesia for Otolaryngology Procedures

Bilateral myringotomy and insertion of ear tubes is one of the most commonly performed ambulatory procedures (Box 10-3). The anesthetic is brief, usually in the range of 5 to 10 minutes. Children are often not premedicated and undergo inhalation induction and maintenance of anesthesia through a facemask. Children with uncomplicated upper respiratory infection can have this procedure performed without a significantly increased risk of perioperative morbidity. Whether children experience significant pain after myringotomy and ear tube placement is controversial.

Commonly used medications for children who are irritable after ear tube placement include acetaminophen (10 to 20 mg/kg by mouth [PO]), and ibuprofen (10 mg/kg PO). Studies comparing acetaminophen and ibuprofen to ketorolac (1 mg/kg PO), all administered 30 minutes preoperatively, found that both ibuprofen and ketorolac were superior to acetaminophen. There are no studies comparing these two nonsteroidal anti-inflammatory medications to higher doses of acetaminophen (15 to 20 mg/kg). Intranasal fentanyl (0.5 to 1 μg/kg), administered while the patient is asleep, has been reported to decrease the incidence of emergence agitation after myringotomy and ear tube placement. Agitation after myringotomy and ear tube placement may be caused by pain or the new perception of louder ambient noise levels.

CLINICAL CONTROVERSY

Do most children have enough pain after ear tube placement to require the administration of opioid analgesic medication, or is their irritability primarily caused by factors other than pain?

Tonsillectomy is performed in children because of recurrent infection, peritonsillar abscess, or obstructive sleep apnea. For any child scheduled for tonsillectomy, it is important to obtain a complete history including the reason for surgery, the presence of snoring at night, apneic episodes at night, the nasal quality of speech, recent upper respiratory infection, and chronic mouth breathing. A child with severe chronic airway obstruction from enlarged tonsils may have pulmonary hypertension. There is no evidence-based guideline to determine which children must have a preoperative sleep study, chest radiograph, electrocardiogram, or echocardiogram. From a number of studies, children at high risk for postoperative respiratory compromise include children with symptoms of obstructive sleep apnea who are under age 3, craniofacial anomalies that decrease the size of the pharyngeal airway, failure to thrive, neuromuscular disorders, cor pulmonale, morbid obesity, high-risk polysomnography criteria, or an oxyhemoglobin desaturation nadir less than 70% on sleep study. Even children with a normal overnight oxyhemoglobin saturation study may have significant postoperative sleep apnea. There is no diagnostic study at this time that can predict which children will have respiratory compromise after surgery. Many freestanding ambulatory surgery centers use the age of 3 or 4 years as the lower limit for outpatient tonsillectomy, although some allow selected children of age 2 and older (Box 10-4).

Premedication of children with obstructive sleep apnea is controversial. Some recommend inhalation induction without premedication. Intravenous induction is another option. Children with obstructive sleep apnea will likely need an oral airway or jaw thrust maneuvers after induction to maintain a patent airway. Rarely, children with preoperative obstructive sleep apnea require rescue intubation or continuous positive airway pressure (CPAP) treatment after tonsillectomy.

Box 10-4 Recommendations for Admission After Tonsillectomy

Age under 3 years (some centers currently allow selected children over age 2 to be included on the outpatient pathway)
Coagulation defect
Other significant systemic medical disorders
Craniofacial abnormality
Acute peritonsillar abscess
Geographic or social conditions that prevent easy and rapid return to an appropriate medical facility for treatment of a complication

Adapted from Brown OE, Cunnigham MJ: Tonsillectomy and adenoidectomy. Inpatient guidelines: Recommendations of the AAO-HNS pediatric otolaryngology committee. AAO-HNS Bulletin, 1996.

During the tonsillectomy, maintenance of an airway is accomplished by intubation (by conventional endotracheal tube or precurved tube) or flexible laryngeal mask airway placement. Some anesthesiologists spray lidocaine (4 mg/kg) inside the larynx and trachea during laryngoscopy. Anesthesia can be maintained with either a potent inhaled agent or intravenous propofol and remifentanil infusion. Nitrous oxide and oxygen or else air and oxygen are commonly used with potent agents. Morphine (0.1 to 0.2 mg/kg) and fentanyl (3 to 5 μg/kg) are the most commonly administered opioids. There are advocates of both deep and awake removal of airway devices in patients undergoing tonsillectomy. Whichever method is preferred, it is probably wise to transport the patient to the postanesthesia care unit with supplemental oxygen in the tonsil position—in a lateral decubitus and slightly-head down position. Studies evaluating the use of ketorolac during tonsillectomy showed an increased risk of postoperative bleeding. Initial studies to evaluate the efficacy of COX-2 drug administration for analgesia were promising, although the removal of rofecoxib from clinical use deleted the only COX-2 liquid available in the United States.

Many patients receive acetaminophen every 4 to 6 hours after tonsillectomy. Nausea and vomiting are more common after tonsillectomy and adenoidectomy than after many other types of surgery, with an incidence of up to 75% in untreated patients. Most practitioners administer at least two antiemetic agents, including dexamethasone, which also may reduce swelling from the surgery site. Subhypnotic doses of propofol have not been effective in children to control postoperative nausea and vomiting after tonsillectomy. The Food and Drug Administration (FDA) has placed a "black box" warning on two antiemetics: a general warning on droperidol because of ECG long QT interval danger and a warning about excessive sedation when using promethazine in children under 2 years of age. Adequate intravenous hydration is important, both because of the risk of bleeding after tonsillectomy and because of the risk of dehydration from postoperative nausea and vomiting or decreased fluid intake.

The optimal duration of postoperative observation of tonsillectomy patients is controversial. The majority of posttonsillectomy bleeds occur in a bimodal distribution, either within the first 6 hours or else much later, at 8 to 10 days after surgery. Many centers are comfortable with 4 to 6 hours of observation after tonsillectomy to ensure that the patient is not having significant airway obstruction, oxyhemoglobin desaturation, or bleeding. Recently, shorter periods of postoperative observation have been suggested as equally safe.

Rigid bronchoscopy in the outpatient setting is usually a diagnostic exam, a routine follow-up exam after tracheal surgery, or a treatment procedure for papillomatosis. Laryngeal papillomas are the most common benign neoplasm of the upper airway in children. Usually, laryngeal papillomas are diagnosed prior to age 5. Symptoms include hoarseness, dyspnea, and stridor. Papillomas commonly recur, and many children with papillomas are regularly scheduled for laser treatment, mechanical excision, or diagnostic bronchoscopy, depending on progression of the disease. Papillomas tend to regress around the time of puberty.

Premedication of children scheduled for bronchoscopy is determined by the estimated likelihood of airway compromise after sedation. If children with symptoms of airway obstruction do require sedation, it should be done with monitoring and immediate availability of the anesthesiologist and oxygen, suction, and ventilation apparatuses. Inhalation technique is the most common method of anesthetic induction for this group of patients. Older children may prefer an intravenous induction. Intravenous access is always obtained after induction so that rapid increase in anesthetic depth can be accomplished by intravenous medication administration. Laryngotracheal anesthesia with lidocaine (4 mg/kg) is helpful to avoid coughing and airway irritability, both during the bronchoscopy and during emergence.

Maintenance of anesthesia with an inhaled anesthetic in 100% oxygen may be accomplished by ventilating through a rigid bronchoscope, either by spontaneous breathing technique using insufflation through the nasopharynx or oropharynx or by jet ventilation with a continuous intravenous propofol infusion, with or without remifentanil. The choice of technique is determined by whether the endoscopist needs to observe the airway with the patient breathing spontaneously or if a quiet airway is needed. For laser treatment of papillomas, it is necessary to decrease the inspired oxygen to less than 25% by diluting it with air or helium. Nitrous oxide is not suitable because it supports combustion.

Depending on the size of the patient, airway maintenance is accomplished with either a Hunsaker tube (i.e., a subglottic jet ventilation device), a metal endotracheal tube, a laser-resistant tube, or supraglottic jet ventilation. If a laser-resistant endotracheal tube is used, the cuff is filled with saline. At times, it may be necessary to secure the airway with an endotracheal tube or a rigid bronchoscope if ventilation becomes difficult by the planned technique. After stabilizing the airway, obstructing papilloma can be resected by mechanical means to enable the use of the preferred airway management technique.

Bronchoscopic procedures always require close cooperation between the anesthesiologist and the surgeon. When using supraglottic and subglottic jet ventilation techniques, it is imperative for both the surgeon and the anesthesiologist to assure appropriate placement of the ventilation device and adequate egress of exhaled gas to avoid pneumothorax and pneumomediastinum. With true rigid bronchoscopy, children should be observed for at least 4 hours after the procedure to watch for signs of airway swelling manifested as croup, stridor, airway obstruction, or oxyhemoglobin desaturation. A quick examination of the airway using a thin, flexible endoscope may require briefer observation time.

Treatment of croup or stridor after bronchoscopy is accomplished with intravenous dexamethasone (0.5 to 1 mg/kg), nebulized 2% racemic epinephrine (0.5 to 1 mL), or reintubation, depending on the severity of airway compromise. The use of racemic epinephrine has decreased in the last few years. If a patient requires any treatment for croup or stridor, he or she should be watched for at least 2 hours after resolution of the symptoms or after the last nebulized epinephrine treatment because of the risk of rebound swelling. Persistent stridor or croupy cough probably necessitates admission to the hospital. Opioid medication is not needed after simple rigid bronchoscopy.

Flexible bronchoscopy may also be performed in the outpatient setting. This can be accomplished through an endotracheal tube, a laryngeal mask airway, or with oropharyngeal or nasopharyngeal insufflation of an anesthetic agent. An inhaled anesthetic with oxygen is probably the most common technique. In this situation, laryngotracheal anesthesia with 1% or 4% lidocaine (4 mg/kg total) may be administered by the endoscopist through the flexible bronchoscope during the course of the examination. Oxygenation may be aided by insufflation of supplemental oxygen through the flexible bronchoscope.

Endoscopic sinus surgery is performed with the patient intubated with either an oral precurved or a conventional endotracheal tube. The anesthesiologist should be aware of the amount and type of intranasal vasoconstrictor agent used by the surgical team to avoid a toxic dose. Patients undergoing functional endoscopic sinus surgery are at risk for retrobulbar hemorrhage, which may lead to blindness. The surgeon may request no tape on the eyes or the use of water-soluble lubricant so that the status of the eyes can be assessed throughout the procedure. Postoperative nausea and vomiting is a common problem after endoscopic sinus surgery, and routine prophylaxis with two antiemetics is reasonable. Opioid analgesic medication is usually needed.

Branchial cleft cysts are fistulous tracts that can present as swelling in specific areas of the face and neck. The most common type presents as cysts in the lateral neck, deep to the anterior sternocleidomastoid muscle. These usually come to medical attention because of swelling or infection. Surgical treatment is planned after the infection is controlled. The cyst can extend into the pharynx near the tonsillar fossa. Airway management with endotracheal intubation provides optimal conditions for the surgery.

Anesthesia for Ophthalmology Procedures

For examination under anesthesia, if intraocular pressure measurements are planned, it is important to remember that intraocular pressure varies with anesthetic depth: more deeply anesthetized patients have lower intraocular pressures. Some surgeons request very low concentrations of inhaled anesthetic or the use of IV or intramuscular (IM) ketamine in order to obtain accurate intraocular pressure readings. Most eye examinations under anesthesia can be performed with the patient spontaneously breathing inhaled anesthetic through a facemask or laryngeal mask airway.

Eye muscle surgery is probably the most common ophthalmologic surgery (Box 10-5) performed in the pediatric population. If an eye muscle forced duction test is planned, the test is not valid within 20 minutes after succinylcholine administration. Two other concerns in anesthetizing this group of patients include stimulation of the oculocardiac reflex and the high incidence of postoperative nausea and vomiting—up to 80% in untreated patients. The oculocardiac reflex is mediated through trigeminal afferent and vagal efferent pathways and is stimulated by traction on the extraocular muscles or pressure on the globe.

Box 10-5 Common Ambulatory Ophthalmology Procedures

Examination under anesthesia
Eye muscle surgery
Lacrimal duct probing
Excision of chalazion
Insertion of lens or prosthesis

The most common response is bradycardia, but other serious arrhythmias can occur. The initial treatment for bradycardia is to ask the surgeon to cease manipulating the eye. Atropine (0.02 mg/kg IV) or glycopyrrolate (0.01 mg/kg IV) may be administered if needed. The incidence of postoperative nausea and vomiting in these patients can be decreased by adequate hydration with intravenous fluids, using at least two antiemetic agents and reducing opioid use by administering 0.5 to 0.75 mg/kg of ketorolac intravenously.

Options for anesthesia include total intravenous anesthetic with propofol, a combination of propofol infusion with a potent agent or nitrous oxide, or a potent agent in oxygen plus or minus nitrous oxide. Airway maintenance during strabismus surgery can be accomplished with either tracheal intubation or a laryngeal mask airway. The surgeon may request muscle relaxant to facilitate the repair.

Lacrimal duct probing can usually be accomplished using an inhaled anesthetic by facemask, laryngeal mask airway, or insufflation. Intravenous catheter placement may not be necessary. If silicone stent placement is necessary, the patient may benefit from an intravenous opioid or ketorolac, and intubation or a laryngeal mask airway may be necessary for surgical access.

Excision of chalazion can usually be accomplished with the child spontaneously breathing a potent anesthetic by insufflation, a facemask, or a laryngeal mask airway. Intravenous access and opioid are not usually required.

Anesthesia for Urology Procedures

Common ambulatory urology procedures are listed in Box 10-6. Cystoscopy and meatotomy are brief procedures that normally do not require opioid administration. Patients can usually receive an inhaled anesthetic with spontaneous ventilation. If a patient requires stenting or a residual urinary catheter, ketorolac (0.5 mg/kg, up to 15 to 30 mg) may be beneficial to decrease bladder spasm. Ketorolac probably should not be administered to patients with renal insufficiency. After meatotomy, local application of lidocaine gel is a reasonable analgesic.

Box 10-6	**Common Ambulatory Urology Procedures**

Cystoscopy
Meatotomy
Orchiopexy
Circumcision
Hydrocelectomy
Testicular biopsy
Hypospadias repair

Orchiectomy and hydrocelectomy are performed under general anesthesia. Airway management is the choice of the anesthesia provider, except in the case of a nonpalpable testis. In patients with nonpalpable testis, a general anesthetic with muscle relaxant may facilitate the surgery, especially if laparoscopy is utilized. Postoperative pain relief can be accomplished in a variety of ways including intravenous opioid, intravenous ketorolac, local anesthetic infiltration by the surgeon, or caudal analgesia with either 0.125% or 0.25 % bupivacaine (maximum dose, 2 mg/kg).

Circumcision is commonly performed in the outpatient setting. A general anesthetic is required, and airway management is determined by the size of the child and the anesthetist's preference. Many practitioners find that a laryngeal mask airway may become malpositioned more easily in children under age 6 months and prefer a conventional facemask or endotracheal tube to maintain the airway. Analgesia after circumcision can be accomplished with a ring block, a dorsal penile nerve block, a caudal block, or an intravenous opioid. Due to the risk of bleeding problems, surgeons may ask that ketorolac not be used.

Hypospadias repair is commonly performed in children under 1 year of age. With this procedure, a popular technique is to combine general anesthesia with a caudal block (Fig. 10-3). The block can be performed at the beginning of the operation to reduce the general anesthetic requirement or at the end of the surgery to maximize the duration of the block for postoperative analgesia. A caudal block with 0.5 to 1 mL/kg of 0.25% bupivacaine will last for 4 to 6 hours after surgery. Ropivacaine can be used instead of bupivacaine. It is important to instruct parents that the child will require pain medication when the block wears off. For children over the age of 1 year, some practitioners add clonidine (1 to 2 μg/kg; maximum dose, 30 μg) to prolong the block; larger doses of clonidine may be associated with sedation or hypotension. Clonidine is acceptable for use in the outpatient setting.

Anesthesia for General Surgery Procedures

Inguinal hernia repair is probably the most commonly performed operation in pediatric outpatients. Other frequently performed general surgery procedures are listed in Box 10-7. Inguinal hernias in children are caused by a patent processus vaginalis. (A hydrocele is an accumulation of fluid in the patent processus vaginalis.) Most inguinal hernias are discovered during the first 6 months of life. Inguinal hernias are more likely to become incarcerated in premature infants than in term infants. This is why many surgeons consider it more urgent to repair a hernia in a former premature infant than in a term infant.

A

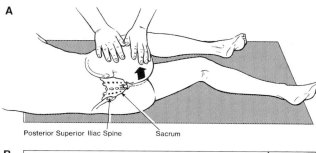

B

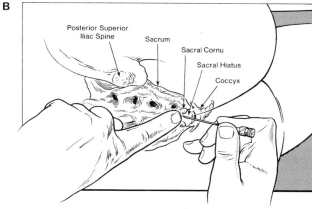

C

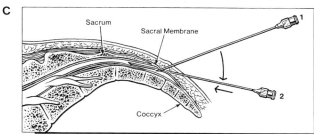

Figure 10-3 Caudal nerve block. (Reprinted from Cousins MJ, Bridenbaugh PO [eds]: Neural Blockade in Clinical Anesthesia and Management of Pain, 3rd ed. Philadelphia, Lippincott-Raven, 1998, p 333.)

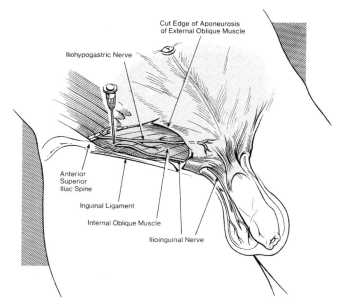

Figure 10-4 Ilioinguinal nerve block. (Reprinted from Cousins MJ, Bridenbaugh PO [eds]: Neural Blockade in Clinical Anesthesia and Management of Pain, 3rd ed. Philadelphia, Lippincott-Raven, 1998, p 630.)

In young infants, many surgeons use a brief laparoscopic examination to check the opposite side after repairing the open hernia. General anesthesia is commonly used for repair of inguinal hernias, although small infants may have spinal anesthesia. Airway management is the choice of the anesthesia provider: facemask, laryngeal mask airway, and endotracheal tube are all acceptable methods. Intravenous cannulation is routinely performed. Analgesia for inguinal hernia repair can be accomplished in a number of ways including caudal block (0.5 mL/kg of 0.25% bupivacaine), ilioinguinal (Fig. 10-4) and iliohypogastric nerve block (1 mL/kg of 0.25% bupivacaine), local infiltration by the surgeon (1 mL/kg of 0.25% bupivacaine), intravenous morphine (0.1 mg/kg), and intravenous ketorolac (0.5 mg/kg). Some centers use a combination of local infiltration by the surgeon and intravenous morphine with or without ketorolac with good results. All methods have been reported as providing effective postoperative analgesia.

Umbilical hernia occurs when abdominal viscera protrude through a stretched umbilical ring. Incarceration is rarely a complication of umbilical hernia. Some surgeons prefer patients to be intubated for umbilical hernia repair for muscle relaxation. Postoperative analgesia can be accomplished with a combination of infiltration of local anesthetic and the use of intravenous opioid or ketorolac. Bilateral intercostal nerve block of the tenth intercostal nerve can also provide good analgesia after umbilical hernia repair.

Excision of superficial skin lesions can be accomplished with inhaled anesthesia and local anesthetic infiltration by the surgeon. Airway management will be determined by patient positioning for the procedure and any special patient issues. Opioids are not necessary.

Esophagoscopy and dilation requires general anesthesia, usually with an endotracheal tube. However, there are reports of using a laryngeal mask airway with acceptable results. Children with a history of esophageal atresia or tracheoesophageal fistula frequently develop esophageal stricture. These children have an increased incidence of obstructive and restrictive lung disease, probably because of recurrent aspiration.

Diagnostic esophagoscopy is frequently performed in children with gastroesophageal reflux disease, swallowing disorders, or recurrent vomiting. Airway management is dictated by patient history. In selected patients, esophagoscopy alone can be performed with a natural airway and insufflation of inhaled anesthetic by oropharynx or nasopharynx, or else it can be performed with an infusion of intravenous anesthetic with propofol with

---

Box 10-7   Common Ambulatory General Surgery Procedures

Inguinal hernia repair
Umbilical hernia repair
Excision of superficial skin lesions
Excision of breast mass or gynecomastia
Esophagoscopy and dilation
Rectal exam and dilation
Insertion or removal of central venous lines

CLINICAL CONTROVERSY

What is the preferred analgesic for inguinal hernia repair or orchiopexy? Options include caudal block, ilioinguinal nerve block, local anesthetic infiltration, intravenous opioid, nonsteroidal anti-inflammatory drugs (NSAIDs), or a combination thereof.

---

insufflation of supplemental oxygen. Many children do not require opioids but do experience sore throat from the passage of the endoscope. Abdominal cramping from gas in the stomach or duodenum can occur if the endoscopist does not remove the insufflated gas prior to removing the endoscope. Antiemetic therapy may be needed.

Rectal examination and dilation can be performed in either the lithotomy or the prone position, depending on the surgeon's preference. Opioids are usually not necessary. Other anal procedures may be managed with local anesthetic and ketorolac.

Patients undergoing Port-a-Cath and central venous line placement or removal will usually require general anesthesia. Some adolescents are candidates for monitored anesthesia care with a local anesthetic. However, many of the younger children will require intravenous pain medication or antiemetic therapy. Airway management is generally the choice of the anesthesia provider; however, if insertion through a neck vein is planned, an endotracheal tube or laryngeal mask airway may be a better choice than a facemask.

Anesthesia for Orthopedic Procedures

Most ambulatory orthopedic procedures (Box 10-8) can be performed under general anesthesia using a facemask, a laryngeal mask airway, or an endotracheal tube. Sometimes open reduction of fractures is necessary, which is why intravenous access should always be obtained when a patient is scheduled for closed reduction. Hip spica casts deserve special mention because the patient is usually positioned on a spica casting table, which does not afford easy access to the patient's airway. Laryngeal mask airways may dislodge more easily in infants, especially in those having hip spica cast changes. Some anesthesiologists prefer an endotracheal tube for airway management when using a spica casting table.

RECOVERY AND OUTCOMES AFTER AMBULATORY PEDIATRIC SURGERY AND ANESTHESIA

There are few outcome studies after ambulatory pediatric anesthesia. A review of ambulatory pediatric tonsillectomy reported an unplanned admission rate of 8.2%.[4] An additional 3.2% of patients were admitted following discharge from the hospital. Another study from the Children's Hospital of Pittsburgh comparing postoperative complications after tonsillectomy in children with Down syndrome to a control group noted that respiratory complications are five times as likely in the Down syndrome group.[5] They recommend inpatient stays for all patients with Down syndrome having a tonsillectomy. Outcomes of interest include unplanned admission rate and postoperative emergency room visit rate.

There is little data available on rates of emergency room visits after pediatric ambulatory anesthesia. Admission rates in reported series range from 0.1% to 5.3%. Most of these series are old. The most common reasons for overnight admission included vomiting, fever, bleeding, croup, and other respiratory complications. At Children's Hospital National Medical Center, the rates of hospital admission after ambulatory surgery decreased from 0.9% in a series from 1983 to 1986 to 0.3% in a series from 1988 to 1991. In the second time period, it was noted that the ASA classification had increased and the complexity of procedures performed had increased. The second series also included tonsillectomies, and the first series did not. Children's Hospital of Eastern Ontario reported an admission rate of 1.7% in a series from 1992 to 1997, with vomiting and respiratory difficulty cited as the most common reasons for unplanned admission. Some authors note that bleeding after tonsillectomies was included and accounted for a significant number of unplanned admissions. In the older series, tonsillectomies were not performed on an outpatient basis. The downward trend in unplanned admissions after ambulatory surgery indicates that pediatric ambulatory surgery is relatively safe and effective.

Fast tracking in ambulatory surgery is just beginning to be utilized for pediatric patients. Selecting pediatric patients for fast tracking may be more difficult than selecting adult patients because of the difficulty in communicating with young children. One report of fast tracking in pediatric patients ages 7 and older stated that

---

Box 10-8   Common Ambulatory Orthopedic Procedures

Cast change
Arthroscopy
Closed reduction of fractures
Hardware removal or insertion

parents reported twice as much restlessness during the early postoperative period in fast-tracked children. This was attributed to inadequate analgesia. More studies are needed to define the role of fast tracking in the pediatric ambulatory population.

CONCLUSION

Children are usually excellent candidates for ambulatory surgical procedures. However, the ambulatory center or office must have equipment, procedures, and personnel appropriate to the age, the size, and the health issues of these patients. Education and preparation of patients and family are essential for a smooth transition into and out of the surgery center. It is important to consider the special needs of children and parents in the ambulatory perioperative period. Further research is needed to determine the age and physical condition limits for children in outpatient surgery and procedures.

REFERENCES

1. Kurth CD, Spitzer AR, Broennle AM, Downes JJ: Postoperative apnea in perterm infants. Anesthesiology 66:483–488, 1987.

2. Liu LM, Cote CJ, Goudsouzian NG, et al: Life threatening apnea in infants recovering from anesthesia. Anesthesiology 59:506–510, 1983.

3. Welborn LG, Hanallah RS, Luban NLC, et al: Anemia and postoperative apnea in former preterm infants. Anesthesiology 74:1003–1006, 1991.

4. Lalakea ML, Marquez-Biggs I, Messner AH: Safety of pediatric short-stay tonsillectomy. Arch Otolaryngol Head Neck Surg 125:749–752, 1999.

5. Goldstein NA, Armfield DR, Kingsley LA, et al: Postoperative complications after tonsillectomy and adenoidectomy in children with Down syndrome. Arch Otolaryngol Head Neck Surg 124:171–176, 1998.

SUGGESTED READING

Baum VC, Yemen TA, Baum LD: Immediate 8% sevoflurane induction in children: A comparison with incremental sevoflurane and incremental halothane. Anesth Analg 85:313–316, 1997.

Cote CJ: The upper respiratory tract infection (URI) dilemma: Fear of a complication or litigation? Anesthesiology 95:283–285, 2001.

Fisher DM: When is the ex-premature infant no longer at risk for apnea? Anesthesiology 82:807–808, 1995.

Fishkin S, Litman RS: Current issues in pediatric ambulatory anesthesia. Anesthesiol Clin North America 21:305–311, 2003.

Green CR, Pandit SK, Schork MA: Preoperative fasting time: Is the traditional policy changing? Results of a national survey. Anesth Analg 83:123–128, 1996.

Kain ZN, Mayes LC, Wang S, et al: Parental presence during induction of anesthesia versus sedative premedication: Which is more effective? Anesthesiology 89:1147–1156, 1998.

Kain ZN, Mayes LC, Wang S, et al: Parental presence and a sedative premedicant for children undergoing surgery: A hierarchical study. Anesthesiology 92:939–946, 2000.

Lalakea ML, Marquez-Biggs I, Messner AH: Safety of pediatric short-stay tonsillectomy. Arch Otolaryngol Head Neck Surg 125:749–752, 1999.

Orr RJ, Ramamoorthy C: Controversies in pediatric ambulatory anesthesia. Anesthesiol Clin North America 4:767–780, 1996.

Skolnick ET, Vomvolakis MA, Buck KA, et al: Exposure to environmental tobacco smoke and the risk of adverse respiratory events in children receiving general anesthesia. Anesthesiology 88:1144–1153, 1998.

Splinter WM, Reid CW, Roberts KJ, Bass J: Reducing pain after inguinal hernia repair in children: Caudal aesthesia versus ketorolac tromethamine. Anesthesiology 87:542–546, 1997.

Tait AR, Malviya SH, Voepel-Lewis T, et al: Risk factors for perioperative adverse respiratory events in children with upper respiratory tract infections. Anesthesiology 95:299–306, 2001.

Tait AR, Pandit UA, Voepel-Lewis T, et al: Use of the laryngeal mask airway in children with upper respiratory tract infections: A comparison with endotracheal intubation. Anesth Analg 86:706–711, 1998.

Weldon BC, Watcha MF, White PF: Oral midazolam in children: Effect of time and adjunctive therapy. Anesth Analg 75:51–55, 1992.

Yentis SM, Levine MF, Hartley EJ: Should all children with suspected or confirmed malignant hyperthermia susceptibility be admitted after surgery? A 10-year review. Anesth Analg 75:345–350, 1992.

APPENDIX 1: SAMPLE POLICY FOR PARENTAL PRESENCE AT INDUCTION OF GENERAL ANESTHESIA

Purpose

To provide a guideline that allows a pediatric patient's support person (including a parent, a guardian, another family member, or another person) to support the child during induction of anesthesia. In the outpatient surgery center, operating room (OR) nursing staff fulfills the same function as Child Life staff.

Policy

Ideally, a calm, comforting environment should be provided for pediatric patients and their families. The patient's family may, if it does not place the child at increased risk, participate in the surgical experience. The goal is to reduce stress caused by separation anxiety and an unfamiliar environment. When appropriate, parental presence at induction (PPI) is permitted. However, this is not an "invitation," nor a requirement, for family members.

Procedure

Steps	Key Points
1. Confirm with anesthesiologist that the child's support person (as defined in purpose statement) wishes to be present during induction of anesthesia. Assess the appropriateness of his or her attendance at induction of anesthesia. The anesthesiologist determines cases with anticipated difficult airway or medical conditions that preclude PPI. Children less than 6 months old are unlikely to have separation anxiety. In these cases, PPI is for the parent's benefit. Surgical Services and/or Child Life should not promise PPI until discussed with anesthesiologist.	1a. Possible contraindications for PPI include: -Child's medical condition, age, or difficult airway: anesthesiologist determines issues. -Support person unable to tolerate viewing medical procedures or environment. -Known infections or illness of the support person. -Support person is not able to attend induction due to presence of patient's siblings without other caregivers. 1b. Surgical and anesthesiology personnel must be informed of support person's presence in the induction room.
2. Educate and orient the support person about what to expect at PPI; give a brief orientation to the room, his or her role in the induction room, and the proper time to be escorted out. A calm and quiet environment is essential during anesthesia induction. Unnecessary conversations by surgical or other personnel should be postponed until the child is anesthetized. Avoid loud noises such a pagers, phone ringers, and equipment rattling.	2a. Educate and orient the support person with verbal and written explanations about what to expect at induction. Include information on transportation to the induction room, positioning of the child and the support person, and monitoring and equipment. Inform the support person about expected events during induction of anesthesia: restlessness followed by sedation, irregular breathing, possible movement during Stage 2, and appearance of child as asleep or limp. 2b. Nursing staff will provide the support person with access to written documentation on "Information for Parents About Anesthesia for Your Children (First Day Surgery or OSC)" during the admission process. 2c. Educate and orient the support person about equipment, alarms, and sounds often heard in the induction room. 2d. The support person's role at induction is to provide reassurance to the child. This may include talking, touching, or other comfort measures. 3. Street attire worn by the support person must be covered while in restricted areas in order to maintain an aseptic and sterile environment. A cap should cover scalp hair; a gown should cover street clothes. Masks are not worn unless determined to be necessary by the anesthesiologist or circulating nurse.
4. A Child Life representative or a member of the nursing staff is required for a support person to be present at induction.	4a. A Child Life and/or registered nurse, an ORSA, or a nursing assistant is responsible for escorting the support person. 4b. The escort will be in attendance during the anesthesia induction. She or he will facilitate proper positioning of the parent and child and will provide assistance to the anesthesia team. 4c. A Child Life representative or a member of the nursing staff is required for a support person to be present at induction.
5. The pediatric patient may walk to the induction room (if not premedicated), may be transported by cart, crib, or wagon, or may be carried by family or medical personnel.	5. If not premedicated, pediatric patients may choose to walk to the induction room. Otherwise, they may arrive in a cart, crib, or wagon, or they may choose to be carried by family or medical personnel.
6. During preinduction, the child may be positioned on a table or bed or held by the support person. The anesthesiologist determines the positioning of the child during induction. If the child is to be held during induction, a stable chair (preferably without wheels) should be provided for the support person.	6a. During the preinduction period, the safety of the support person and child should be foremost. 6b. A chair may be provided for the support person. The chair should have a back and should be stationary. (The anesthesiologist decides if the child should be held or should be placed on the bed during induction.) 6c. The position of the child during induction should provide comfort, security, and safe airway management.
7. In case of difficult induction or unexpected change in patient condition, the support person should be expeditiously escorted out of the induction room. When the child is stable, medical personnel should inform the family about the child's condition.	7. During difficult situations, medical personnel provide the best care when not distracted. In case of an unexpected adverse change in the child's condition, the support person should be expeditiously escorted out of the room by medical staff and, as soon as possible, provided with information and support.
8. The support person should be escorted back to the child's room, the preoperative preparation area, or the surgical waiting area after the patient is anesthetized or at the order of the anesthesiologist. Family should be informed about the estimated length of the procedure, and they should be given information about the child's condition and what events to expect.	8. The support person should usually be escorted out of the induction room before invasive procedures are initiated. Medical personnel should provide comfort, answers to questions and concerns, reassurance regarding the child's condition, and estimates of the procedure's duration. Family should be informed that some of them might be allowed at the child's side when the child is awake and stable in the postanesthetic care unit (PACU). PACU staff or the Child Life specialist should notify the family when they are allowed to visit the PACU. A Child Life specialist or medical personnel should escort the family to the PACU.

9. Family (including parents, guardians, other family member, or other support persons) should be informed about the child's condition if the operative procedure is longer than anticipated.

10. PACU staff should be informed that the child's family desires to be present in the PACU during Stage 1 recovery. All patients under 18 should be identified, and Child Life should be contacted to act as escorts for family members for the PACU.

9. The circulating nurse should inform appropriate medical staff about any procedural delays or problems. Medical personnel should then inform and reassure the family.

10a. Inform PACU staff that the family wishes to be present during recovery in the PACU.

10b. Family members may be allowed to be with the child in the PACU if the child is stable or at the discretion of the anesthesiologist.

ORSA, Operating room surgical assistant; *OSC,* outpatient surgery center; *PACU,* postanesthetic care unit.

APPENDIX 2: INFORMATION FOR PARENTS ABOUT PRESENCE DURING THE START OF ANESTHESIA

The anesthesiology department wishes to make the process of going to sleep as pleasant as possible for you and your child. (Of course, anesthesia is far more complex than simple sleep, but many often use the term "sleep.") One way to reduce preoperative anxiety is to give your child a sedative medication to make him or her more relaxed. Usually, these medications are given by mouth, but, in certain circumstances, they may be given as an injection. Not every child needs a sedative, especially if you will be present during the start of anesthesia, but we will discuss this with you. Your presence at the start of anesthesia can involve you, as much as possible, in your child's care, but you are not required to participate. We usually allow you (or another adult) the opportunity to stay with your child until he or she is asleep under anesthesia. This will be a decision made only by the anesthesiologist and you. There may be circumstances where the anesthesiologist prefers you not to be present so that all attention can be focused on your child. Children older than 9 months of age might benefit the most from your presence. Again, you are not required to accompany your child to the operating room. Importantly, we must have an extra person accompany each parent in the operating room, so we ask only one person to come back with the child.

Points to consider:

- If you are a bit squeamish about hospitals or the sight of medical equipment, you may wish to have your spouse or another adult, if available, accompany your child into the operating room.
- If you go with your child and are standing close during the start of anesthesia, you may smell the anesthesia gas. It has a rather strong, pungent odor, but the amount you breathe will not be enough to cause you to become sleepy.
- Some women who are in the first 3 months of pregnancy like to avoid any exposure to any medications. There is no evidence that brief exposure to very dilute anesthetic gases will cause any harm to you or your developing baby. However, if you are concerned about this issue, let us know.

If you decide to accompany your child, you will be given a gown to put over your clothes. Your child can sometimes sit in your lap during the start of anesthesia, but if he or she is a small infant or is more than about 3 years old, it may be best to have your child sit or lay on the operating room bed. The anesthesiologist will talk to you about the best positioning. Children can go off to sleep breathing the anesthetic gas mixture through a clear mask, which we can often flavor with a fruity smell (although it never totally covers the smell of the anesthetic). Sometimes we just hold the tubing near the child's mouth. We also may tell your child a story and talk to him or her in a low, soothing voice. You are an important part of this process since your presence should have a calming influence. You can help us, too, by reassuring your child that all is well and by holding your child's hands as he or she drifts off to sleep.

The process of becoming anesthetized takes about a minute, but it is not like the movies, where anesthesia takes only a few seconds. Often, in between being awake and asleep, your child may become disoriented and talk or reach out, his or her eyes may roll back, and he or she may even try to sit or stand up. Your child's breathing may be fast or irregular, and may become noisy. This is *normal* and is nothing to be worried about. The child usually remembers very little of this. You can help by being calm and by gently restraining your child's hands if necessary.

As your child falls further asleep, he or she will become relaxed and quiet. At this point, we will let you know that your child is now asleep, and a nurse will escort you out of the operating room and back to your child's room. Please ask if you have questions about this process. We do require you to leave at this point.

If, at any point in the process of falling asleep, there is an unexpected event, we may ask that you leave the room immediately. We appreciate your *immediate and complete cooperation, and we will allow you to be present in the operating room only by agreeing to this.* We will only ask you to leave to ensure the safety of your child, especially if we need to focus all of our attention on some unexpected event.

Older children (8 years or older) or those with certain medical problems may go to sleep more quickly and comfortably with an intravenous injection through a small plastic tube placed in a vein on the back of the hand or arm. This is called an IV. This may be placed while still in the child's room, with your presence. We often use a local anesthetic (applied as a cream or through an injection) to numb the skin before this tube is inserted. We will discuss which method will work best for your child.

After the anesthetic, we will let you know when you are allowed to see your child in the recovery room. Almost all children are disoriented and upset for at least 15 to 20 minutes after awakening. This is not always related to the amount of pain they are experiencing.

One last important point: the possibility always exists that the anesthesiologist or surgeon might need to consult with you during the procedure. Therefore, we ask that you remain inside the hospital or surgery center, preferably close to the waiting area. If you decide you must leave the waiting area, first please stop at the nursing station.

CHAPTER 11

Geriatric Ambulatory Anesthesia

BRIAN K. BEVACQUA

Most developed nations have a steadily growing percentage of geriatric (i.e., aged 65 and older) citizens. In the United States, the geriatric group is the fastest growing age group, predicted to be over 20% of the total population by 2025. In addition, within this group, the population at age 85 and older is increasing the fastest. The geriatric population surge will have an important impact on the consumption of medical resources. Older patients, currently 15% of the population, utilize a disproportional amount of medical resources. The geriatric group consumes 30% of all prescription medications, 40% of over-the-counter medications, 40% of physician office time, and 33% of hospital time. Of importance to medical providers in anesthesiology and surgery is the increase in the number of invasive procedures and the complex medical management often needed for older patients. Currently, one-third of all surgeries in the United States are performed on patients aged 65 and older. About 50% of the geriatric group will undergo surgery in the latter part of their life.

There is a shift in the type of surgery performed as patients age, with less emergency trauma surgery than in younger patients. Operations to preserve and to improve an individual's functional status (e.g., joint repair and replacement or cataract surgery) will increase in frequency and will be offered to older and sicker patients. Given the financial realities of medical care in the United States and the expected costs associated with care for the geriatric surgery patient, cost savings offered by the ambulatory process will continue to be attractive to government and third-party payers. Providers can anticipate pressure to perform more invasive ambulatory procedures for older patients. Despite all of these concerns, studies have shown that patients in their 80s, 90s, and older can, and do, usually survive surgery with adequate return to baseline daily activities.

Chronological age alone is a predictor of postoperative complications, including death. However, age criteria are not included in the American Society of Anesthesiologists Physical Status classification. Although this appears inconsistent, it is helpful to understand that the effects of aging are not the same for each individual and may be different for each organ system within individuals. Any concurrent diseases will further add to loss of functional reserve. Preoperative assessment must be performed carefully in order to give realistic predictions of fitness for surgery and anesthesia.

Geriatric patients more often present for emergency surgery than do younger patients, and with markedly increased morbidity and mortality. In contrast, elective ambulatory surgery, by careful planning and attention to detail, should be associated with significantly lower perioperative risk. In addition, refinements in minimally invasive surgery and anesthetic management can result in rapid recovery. For example, a study of laparoscopic cholecystectomy showed no increase in major or minor morbidity for those in a population older than age 80 when compared with a geriatric group younger than 80. The ambulatory process stresses rapid return to a familiar environment and a stable social situation, thereby avoiding the physical (e.g., nosocomial infections) and cognitive risks of inpatient hospital stays for the older population.

Some have expressed the opinion that the elderly have been subjected to a massive experiment in mandatory outpatient surgery in the last 3 decades. Although this appears to be an overstatement, the experiment may have been quite useful. At its core, the ambulatory process should provide for careful patient preparation across all age groups. The geriatric population may benefit the most from a process that minimizes unexpected outcomes by careful preoperative preparation.

PHYSIOLOGIC AND CLINICAL CHANGES ASSOCIATED WITH AGING AND CHRONIC DISEASE

Aging is associated with a loss of functional reserve and a reduced maximal performance capacity of all organ systems. In the normal nonstressed state, these changes are not usually noticeable on a screening physical exam or in laboratory tests. The reserve capacity of important organ systems is sufficient for continued daily function. Estimating perioperative risk requires a realistic estimate of how well each organ system and the entire patient will function when faced with the cascade of surgical stress. Preparation of the geriatric patient begins with an understanding of the physiologic changes caused by aging and the presence of chronic disease.

Cardiovascular Aging

Myocardial cells begin to die in infancy at an estimated rate of 38 million per year. The remaining myocardial cells hypertrophy, resulting in an increase in left ventricular mass with aging. Increased fibrosis is observed in the myocardium and conduction system with advanced age. Systolic function is preserved over time despite these changes, and there is no change in resting cardiac function.

There is a decrease in autonomic responsiveness with aging, both at rest and during stress. This occurs despite elevated plasma levels of epinephrine and norepinephrine. This change in response results in a progressive decrease in maximal heart rate and a decrease in heart rate response for any given stimulus compared to younger adults. In addition, there is a 1% drop in maximal cardiac output per year after age 30. This decline in maximal cardiac work becomes significant with exercise and during stressful periods such as surgery. Some of

these changes can be slowed, or at least compensated for, by physical conditioning in older people.

Arteries become stiffer and less compliant with advancing age. This is due to the progressive disorientation, fragmentation, and degeneration of the elastin fibers in the media of the arterial walls. This process results in collagen deposition, calcification, and cystic degeneration. Central arteries such as the aorta become dilated and tortuous. These changes are not seen in the peripheral arteries. Resting right atrial, pulmonary arterial, and pulmonary capillary wedge pressures will be unchanged with age. However, pulmonary vascular resistance will increase with exercise as people age.

Total body water and intracellular volume decreases with age; however, plasma and blood volume do not change with aging. In addition, older patients respond less appropriately to volume depletion. They have a diminished sense of thirst, have less ability to concentrate urine, and respond less to aldosterone than younger adults. Older patients often react as if they are hypovolemic when faced with the stresses of surgery and anesthesia.

Systolic blood pressure rises about 6 to 7 mm Hg per decade. Therapy for hypertension is more common in older adults. Diastolic pressure may remain unchanged or may decrease with age. In addition, accurate blood pressure reading may be more difficult with a cuff sphygmomanometer due to stiffer and less compressible arteries. Clinically, these changes lead to a less compliant myocardium that is more intolerant of sudden increases and decreases in intravascular volume. Ventricular performance will also be more dependent on atrial systole for optimal filling of the stiffer ventricle. Changes in the conduction system and in ventricular function make the geriatric patient more likely to suffer from atrial fibrillation and less likely to tolerate it. Changes in diastolic function (i.e., active relaxation), combined with fibrosis and ventricular hypertrophy, lead to the need for increasing filling pressures. The geriatric patient will be more sensitive to loss or dyssynchrony of atrial systole. Loss of atrial "kick" or the presence of tachycardia will make it more difficult to achieve optimal diastolic filling pressures. Congestive heart failure is more common in the perioperative period in the geriatric population, especially in situations in which there are large or sudden changes in intravascular volume. Compensatory mechanisms that would be expected to preserve cardiac output, such as an increase in heart rate, become less vigorous with aging. Intravascular volume expansion may make the situation worse by dilating cardiac chambers beyond their optimal size. Decreases in blood pressure during induction of neuraxial or general anesthesia may be best treated in the geriatric population with vasopressors and smaller amounts of intravenous fluids.

In addition to an altered response to volume loading, there is a reduced response to inotropic, chronotropic, and vasopressor medications. Larger-than-expected doses of atropine, ephedrine, and phenylephrine may be needed to achieve an adequate effect. The negative consequences from hypotension in the geriatric population include decreases in postoperative mental status, reduced renal function, and myocardial injury. There is a rightward shift of vascular autoregulation. Consequently, more careful cardiovascular monitoring is often needed. It has been suggested that more routine use of arterial cannulation for blood pressure monitoring is indicated in the oldest group of patients—those age 80 and above—during the perioperative period.

CURRENT CONTROVERSY: IS MORE MONITORING BETTER?

Despite the expected problems that geriatric patients will have dealing with fluid shifts in the perioperative period, there is little evidence that invasive monitoring will change treatment or outcome. The routine use of arterial catheters has been advocated in those 80 years old and older having major surgery. Is more aggressive monitoring indicated in elderly outpatients for some outpatient surgeries?

Knowledge of age- and disease-related issues could be used to estimate cardiac risk during elective surgeries. Clinical predictors, functional status, and surgery-specific risk should be considered in calculating perioperative cardiac risk according to the American College of Cardiology guidelines (Boxes 11-1, 11-2). Some interventions may reduce overall risk. In a population at high risk for postoperative cardiac complications, β-blocker medications have been shown to reduce the incidence of postoperative myocardial ischemia and cardiac death. The timing, the route of administration, and the choice of medication may be less important than the initiation of the therapy itself. All of the following have produced significant reductions in cardiac morbidity and mortality: oral or intravenous β-blockers, initiation of therapy several weeks prior to or immediately prior to surgery, β-blockers given for 48 hours (versus 30 days) postsurgery, and medications titrated to heart rates from 50 to 80 beats per minute. The optimum plan has not yet been determined.

It is recommended that perioperative β-blocker therapy be initiated for patients with one major or two minor risk factors at least 7 days before surgery (Table 11-1). Initiation of preoperative β-blockade may reduce the need for noninvasive cardiac testing. This may not hold true for populations at higher risk who might benefit from further risk assessment and further evaluation. In addition, preoperative oral clonidine (2 μg/kg) may also be cardioprotective in patients who cannot tolerate β-blockers (Box 11-3).

Box 11-1 Perioperative Clinical Risk Factors

MAJOR RISK FACTORS

Acute or recent myocardial infarction with evidence of important ischemic risk by clinical symptoms or noninvasive study
Unstable or severe angina (Canadian class III or IV)
Decompensated heart failure
Significant arrhythmias
Severe vascular disease

INTERMEDIATE RISK FACTORS

Mild angina (Class I/II)
Previous myocardial infarction by history or pathological Q waves
Compensated or previous heart failure
Diabetes mellitus (particularly insulin-dependent)
Renal insufficiency

MINOR RISK FACTORS

Advanced age
Abnormal ECG (i.e., left ventricular hypertrophy, left bundle-branch block, or ST-T abnormalities)
Rhythm other than sinus (e.g., atrial fibrillation)
Low functional capacity (e.g., inability to climb one flight of stairs with a bag of groceries)
History of stroke
Uncontrolled systemic hypertension

Adapted from Eagle KA, Berger PB, Calkins H, et al: ACC/AHA Guideline Update for Perioperative Cardiovascular Evaluation for Noncardiac Surgery—Executive Summary. Anesth Analg 94:1052–1064, 2002.

Box 11-2 Perioperative Surgical Risk Factors

MAJOR RISK FACTORS

Emergency major surgery, especially in the elderly
Vascular surgery
Complex surgeries longer than 3 hours or with large fluid shifts

INTERMEDIATE RISK FACTORS

Carotid endarterectomy
Head and neck surgery
Abdominal surgery
Chest surgery
Orthopedic surgery
Prostate surgery

LOW RISK FACTORS

Endoscopic procedures
Superficial procedure
Cataract surgery
Breast surgery

Adapted from Eagle KA, Berger PB, Calkins H, et al: ACC/AHA Guideline Update for Perioperative Cardiovascular Evaluation for Noncardiac Surgery—Executive Summary. Anesth Analg 94:1052–1064, 2002.

Table 11-1 Indications for Initiation of Perioperative β-Blockers

Patients with One Risk Factor:

- CAD (including history of MI, history of current angina, use of sublingual nitroglycerine, positive exercise test results, Q waves on electrocardiogram, patients who have undergone angioplasty or coronary stenting or CABG who have angina)
- Cerebrovascular disease (history of CVA or TIA)
- Symptomatic cerebrovascular disease
- Serum creatinine level ≥2.0 mg/dL
- Diabetes mellitus (insulin-requiring)
- High-risk surgical procedure defined as intraperitoneal, intrathoracic, or suprainguinal vascular procedure

Patients with Any Two Risk Factors:

- Age ≥65
- Hypertension
- Current smoker
- Serum cholesterol level of at least 240 mg/dL
- Diabetes mellitus (noninsulin type)
- Positive family history of coronary artery disease

CABG, coronary artery bypass grafting; CAD, coronary artery disease; CVA, cerebrovascular accident; MI, myocardial infarction; TIA, transient ischemic attack.
Adapted from Auerbach AD, Goldman L: Beta-blockers and reduction of cardiac events in noncardiac surgery: Scientific review. JAMA 287:1435–1444, 2002.

Box 11-3 Clonidine

Clonidine (2 μg/kg, orally) can be used for patients who would benefit from β-blockers but might not tolerate them.

Preoperative coronary angioplasty, similarly to coronary bypass surgery, may reduce perioperative cardiac complications. However, both angioplasty and cardiac surgery groups may have restenosis of coronary arteries or grafts in the years after the procedures. The risk of cardiac complications after noncardiac surgery starts increasing 4 to 5 years after both coronary artery bypass surgery and coronary angioplasty. The medical history and preoperative physical exam should be used to assess the need for additional diagnostic testing. Patients may not be protected from coronary events if the interval between coronary intervention and surgery is prolonged. In addition, proceeding too soon after coronary intervention can also be dangerous. It is currently recommended to delay surgery at least 1 week after coronary angioplasty and 2 to 6 weeks after coronary artery stenting while continuing antiplatelet therapy. Early instability of coronary artery wall architecture may cause myocardial ischemia and infarction during perioperative stress. Drug-eluding coronary artery stents may require longer use of antiplatelet agents (3–6 months) after placement, further delaying effective surgery.

Chronic lipid-lowering therapy makes a significant difference in postoperative mortality in patients with elevated cholesterol. This may be due, in part, to the anti-inflammatory effects of 3-hydroxy-3-methylglutaryl coenzyme A (HMG-CoA) reductase inhibitors, also known as statins. Statin agents should usually be continued throughout the perioperative period since these drugs may reduce the incidence of perioperative myocardial infarction, similarly to β-blockers. It is unknown if anesthetics influence the occurrence of hepatic damage and myopathy, the known side effects of these drugs. Patients should be screened for statin myopathy syndromes preoperatively. Serum creatine kinase levels should be checked preoperatively in patients who are taking statins and who have myalgia symptoms.

Pulmonary Aging

With age, the thorax loses elasticity and becomes stiffer and rounder. These factors contribute to a marked increase in the work of breathing and increased expiratory time. Respiratory muscles become weaker and have less endurance and are not able to meet the increased demands expected during exercise or surgery. Forced expiratory volume in 1 second decreases about 9% per decade of life. The nongas exchange conducting airways increase in size with aging, and this contributes to an increase in dead space ventilation. The extent of these changes is highly variable.

Total lung capacity remains unchanged or decreases slowly with aging. Vital capacity will decline about 40 mL/yr in men and 31 mL/yr in women. Residual volume increases with age. Closing volume increases from 10% of total lung volume at age 20% to 30% at age 70. Therefore, in the fourth decade, closing volume will encroach on tidal volume breathing while supine and while upright beyond age 65. These adverse changes will be increased by anesthetic agents, postoperative narcotics, surgical positioning, and operations on the abdominal and thoracic cavities. Airway collapse and atelectasis must be anticipated and treated in elderly surgical patients. These unfavorable changes will be further accentuated by the existence of obesity, smoking, or airway disease.

There are age-associated decreases in the number of gas-exchange units, resulting in a decrease of 15% in functional alveolar surface area by age 70. Alveolar surface tension and forced expiratory flow are reduced. These changes, along with ventilation perfusion mismatching and increased physiologic dead space, are associated with an age-related decline in arterial oxygen tension. In addition, supplemental oxygen will be less effective at correcting this defect with aging. Arterial partial pressure of CO_2, owing to its greater solubility, will be unchanged. Ciliary function also decreases with age and contributes to the greater risk of postoperative pneumonia noted with increasing age.

Control of breathing is significantly altered with aging. Older patients have a diminished response to hypoxia and hypercapnia. This decrease in tidal volume is multifactorial but is believed to be due to altered receptor function. The perception of dyspnea remains intact, but the compensatory response seen in younger adults is reduced with aging.

Despite all of these unfavorable pulmonary changes seen with aging, chronologic age alone is considered a minor risk factor, conferring a two-fold increase in risk of pulmonary complications when compared to younger adults. Comorbidities, emphysema and bronchitis, current tobacco consumption, and poor functional status are important pulmonary risk factors for all age groups. In addition, the surgical site alone will be the single most significant risk factor, with thoracic and upper abdominal surgeries having the highest incidence of postoperative complications in all age groups.

Routine spirometry is not indicated. It may be useful in patients with known lung disease in whom new spirometry can be compared with previous test results. Pulmonary function testing may also be helpful in patients with unexplained dyspnea and exercise intolerance. Incentive spirometry, coughing and deep breathing, and optimization of anti-inflammatory and bronchodilator agents are allimportant for patients at high risk for postoperative pulmonary complications. Perioperative medications such as opioids and muscle relaxants will diminish the older patient's pulmonary reserve.

Elderly patients who are dyspneic may have difficulty lying supine. If there is any question whether an elderly patient can undergo even a simple procedure such as cataract extraction under local anesthesia, ask the patient to lie in the supine position for the expected duration of the procedure.

Gastrointestinal and Nutritional Issues

There is a 40% loss in hepatic mass by age 80, with a corresponding decrease in hepatic and splanchnic blood flow. A decrease in hepatic regenerative capacity is seen

with aging, making the older patient less likely to recover after a viral, medication-related, or toxic liver injury. There should normally be no age-related change in hepatic function, but the geriatric surgery patient will have less reserve and will be more sensitive to medications that are metabolized and excreted by the liver.

The elderly may have decreased food intake involving both micro (e.g., vitamin E and calcium) and macro (i.e., protein) nutrients. This may be due to living alone or to inadequate income as well as to associated disease such as cancer or diabetes mellitus. Polypharmacy may affect appetite and, combined with age-related reduced taste sensation and a decreased ability to chew, may further reduce food intake. Activity level often decreases with age and infirmity; there will be an associated gain in weight and in the proportion of fat in the geriatric patient. Basal metabolic rate is estimated to decline 1% per year after age 30. Although baseline nutritional deficiency and subsequent low serum albumen levels are associated with poor operative outcomes, there is not yet convincing evidence that acutely correcting these problems before a planned surgery leads to better outcomes.

CURRENT CONTROVERSY: SHOULD NUTRITIONAL ABNORMALITIES BE CORRECTED BEFORE ELECTIVE SURGERY?

Despite evidence that nutritional deficits (e.g., low serum albumin) are correlated with poor operative outcomes, there is no convincing evidence that delaying surgery to correct this problem improves outcomes. Should we consider delaying minor surgery while correcting nutritional deficits?

Body stores of calories (i.e., fat and muscle), protein (i.e., muscle), and calcium (i.e., bones) should be considered when deciding how to handle starvation in the perioperative period. Catabolism should be anticipated and treatment initiated early and aggressively. Patients in poor health may have problems if oral intake is restricted. Dehydration from prolonged fasting may also be a problem.

The National Surgical Quality Improvement Program, an ongoing study of surgical outcomes in the Veterans Administration Healthcare System, has shown that as preoperative albumin levels decrease, there is an exponential increase in morbidity (10% to 65%) and mortality (1% to 29%). A 1.0-mg/dL drop in serum albumin concentration was associated with a two-fold increase in the risk of postoperative complications and death. Hypoalbuminemia was a better predictor of perioperative sepsis and major infections than other risk factors such as American Society of Anesthesiologists (ASA) physical status, blood urea nitrogen (BUN) level, functional status, or age, even in a low-risk population. A low total serum cholesterol level has also been identified as a predictor of postoperative morbidity.

Assessment and postoperative correction of nutritional deficits may have a significant effect on outcomes. An aggressive multidisciplinary approach to perioperative nutrition may reduce postoperative complications, even in the outpatient surgery setting.

Genitourinary Aging

There is a progressive 0.5% to 1.0% per year loss of cortical nephrons beginning at age 30. This decline in functioning glomeruli and glomerular filtration rate is not reflected in serum creatinine levels despite a 30% to 50% drop in creatinine clearance by age 65. The unchanged serum creatinine level is attributed to a decline in skeletal muscle mass and reduced excretion of muscle breakdown products that parallels the loss of kidney function. While moderately decreased renal function ordinarily has little effect on the geriatric patient, it can have significant implications when using medications in the perioperative period. It is recommended that estimated or measured creatinine clearance be used as a guide in dosing medication eliminated by the kidneys.

There is a slower and less complete renal and pituitary response to dehydration. The ability to concentrate urine, to conserve free water, and to handle fluid and electrolyte administration is altered. In addition, thirst is not as accurate an indicator of dehydration in the geriatric population. Younger patients without cardiovascular disease can tolerate significant and sudden changes in blood volume without obvious hemodynamic perturbation. This is not true for older patients, who are less able to compensate for intraoperative and postoperative volume shifts. Careful monitoring of volume status is necessary to avoid hypovolemia or hypervolemia. Finally, there may not be adequate renal reserve function to meet the increased metabolic demands of the perioperative period, with acute renal failure responsible for at least 20% of postoperative mortality in the geriatric population.

Bladder capacity is diminished in the aged individual, causing problems with nocturia and sleep dysfunction. Incontinence is not considered a normal part of aging, and its presence should be investigated. Urinary tract infections are more common and may present in more subtle ways, including mental status changes, in older populations. Routine urinalysis and urine cultures are not justified in the elderly, despite this age group having more frequent infections. A major goal of ambulatory anesthetic and surgical planning should be the preservation of urinary continence.

Nervous System Aging

There is a gradual and inexorable loss of neurons with aging, with a decline of up to 30% of gross brain weight by age 80. The proportion of the cranial vault occupied by the brain drops from 92% to 82%. The extra volume is replaced by cerebral spinal fluid, but this makes the aging population particularly susceptible to acute and chronic subdural hematoma formation after even minor trauma. Cerebral blood flow also decreases by 15% to 20%. There is a generalized depletion of neurotransmitters due to a reduced synthesis and an accelerated destruction. The more metabolically active and specialized neurons are the most susceptible to age-related loss. There is reported to be a 50% loss of neurons in the cerebral and cerebellar cortices, the locus ceruleus, the thalamus, and the basal ganglion, with the remaining synapses becoming markedly simplified. Peripheral nerve fibers, axons, and afferent and efferent nerve conduction velocity all decrease. Plasma epinephrine and norepinephrine levels decline in association with a reduction in autonomic activity. Efferent motor pathway signal velocity declines by 0.15 m/sec/yr. This, combined with slower corticospinal transmission, yields a slower initiation of voluntary motor activity.

Despite these changes, intelligence and memory should be grossly unchanged in healthy patients well into the geriatric period. The progressive decline in nervous system function associated with age will compromise reserve capacity but generally may not be apparent during normal daily function. It has recently been shown that chronic hypertension is associated with cognitive decline in the elderly. Since the brain is the target organ system for many of the anesthetic agents and medications given in the postoperative period, including opioids, changes in nervous system reserve and function with aging are important.

CLINICAL CAVEAT

Memory and intelligence do not change as a function of aging in healthy patients. Therefore, problems with mental function should be considered pathologic and need to be investigated.

Functional Status

While there is no specific biochemical or genetic marker that can be used to quantify the condition of aging, it is the decline in functional status that is most readily apparent. All the senses become less acute with increasing age. Short-term memory, new learning, visual and auditory reaction times, and visual-spatial coordination also become slower with aging. Maximal exercise capacity decreases, but this decline can be attenuated with conditioning, diet and medication, or nutritional supplement therapies. Diseases that compromise function, such as rheumatoid arthritis, osteoarthritis, or Parkinson's disease, are more frequent. It is important that the anesthesiologist has a realistic assessment of the reserve capacity required to meet the stress of surgery.

Poor preoperative functional status has been shown to be a more significant risk factor for postoperative complications than age alone. Patient self-reporting of exercise capacity in a preoperative evaluation clinic can predict cardiac and other major complications. In addition to patient self-reporting, simple testing (such as maximal hand grip) may correlate with postoperative outcome. In a study relating preoperative function with postoperative outcome, patients were asked to climb a hospital stairway as far as possible. The number of stairs climbed was a stronger predictor of 30-day postoperative cardiopulmonary complications than age, preexisting pulmonary disease, weight, or spirometry. No patient who could climb seven flights of stairs had a complication, while eight of nine patients who could not climb one flight of stairs did have a complication (Table 11-2).

Immune System Aging

There is a decline in immunologic function associated with aging, but these changes are difficult to quantify. Depressed immune and inflammatory function has a number of clinical implications, including an increased incidence of cancer, a delayed presentation of a myocardial infarction, an infection, or a ruptured abdominal organ. There is no simple way to measure the reserve capacity of the immune system or the expected response to the stress of surgery. The presence of malnutrition may be indirectly reflected in low serum albumin, prealbumin, or cholesterol blood levels. Unfortunately, short-term correction of the nutritional deficit has not been shown to produce improved operative outcomes.

Dietary antioxidants such as vitamin E and polyphenol may enhance immune response, delay the onset of Alzheimer's disease, reduce viral titers, and reduce the expression of proinflammatory cytokines by endothelial cells. These agents may promote immune responses and may have favorable effects on both the development and the course of cardiovascular disease and cancers. Patients may be self-administering large amounts of vitamin E, vitamin C, and nutraceuticals such as turmeric, ginger, and green teas. Consumption of these substances will be on the rise as baby boomers age and search for mechanisms to slow or reverse the aging process. Current preoperative practice recommends discontinuing herbal agents and vitamins 7 to 14 days before surgery. In the future, some of these agents may actually play a role in promoting better outcomes and, rather than being discontinued, could be part of perioperative care.

PREOPERATIVE PREPARATION AND OPTIMIZATION

During the ambulatory preoperative preparation period, special emphasis should be placed on the cardiovascular, pulmonary, and nervous systems. These are the systems most directly affected by anesthetic agents and medications in the perioperative period. The preoperative evaluation process is an excellent opportunity for health screening and a key time to counsel patients concerning lifestyle risk modification. However, long-term health maintenance is not the primary focus of the preoperative process. While chronic medical problems must never be ignored, resources should be directed toward issues that will make a difference in the planning for anesthesia and surgery. For

---

Table 11-2   Evaluation of Functional Status: The Duke Activity Status Index

Activity: Can you . . .	Estimated Metabolic Cost of Each Activity (MET Units)
Walk indoors (e.g., around your house)?	1.75
Do light work around the house, such as dusting or washing dishes?	2.70
Take care of yourself in terms of eating, dressing, bathing, and using the toilet?	2.75
Walk a block or two on level ground?	2.75
Do moderate work around the house, such as vacuuming, sweeping floors, or carrying in groceries?	3.50
Do yard work, such as raking leaves, weeding, or pushing a power mower?	4.50
Have sexual relations?	5.25
Climb a flight of stairs or walk up a hill?	5.50
Participate in moderate recreational activities, such as golf, bowling, dancing, doubles tennis, or throwing a baseball or football?	6.00
Participate in strenuous sports, such as swimming, singles tennis, football, basketball, or skiing?	7.50
Do heavy work around the house, such as scrubbing floors or lifting or moving heavy furniture?	8.00
Run a short distance?	8.00

Adapted from Hlatky MA, Boineau RE, Higginbotham MB, et al: A brief self-administered questionnaire to determine functional capacity (The Duke Activity Status Index). Am J Cardiol 64:651, 1989.

example, while long-term health and quality of life will be assisted by testing for hyperlipidemia, an abnormal result is unlikely to change anesthesia planning for a scheduled procedure. It is controversial whether to perform preoperative testing based on chronologic age alone. An exception may be the electrocardiogram, which appears to be cost-effective as a screening tool in a population over 40 to 50 years old. The primary principle is that positive findings during the medical history and physical exam should guide the choice of laboratory and diagnostic testing.

The anesthesia preoperative process is most focused on short-term perioperative stability. Limited resources must be directed to maximizing good outcomes in the first days to weeks. A patient with stable angina and well-preserved exercise tolerance (i.e., 5 metabolic equivalents [METS] or more) may eventually need a follow-up cardiac stress test, although perhaps not before a cataract procedure under local anesthesia. The preoperative process should be concerned with a realistic estimation of risk and optimization of comorbid conditions. Guidelines such as those published by the American Society of Anesthesiologists, the American College of Cardiology, the American Heart Association, and the American College of Physicians are helpful in directing patients into groups requiring more cardiac evaluation.

Laboratory and Diagnostic Workup

An electrocardiogram (ECG) is a generally agreed-upon useful screening tool for surgical patients older than 40 to 50 years of age. In the geriatric population, as many as 25% of resting ECGs will show new changes when compared with previous normal tracings. ECGs are neither sensitive nor specific without clinical correlation, however. For example, 25% of ECGs will be normal in an older population with other clinical evidence of ischemic myocardial disease. There may be an unacceptable high rate of interpreted errors when anesthesiologists, not cardiologists, interpret ECGs.

There is up to a 30% incidence of chest x-ray abnormalities in asymptomatic older patients. Despite this high rate of abnormal findings, screening chest radiography is rarely indicated if the medical history and physical exam do not yield evidence that underlying pulmonary pathology would change the anesthetic or surgical plan of care. Spirometry appears to be useful only for surgery directly involved with lung resection or when following significant chronic obstructive pulmonary disease (COPD) and other airway diseases.

Smoking Cessation

Although current cigarette smoking is a major risk factor for postoperative pulmonary complications, causing as much as a four-fold increase in risk, smoking cessation pre-

operatively may not change these risks. One study of relatively healthy patients for hip and knee surgery with a mean age of 65 showed that interventions that began 6 to 8 weeks before surgery did not reduce postoperative pulmonary complications.[1] Other studies have shown smoking cessation within 1 to 2 months of surgery may paradoxically increase pulmonary complications.[2,3] Smoking is a chronic inflammatory disease; months of tobacco abstinence are required before a favorable change in preoperative risk is observed.

CLINICAL CAVEAT

The preoperative process should be used as an additional counseling opportunity for smoking cessation. When making interventions before scheduled surgery, however, both the patient and the operative team should realize that several months of smoking cessation are needed to see a difference in surgical outcomes.

Coagulation Changes

Imbalances in the coagulation cascade associated with the perioperative period cause increased morbidity and mortality. Aging is associated with a relative increase in coagulation risk, manifested by myocardial infarction, venous thrombosis, and pulmonary emboli. Dietary consumption of fish and fish oil, vitamins, herbs, and medications may modify coagulation risk. The perioperative period is often associated with a hypercoagulable state. However, pharmaceuticals and nutraceuticals that interfere with coagulation are commonly stopped in the preoperative period. With the elderly, a risk-to-benefit approach should be taken, considering individual patient needs and procedure requirements before discontinuing all substances that slow coagulation. For example, case reports have documented coronary stent blockage and fatal postoperative myocardial infarction after antiplatelet agents were prematurely discontinued. In addition, recent research shows that aspirin that is continued up to the time of coronary artery surgery might better preserve neutrophil function. Of course, the favorable effects of these drugs must be balanced against the increased risk of surgical bleeding and the need to discontinue some anticoagulants prior to neuraxial anesthesia. Ambulatory surgery would likely have more types of minor surgery that may allow continuation of at least some anticoagulant and antiplatelet medications throughout the perioperative period.

Diabetes Mellitus

Most patients with diabetes mellitus (DM) in the geriatric population are insulin-resistant or type 2, with native insulin secretion adequate to avoid ketoacidosis. A newer trend is insulin treatment of an increasing number of type 2 patients. Evidence is accumulating that improved serum glucose control will limit long-term diabetic complications. In addition, tighter perioperative serum glucose control has been shown to significantly reduce complications after high-risk surgeries. The presumption is that patients having lower-risk surgeries may benefit as well. It has traditionally been recommended to withhold morning oral diabetes medications and to use half the usual intermediate duration insulin amount on the day of surgery. More aggressive therapy, including the use of insulin infusions or full amounts of long-acting glargine insulin and frequent glucose monitoring, is necessary to achieve normal serum glucose levels. Short ambulatory procedures, with rapid return of oral food intake, probably allow less disruption of antidiabetic medication schedules and drug amounts. It is important, however, that providers understand that a rapid discharge home puts the burden of postoperative diabetes management entirely on the elderly diabetic patient.

Medication Management

If elderly patients have had the treatment of their medical problems optimized before surgery, then almost all of their usual medications should be dosed as per the regular schedule. In general, antihypertensive medications should be continued to ensure blood pressure control and to avoid rebound effects with abrupt drug discontinuation. However, long-acting angiotensin-converting enzyme inhibitor and angiotensin receptor blocker medications increase the incidence of intraoperative hypotension. Some practitioners prefer to withhold these medications prior to general anesthetics. Adverse rebound effects are associated with withdrawal of medications such as clonidine and β-blockers, and this effect may also be present after discontinuation of cholesterol-lowering statins. It has been reported that patients hospitalized after myocardial infarctions have increased mortality if statins are withdrawn.

CLINICAL CAVEAT

If elderly patients have been optimally prepared for surgery, continue their medication management with as little disturbance as possible during the perioperative period.

ANESTHETIC CONSIDERATIONS

The aging nervous system requires smaller amounts of anesthetic agents. This is true with sedation, general, or regional anesthesia. Individualized ambulatory anesthetic plans should be based on an understanding of how current comorbidities and therapies affect each geriatric patient. Specifically, the goals for the ambulatory geriatric patient are to avoid detrimental cardiorespiratory complications, to prevent postoperative delirium and postoperative cognitive dysfunction (POCD), to maintain urinary continence, to provide postoperative analgesia, and to return the patient to baseline function at home as soon as possible.

What is the ideal anesthetic technique for ambulatory surgery in the geriatric patient? There is little evidence-based information that indicates a clear preference for one anesthetic technique over another. Many anesthesiologists, internists, and surgeons have a bias toward local anesthesia with sedation, when possible, in frail patients. Neuraxial and regional anesthesia has also often been promoted as a better option for improved outcomes and a rapid return to baseline functioning. There is some limited evidence to support the use of regional anesthesia in high-risk groups, including older patients, for peripheral surgery. More studies are needed to define the optimum anesthetic for geriatric ambulatory patients.

Increased latency of effect and increased effect of almost all intravenous anesthetic agents should be expected. In the elderly, propofol and thiopental may produce similar changes in heart rate and blood pressure during induction of general anesthesia, but these changes are of greater magnitude than in the young. Postoperative wakefulness, mental orientation, and return to baseline Aldrete recovery scores are faster after propofol. However, total postanesthesia recovery time after propofol induction is comparable to that after thiopental use. Etomidate has less effect on the cardiovascular system but has more emetic events.

Metabolism of longer-acting benzodiazepines increases with age. This will make certain agents, especially those with active metabolites such as diazepam, less suitable in the older patient. Midazolam can be useful when rapid return to baseline function is desired, but it should be titrated slowly to avoid overdosage.

The initial dose of muscle relaxants does not change with age, but the dosing interval often increases, especially if relaxant elimination is based on hepatic or renal clearance.

Likewise, smaller amounts of intra- and postoperative opioids will be needed due to slower metabolism and excretion. Long-acting opioids and opioids combining agonist and antagonist activity increase the risk of delirium and problems with balance and ambulation. Dosing of remifentanil and alfentanil should be started at 50% of the dose used in younger adults.

Hypotension after spinal anesthesia is more common in the geriatric population than in younger adults. Hypotension is more dramatic and may cause more problems due to the presence of coronary artery and other vascular disease. Intravenous fluid loading before spinal anesthesia does not reliably prevent blood pressure decline. Early intervention with vasoactive drugs is often necessary. Peripheral nerve blocks result in lowered perioperative stress than general anesthetics and have the advantage of providing prolonged analgesia into the postoperative period, facilitating early discharge home.

CURRENT CONTROVERSY: IS REGIONAL ANESTHESIA BETTER FOR OLDER PATIENTS?

After decdes of investigation, there is still not convincing proof that regional anesthesia and postoperative analgesia have improved outcome over general anesthesia and parenteral or oral analgesia anesthesia to make the ambulatory process smoother and perhaps, safer for geriatric patients

---

Reduced cardiac output shortens uptake time for volatile anesthetics and, combined with positive pressure ventilation, could produce greater hypotension. There may be prolonged recovery from volatile anesthetics, and even nitrous oxide can have a prolonged effect on memory and cognition. However, one study failed to demonstrate decreased recovery time or a reduction in POCD when seroflurance was supplemented with incremental doses of remifentanil for geriatric patients.[4]

General anesthesia performed with both volatile anesthetics and intravenous medications seems safe for the geriatric patient. In a large study, total intravenous anesthesia using fentanyl, ketamine, and propofol was administered to patients as old as 92 years of age. No cardiac complications that could be directly attributed to the anesthetics alone were noted after following 26,079 patients for 3 months postoperatively.[5] In another study, postanesthesia care unit (PACU) stay was not shortened when remifentanil was compared with isoflurane for maintenance of general anesthesia in patients older than age 75.[6] However, isoflurane was associated with significantly lower Mini-Mental Status scores for the first 12 hours after surgery than was remifentanil. Small studies have shown early and transient cognitive dysfunction after general anesthesia that returned to baseline by the second or third postoperative day. However, these differences were only apparent after complex mental testing and were not easily detected on casual exam.

There may be a role for neurologic level-of-consciousness monitoring in the geriatric population having general anesthesia. One study linked significantly greater long-term postoperative mortality after general anesthetics when Bispectral Analysis Scores were below 40 than in patients whose intraoperative scores were in the 40 to 60 range.[7]

No cause-and-effect relationship has yet been determined, and this study has been criticized for methdological flows. Nonetheless, the altered autonomic response to surgical stimulation in the elderly may make level-of-consciousness monitoring more useful than in other age groups.

INTRAOPERATIVE AND POSTOPERATIVE CONSIDERATIONS

Older patients are more likely to lose heat and to have less ability to regenerate lost heat during the perioperative period. The rate of intraoperative core body temperature loss in older adults, 1° C/hr, is twice that of younger adults. Adequate body covering should be combined with active convection warming systems when needed. Keeping patients warm should be a multidisciplinary concern. Intraoperative hypothermia increases the risk of infection, altered drug metabolism, and cardiac complications.

Careful perioperative positioning is critical to prevent skin, nerve, muscle, and bone injuries in the elderly. Fragile tissue and bones can be more easily injured when positioning the older patient.

Early ambulation is essential when attempting to return geriatric ambulatory patients to their home environment. Immobility after surgery will increase the likelihood of pressure ulcer formation. Immobility also increases bone resorption and the risk of future fractures. There is an increased risk of atelectasis, aspiration, and pneumonia. In addition, the risk of venous stasis, clot formation, and embolization will increase. Generalized deconditioning, anorexia, and constipation in the postoperative period will also improve with ambulation. Allowing retention or early return of glasses, hearing aids, and dentures can facilitate ambulation and communication, preserve cognitive orientation, and enhance a sense of dignity in the postoperative period.

A rapid return to baseline bowel and bladder function is important to the elderly. Opioids can produce debilitating constipation. Many perianesthetic medications can cause urinary retention, especially in males with prostatic hypertrophy. Although there has been a trend to not require postoperative voiding in outpatients, the elderly may not be appropriate candidates for this practice in many situations.

Delirium and Postoperative Cognitive Dysfunction

Alterations in mental function are often significant issues in the geriatric patient. Medications such as cholinesterase inhibitors are often used in the memory-impaired patient. These agents can interact with medications used during anesthesia and for postoperative pain control. Even if the patient does not have a preexisting cognitive deficit, both short- and long-term mental status changes may occur after surgery and anesthesia. There is evidence that elderly outpatients tend to have better mental function than elderly inpatients. In patients who were judged to be functioning normally before surgery, POCD and new-onset postoperative delirium occurred in 5% to 20% of patients over age 70 and in 30% to 50% of those over age 80. As many as 10% to 13% of surgical patients older than 60 experience POCD 3 months after noncardiac surgery, with an incidence of over 41% after orthopedic surgery.

Both short- and long-term mental status changes are associated with increased postoperative morbidity and mortality, as is the lowered likelihood of returning to independent functioning. These deleterious changes represent a potential problem with ambulatory surgical and anesthetic management. In addition, many patients judged as functioning normally at home may have been living on a functional cliff that was uncovered by the stress of surgery and anesthesia. A 2004 multicenter report by Canet et al.[8] showed less cognitive dysfunction for elderly patients undergoing minor surgery under general anesthesia as outpatients versus as inpatients.

Delirium is defined as an acute disruption of attention and cognition, a reduced ability to concentrate, and impaired consciousness. Postoperative delirium is positively associated with age greater than 70 years, preexisting cognitive and functional impairment, a history of delirium in the past, and preoperative alcohol or opioid use. Postoperative delirium is associated with increases in major complications such as myocardial infarction, pneumonia, respiratory failure, and death. Significantly greater surgical facility and nursing resources will be needed to care for these patients. Postoperative delirium will also significantly increase total care charges because of extended stays and increased use of consultant services. Studies have shown an increased incidence of delirium after receiving volatile anesthetic agents (especially high levels) and centrally acting anticholinergic medications. Previous associations of delirium with intraoperative and postoperative hypotension and hypoxia have been challenged.

The best prevention may be preoperative recognition of high-risk individuals and early intervention. Preventive measures should include frequent orientation to time, place, and circumstance, including the use of larger clocks and calendars. Minimizing physical and chemical restraints, rapid mobilization and feeding, and the immediate postoperative use of glasses and hearing aids may assist in the prevention of delirium. The use of drugs such as droperidol that impair early mobilization will delay return to preoperative functioning, especially for patients with Parkinson's disease.

Cognitive dysfunction describes the spectrum of changes in mental functions ranging from subtle changes in memory and personality to a complete loss of the skills that are needed to live independently. It is easier to define and quantify POCD in studies that use formal mental status exams. Geriatric patients may only appear confused due to hearing and visual defects secondary to the removal of glasses and hearing aids. In addition, older patients may need more time to recall and describe events. POCD significantly increases perioperative costs by increasing the length of stay and increasing consultant and nursing costs. POCD increases with age, affecting more than a quarter of those age 90 or older. It appears to be transient in younger adults, resolving within 3 months in the 40 to 59 age group, but is more persistent in older patients. At 1 week, 26% of older patients have POCD, 10% have it after 3 months, and, in 1%, it is permanent.

There are specific and easily applied tests (i.e., the Activity Scale, the Confusion Assessment Method, and the Mini-Mental State) that can be used to evaluate patients for POCD in the preoperative period if needed. In addition, computerized testing may be faster and better in assessing preoperative baseline functioning. The preoperative anesthesia visit is an excellent opportunity to obtain a picture of the patient's level of function, both from patient self-reporting and from family members.

Just as the level of the patient's preoperative physical condition helps estimate the patient's functional reserve for postoperative stresses, preoperative mental assessment can assist in predicting if the ambulatory geriatric patient will be able to recover with a return to his or her preoperative cognitive level. After this assessment, a decision should be made about the patient's suitability for the ambulatory pathway (Box 11-4).

A presumed link between postoperative hypotension and hypoxia with POCD has been questioned. One group found that the presence of abnormally low blood pressure and pulse oximetry reading in the initial 72 hours after surgery failed to correlate with long-term cognitive dysfunction.[9] A study reported using hypoten-

---

Box 11-4   Drugs to Treat Alzheimer's Disease that Are Being Increasingly Used in the Elderly

Aricept (donepezil): Inactivates acetylcholinesterase
Cognex (tacrine): Inactivates acetylcholinesterase
Exelon (rivastigmine): Inactivates acetylcholinesterase
Reminyl (galantamine): Inactivates acetylcholinesterase
Namenda (Memantine): N-methyl-D-aspartate receptor antagonist

sive epidural anesthesia with a mean blood pressure as low as 45 to 55 mm Hg; they showed no increase in expected rates of POCD in a hip replacement surgery population with a mean age of 72 years.[10] These patients also had central venous monitoring or pulmonary artery catheters in place and low-dose epinephrine infusions to preserve cardiac output, therapy not likely to be used in outpatients.

A recent meta-analysis found that intraoperative use of neuraxial anesthesia did not reduce the incidence of POCD when compared with general anesthesia.[11] Despite these findings, regional anesthesia and analgesia is still often recommended as a favorable anesthetic alternative in a population with baseline cognitive dysfunction or for those who are at high risk for delirium in the postoperative period.

Do-Not-Resuscitate Status

Many older patients have decided they do not want extraordinary interventions that might prolong a poor

---

CLINICAL CAVEAT

There is no way to eliminate the risk of postoperative delirium and POCD. However, the following can be recommended:

Avoid:	Use:
• Long-acting medications	• Local anesthesia (when possible)
• Anticholinergic medications that cross the blood-brain barrier	• Regional anesthesia and analgesia
• Agonist/antagonist opioids	• Shorter-acting medications (e.g., remifentanil, sevoflurane, and desflurane)
• Meperidine	
• Long-acting opioids (when possible)	

---

quality life. Any care-limiting decision must be discussed with the geriatric patient (or, as appropriate, their guardian or family) during the preoperative process, and a specific plan for acceptable treatment must be defined. As a rule, it is reasonable to ask permission to treat problems that are temporary, that are related to the procedure, and for which acute interventions have a reasonable chance of returning the patient to preoperative quality of life. Patients with do-not-resuscitate (DNR) orders in place preoperatively should not be denied surgery. However, it is essential to have a preoperative plan since studies have shown that patients with DNR decisions appear to have an increased risk of cardiopulmonary arrest in the perioperative period. The discussion that takes place between the surgeon, the anesthesiologist, and the patient must

be clearly documented in the medical record before proceeding with surgery.

Postoperative Pain Management

Age by itself does not lessen the pain associated with surgery. Postoperative pain is of the same intensity in the geriatric population as it is after surgeries in younger adults. Dementia and difficulty with patient communication do not lessen the physical and mental burden that postoperative pain places on the older patient. Pain should be anticipated and treated.

There are many physiologic concerns after ambulatory surgery in the geriatric population that argue for effective pain control. Untreated or undertreated postoperative pain is an important issue in older patients with limited functional reserve. For example, pain can increase myocardial oxygen consumption and decrease coronary perfusion in a population already at risk for myocardial ischemia. Pain increases sympathetic output, and this can lead to cardiac arrhythmias, peripheral vasoconstriction, and enhanced platelet aggregation. In addition, acute pain, such as seen after surgery, frequently leads to the development of persistent pain that could be avoided by aggressive efforts to provide analgesia in the immediate postoperative period.

As they are with younger adults, opioids are a mainstay of treatment for pain in the geriatric population. In an ambulatory setting, however, opioid-associated side effects of nausea and vomiting, urinary retention, problems with balance and ambulation, and respiratory depression may delay discharge or necessitate inpatient admission. A multimodal plan that judiciously uses opioids but includes surgical-site local anesthetics, nonsteroidal anti-inflammatory drugs (NSAIDs), and regional analgesia allows for the rapid return of older patients to their ambulatory baseline status.

NSAIDs, either alone or as part of a multimodal approach to pain control, are effective analgesics after both major and minor surgery. NSAIDs can significantly reduce the requirement for opioid analgesics. In one study, discharge time was shortened after anorectal surgery or hernia repair by the use of postoperative NSAIDs. Preoperative administration of NSAIDs has been shown to reduce postoperative pain and to shorten significantly the time to discharge. However, preoperative use has not been shown to lead to speedy return to baseline activity after surgery. As a caution, elderly patients may have diminished renal function, which may be further decreased with NSAIDs. Increases in intravascular volume, secondary to NSAID effects on sodium and water excretion, may exacerbate hypertension or precipitate congestive heart failure.

NSAID use in the elderly also increases the risk of gastrointestinal bleeding.

The use of cyclooxygenase-2 (COX-2) selective inhibitors has several theoretical advantages over nonselective NSAIDs. COX-2 agents do not interfere with platelet function, unlike nonselective NSAIDs; this difference may decrease intra- and postoperative bleeding with COX-2 drugs. Gastrointestinal bleeding associated with nonselective NSAIDs may also be reduced with COX-2 agents. Potential problems with COX-2 use include increased costs, lack of a parenteral preparation in the United States, and a possible increased incidence of thrombotic events.

A meta-analysis comparing COX-2 inhibitors to nonselective NSAIDs found that rofecoxib (50 mg) and parecoxib (40 mg) were equipotent. The COX-2 agents were at least as effective as nonselective NSAIDs but appear to have a longer duration of analgesia after dental surgery. Celecoxib (200 mg) and lower doses of parecoxib (20 mg) were not as effective as analgesics compared to other COX-2 agents. In addition, rofecoxib (50 mg) was judged more effective than even 200 mg of celecoxib. The withdrawal of rofecoxib from the world market has caused concern that COX-2 inhibitor agents, as a class, may have adverse thrombogenic consequences, at least during chronic use. COX-2 use after cardiac surgery may actually increase complications, including death. It is uncertain if short-term COX-2 use will remain an acceptable indication.

Continuation of central neuraxial anesthesia used for surgery provides excellent postoperative analgesia but will not usually be an option in the ambulatory setting. Local anesthetics can interfere with ambulation and hemodynamic stability. Urinary retention and respiratory depression are risks when neuraxial opioids are used. Peripheral nerve blocks, by either single injection or continuous infusion, are an excellent alternative for postoperative analgesia. For example, a femoral nerve block using a single injection or catheter technique can provide effective analgesia after knee surgery. These techniques can reduce the use of systemic medications that often cause sedation, ambulation difficulty, and confusion in the elderly.

FUTURE ISSUES

Just as pediatric patients are now seen as more than small adults, geriatric patients should not be viewed simply as older adults. The increasing numbers of elderly patients, combined with expanding surgical options, argue for consideration of geriatrics as a separate subspecialty of both anesthesia and surgery. Other disciplines, including internal medicine and psychiatry, have already established expertise in the area of geriatric practice. One of the roadblocks to selective care of geriatric patients is the nature of scheduling operative patients. A study examined the distribution of physiologically complex surgeries in patients aged 80 and older in Iowa, comparing these to similar surgical care for infants and young children. The authors noted that while pediatric surgery in Iowa was concentrated in three hospitals, geriatric care was administered in most centers throughout the state.[12]

Even patients 100 years old and older can be expected to survive without major complications when they are carefully selected and prepared for certain surgeries. Surgery should not be denied due to age alone. While the decline in organ function associated with aging has been judged as both natural and inexorable, this may not always be true. Studies involving long-term calorie restriction in animals have shown that some of the natural changes seen with aging can be slowed or avoided. The promotion of anti-aging and wellness with both traditional and complimentary medical therapy is increasing as the population ages. These techniques often use diet and exercise, as well as vitamin, herbal, and pharmaceutical therapy, to reduce the internal and external manifestations of aging. Risk modification in older age groups may reduce the unfavorable changes of what is considered normal aging.

Ambulatory surgery for the geriatric patient may have once been considered a radical experiment, but now, with proper patient and procedure selection, it has been shown to be acceptably safe and effective.

CLINICAL CAVEAT

When selecting an opioid analgesic for the older surgical patient, consider the following:

- Hydromorphone is more potent than morphine and may be better tolerated (in the long-term) in the older patient.
- Oxycodone has fewer metabolites and side effects than codeine.
- A subset of patients (10%) may be deficient in CYP2D6 enzymes and may not metabolize codeine and codons to their active forms.
- Propoxyphene has a long half-life and a problematic metabolite, nor-propoxyphene.
- Meperidine should be avoided since its neurotoxic metabolite, nor-meperidine, can cause tremors and seizures.
- Agonist/antagonist use is associated with a high incidence of delirium in the geriatric population.

REFERENCES

1. Moller AM, Villebro N, Pedersen T, Tonnesen H: Effect of preoperative smoking intervention on postoperative complications: A randomized clinical trial. Lancet 359:114-117, 2002.

2. Sorensen LT, Jorgensen T: Short-term preoperative smoking cessation intervention does not affect postoperative complications in colorectal surgery: A randomized clinical trial. Colorectal Disease 5:347-352, 2003.

3. Vaporciyan AA, Merriman KW, Ece F, et al: Incidence of major pulmonary morbidity after pneumonectomy: Association with timing of smoking cessation. Ann Thorac Surg 73:420-425; discussion 425-426, 2002.

4. Breslin DS, Reid JE, Mirakhur RK, et al: Sevoflurane—nitrous oxide anaesthesia supplemented with remifentanil: Effect on recovery and cognitive function. Anaesthesia 56:114-119, 2001.

5. Matsuki A, Ishihara H, Kotani N, et al: A clinical study of total intravenous anesthesia by using mainly propofol, fentanyl and ketamine—with special reference to its safety based on 26,079 cases. Masui—Japanese Journal of Anesthesiology 51:1336-1342, 2002.

6. Bekker AY, Berklayd P, Osborn I, et al: The recovery of cognitive function after remifentanil-nitrous oxide anesthesia is faster than after an isoflurane-nitrous oxide-fentanyl combination in elderly patients. Anesth Analg 91:117-122, 2000.

7. Monk TG, Saini V, Weldon BC, Sigl JC: Anesthetic management and one-year mortality after noncardiac surgery. Anesth Analg 100:4-10, 2005.

8. Canet J, Raeder J, Rasmussen LS, et al: ISPOCD2 investigators. Cognitive dysfunction after minor surgery in the elderly. Acta Anaesth Scand 47:1204-1210, 2003.

9. Moller JT, Cluitmans P, Rasmussen LS, et al: Long-term postoperative cognitive dysfunction in the elderly ISPOCD1 study. ISPOCD investigators. International Study of Postoperative Cognitive Dysfunction. Lancet. 351:857-861, 1998.

10. Williams-Russo P, Sharrock NE, Mattis S, et al: Randomized trial of hypotensive epidural anesthesia in older adults. Anesthesiology 91:926-935, 1999.

11. Wu CL, Hsu W, Richman JM, Raja SN: Postoperative cognitive function as an outcome of regional anesthesia and analgesia. Reg Anesth Pain Med 29:257-268, 2004.

12. Wachtel RE, Dexter F: Differentiating among hospitals performing physiologically complex operative procedures in the elderly. Anesthesiology 100:1552-1561, 2004.

SUGGESTED READING

Auroy Y, Narchi P, Messiah A, et al: Serious complications related to anesthesia: Results of a prospective survey in France. Anesthesiology 87:479-486, 1997.

Chen X, Zhao M, White PF: The recovery of cognitive function after general anesthesia in elderly patients: A comparison of desflurane and sevoflurane. Anesth Analg 93:1489-1494, 2001.

Cook DJ, Rooke GA: Priorities in perioperative geriatrics. Anesth Analg 96:1823-1836, 2003.

Kaplan GA, Haan MN, Wallace RB: Understanding changing risk factor associations with increasing age in adults. Annu Rev Public Health 20:89-108, 1999.

Lieber CP, Seinige UL, Sataloff DM: Choosing the site of surgery: An overview of ambulatory surgery in geriatric patients. Clin Geriatr Med 6:493-497, 1990.

Meydani M: The Boyd Orr lecture: Nutritional interventions in aging and age-associated diseases. Proc Nutr Soc 61:165-171, 2002.

Muravchick S: Preoperative assessment of the elderly patient. Anesthesiol Clin North America 18:71-89, 2000.

Oskvig RM: Special problems in the elderly. Chest 115:158S-164S, 1999.

Raja SN, Haythornthwaite JA: Anesthetic management of the elderly: Measuring function beyond the immediate perioperative horizon. Anesthesiology 91:909-911, 1999.

Ruzicka S: The impact of normal aging processes and chronic illness on perioperative care of the elderly. Semin Perioper Nurs 1:3-13, 1997.

Smetana GW: Preoperative pulmonary assessment of the older adult. Clin Geriatr Med 19:35-55, 2003.

Smetana GW, Cohn SL, Lawrence VA: Update in perioperative medicine. Ann Intern Med 40:452-461, 2004.

Thomas DR, Ritchie CS: Preoperative assessment of older adults. J Am Geriatr Soc 43:811-821, 1995.

Tonner PH, Kampen J, Scholz J: Pathophysiological changes in the elderly. Best Pract Res Clin Anaesthesiol 17:163-177, 2003.

Wertheim WA: Perioperative risk. Review of two guidelines for assessing older adults. Geriatrics 55:61-66, 2000.

Wu CL, Hsu W, Richman JM, Raja SN: Postoperative cognitive function as an outcome of regional anesthesia and analgesia. Reg Anesth Pain Med 29:257-268, 2004.

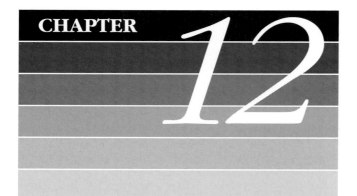

Ambulatory Anesthesia for Dentistry and Office-Based Surgery

ANDREW HERLICH

AMBULATORY ANESTHESIA FOR DENTISTRY

With the aid of anesthesia, modern dentistry and oral surgery have been performed on outpatients for well over 150 years. This dates back to the barber-dentist who extracted, or at least removed, the crown of an offending tooth under the influence of alcohol-induced alteration of consciousness. Anesthetic techniques advanced after the public demonstration of nitrous oxide in Hartford, Connecticut, when a tooth was extracted intact without the patient complaining of pain. Since then, more sophisticated techniques have been developed to anesthetize patients for dental and oral surgical procedures.

Anesthesia Caregivers in the Dental Office

Who is providing ambulatory anesthesia for dental and oral surgical patients? The types of practitioners who are providing these services are quite diversified. In addition to physician anesthesiologists and Certified Registered Nurse Anesthetists, the dental profession has four provider classes who provide anesthesia services for dental therapy. The first two classes, oral surgeons and dentist anesthesiologists, have the most extensive training and spend the greatest proportion of their training in the hospital environment. These practitioners have good airway skills and have had training in anesthesia.

The third provider class is the pediatric dentists. They serve at least 1 month during their training on the anesthesia service of their institution, learning the basics of anesthesia, including intravenous access techniques, sedation and pharmacology issues, principles of monitoring, and the basics of airway management. At most institutions, they are required to take the Pediatric Advanced Life Support course as part of their training. Pediatric dentists are frequently responsible for the care of the physically and emotionally challenged adult patients. Consequently, they are comfortable with the use of a variety of sedation techniques in their office. In spite of this, the anesthesia care team should also learn how to handle patients with complex medical problems.

The fourth type of provider class usually has only a modicum of formal anesthesia and analgesia training. This group includes general dentists, periodontists, and nonoral surgery implantologists. They tend to use oral sedation or single-dose intramuscular techniques. Despite having Advance Cardiac Life Support (ACLS) certification, these practitioners rarely have to use rescue techniques. Consequently, their skills in intravenous access, airway management, and resuscitation are not reinforced by practice and are not likely to be reliable.

The regulation of the administration of anesthesia and sedation in the dental office primarily rests with the laws of the state in which the dentist or physician practices. During the past 10 years, tighter controls have been placed over office-based anesthesia and surgical practice due to a few well-publicized catastrophic outcomes. Therefore, approval to practice sedation and anesthesia is now based on the dental practitioner's previous experience, breadth and depth of formal education prior to practice, and maintenance of continuing education. These regulatory restrictions are intended to prevent adverse outcomes in the dental office that are the result of provider inadequacy.

The Patient Spectrum

Several different groups of patients require anesthesia and sedation in the dental office. Dental-phobic adults requiring some form of anesthesia or sedation are the largest proportion of patients seen in the general dentist office. The anesthesiologist or Certified Registered Nurse Anesthetist (CRNA) rarely encounters these patients because they are managed with only preoperative oral sedation. However, there are many other types of adult patient who may require the presence of an anesthesiologist or CRNA. Patient care may be moved from the dental office to an ambulatory surgicenter, or even to the hospital operating room, if the care is too complex.

Medically compromised patients often require their dental care in the surgicenter or operating room environment. Do these patients really require the administration of anesthesia for routine dental care? The answer is a qualified "yes." Frequently, the dental care rendered to these patients requires that all of the care be completed in a single visit, which may take several hours. Complex patients include those undergoing chemotherapy; patients who are heart, lung, and liver transplant candidates; and those with severe cardiac or respiratory compromise. Urgent surgery plans, including imminent transplantation or valvular heart surgery, frequently require a single dental visit so as not to delay the major surgical care. Another group of patients, those who have the physical inability to cooperate, secondary to pain, restlessness, and movement disorders, frequently require an anesthesiologist. Anesthesiologists are able to provide sedation, analgesia, or general anesthesia to prevent patient motion and to relieve pain. The physically challenged patient who requires a wheelchair adaptor may not be able to undergo such care in the dental office, which may not have equipment to adequately position the patient. Patients with blood dyscrasias, coagulopathies, or those undergoing aggressive chemotherapy, in whom immunocompromise is a significant concern, are more likely to have their dental care administered in the hospital or surgicenter environment. In addition, patients undergoing chemotherapy may have hematological nadirs that render dental care unwise and potentially dangerous without the presence of an anesthesiologist. Therefore, patients in this group are candidates for monitored anesthesia care (MAC) or general anesthesia.

Who Are the Dental Practitioners?

A number of dental specialists, especially oral surgeons and pediatric dentists, require the services of an anesthesiologist for specific dental care. Both practitioners have extensive training in the hospital and clinical environment, which requires knowledge of the medically, emotionally, and physically compromised patient. They also have training in the administration of oral, intramuscular, and intravenous sedation, as well as advanced life support training (Box 12-1).

However, there are other dental practitioners who may also require an anesthesiologist's service. These include periodontists, endodontists, maxillofacial prosthodontists, and implantologists (Box 12-2).

The prosthodontist who requires functional full-arch impressions would have difficulty when patients undergo general anesthesia. Functional impressions of the dental arch require the cooperation of patients to move their tongue and mandible in specific directions while the impression is setting up. At best, these patients may only be able to receive light sedation or true conscious-sedation, as described by Bennett.[1] Bennett describes conscious-sedation as the state in which the patient is calm and fully responsive to either the dentist's or the anesthesiologist's directives. Taking an impression as described above is completely different from the rapid and static impression of a cleft palate arch in an

> ### Box 12-1 Patients Requiring Anesthetic Care for Dental Procedures
>
> **ADULTS AND CHILDREN**
>
> Patients with severe or life-threatening cardiopulmonary disease (i.e., cardiac surgical candidates)
> Patients with movement disorders such as Huntington's disease, cerebral palsy, postencephalitis syndromes, or poorly controlled seizures
> Patients undergoing chemotherapy who have significant physiologic nadirs
> Patients with blood dyscrasias, including coagulopathies
> Patients with severe phobias, impulse control problems, or autism
> Patients with severe orofacial infections or trauma
> Patients who are candidates for major organ transplantation and who require extensive dental therapy
> Patients who are bedridden or wheelchair bound who cannot receive care at bedside
>
> **CHILDREN**
>
> Children of any age with severe bottle mouth caries
> Neonates requiring cleft palate impressions

Box 12-2   Dental Practitioners and Their Specialties

Endodontist: Root canal specialist; also cares for patients who require surgical endodontics

Implantologist: A new specialty; performs dental implants into mandible or maxilla to replace missing teeth on a permanent basis

Maxillofacial prosthodontist: Creates head and neck prostheses after cancer surgery, burns, or congenital anomalies

Oral surgeon: All aspects of oral surgery including surgical endodontics, implantology, facial cosmetic surgery, and dental extractions

Orthodontist: Corrects malocclusions with fixed, removable, or both types of orthodontics; active in cleft palate correction

Pedodontist: Pediatric dentist; most familiar with dental problems of medically compromised children and medically or physically challenged adults

Periodontist: Gum specialist; may perform dental implants as well

Prosthodontist: Designs and fabricates crowns, bridges, and partial and complete dentures; may be involved in implants as well

---

infant, who may require an intraoral obturating prosthesis to improve feeding. Taking this type of impression requires the presence of an anesthesiologist, who must be available to rescue the airway.

Dental Primer: Anatomy, Physiology, Growth, Development, and Iatrogenic Problems

In order to adequately care for dental patients, the anesthesiologist should have a working knowledge of dental anatomy, physiology, growth, and development. The anesthesiologist should also be aware of complications that may arise during dental surgery.

Primary teeth, also known as baby or milk teeth, start to calcify *in utero* at approximately the fourth postconceptual month. The term "milk tooth" comes from the milky white appearance of the enamel. Starting with the mandibular central incisors, the teeth will generally erupt in pairs, starting approximately at the age of 6 months postnatal. The maxillary counterparts may lag in appearance by several months. The entire complement of 20 primary teeth will completely erupt by approximately 24 to 30 months of age. The last tooth to erupt is the second primary molar, also known as the 2-year molar for the timing of its appearance.

The primary teeth do not abut their adjacent teeth. There are natural spaces, or diastemata, that permit the eruption of the permanent or succedaneous teeth without gross malocclusion. This highlights the importance of maintaining good dental care during early childhood. Primary teeth that are lost prematurely may be replaced by using a variety of techniques by either pediatric dentists or orthodontists. The entire primary dentition acts as a space maintainer. Most artificial space maintainers consist of delicate metal wires. These wire devices are cemented to teeth either in the line of the dental arch or across the dental arch, such as a palatal prosthesis. The anesthesiologist must take precautions while examining or manipulating the airway for these patients. Dental cement is strong, but with inattentive airway manipulation, it is possible to avulse a prosthesis.

Between the ages of 6 and 7 years, permanent teeth start to erupt, beginning with the mandibular central and lateral incisors. The maxillary central and lateral incisors erupt as much as 1½ years later. During this stage, the primary teeth become loose due to the eruption of the permanent teeth migrating through the alveolar tissues. Roots of primary teeth resorb secondary to vertical pressure from the erupting tooth. The only portion of the primary tooth remaining during exfoliation is the anatomical crown and, perhaps, a nubbin of the root. The exfoliative process, or the mixed-dentition phase of dental development, takes place until the last primary tooth has been lost.

The full complement of permanent teeth is 32 teeth. However, the third molars, or wisdom teeth, which erupt between early adolescence and early adulthood, are highly variable in the eruption sequence and presence, if they erupt at all. They may be impacted in soft tissue or bone. Their probability of impaction is somewhat proportional to the presence and severity of dental malocclusion and genetic propensity.

Three types of teeth may be congenitally missing singly or in arch pairs. In order of frequency, any or all of the third molars, the mandibular premolars, and maxillary lateral incisors may be missing. Interestingly, the possibility of supernumerary teeth exists. These teeth include a midline tooth called a mesiodens, as well as multiple wisdom teeth at any of the third molar positions in the dental arch.

A tooth consists of three layers. The outermost layer is the enamel, which is reasonably impervious to fluids, microorganisms, and thermal stimuli, but only if good dental care occurs. Enamel is devoid of neurovascular tissue and, when intact, will unlikely transmit painful stimuli. Enamel is the hardest tissue in the body. Compared to permanent teeth, the enamel layer for primary teeth is thinner.

Immediately deep to the enamel is the dentin. Dentin consists of live cells and microtubules that easily transmit materials and sensation to the dental pulp. The dental pulp is the neurovascular supply of the tooth. All nociceptive stimuli are transmitted through the dental pulp into the roots and the sensory nerves attached to the teeth. The pulp tissue in primary teeth is more superficial. Consequently, iatrogenic pulp entry by a dental drill is more likely in primary teeth than in the permanent teeth.

The roots of the teeth are covered by the cementum, which separates the crown from the roots. The cementum is anchored to the alveolar bone by the periodontal ligament. The alveolar bone is covered by gingival and alveolar mucosa. Alveolar bone is a specialized bone that surrounds only teeth. If a tooth or teeth are missing for prolonged periods of time, alveolar bone resorbs. Edentulous areas have alveolar mucosa covering basal bone, upon which removable or fixed dentures rest.

Permanent teeth have stronger and thicker roots than their primary analogues. The incisors and canine teeth (anterior and toward the midline) have a single root and are more subject to iatrogenic trauma and fracture than the premolar and molar teeth (posterior and away from the midline), which have either multiple roots or bifurcated roots. Premolars and molars are more stable and less likely to be avulsed during airway manipulations. Anesthesiologists should direct their attention to the posterior teeth when opening the mouth with the classical "scissors" finger motion. The mandible will open wider and the teeth will not be avulsed. If desired, rather than using an oropharyngeal airway that rests against the anterior incisors, a gauze bite block should be placed along the occlusal plane of the posterior teeth. With use of an oropharyngeal airway as a bite block, the vector forces are 90 degrees to the single rooted teeth and are more likely to fracture or to avulse the teeth. These events become more problematic during the mixed dentition phase, when there are naturally mobile teeth.

If a tooth is avulsed and cannot be found, a lateral and anteroposterior chest radiograph should be taken to locate the tooth. If the tooth is located in the esophagus, it will likely pass through the gastrointestinal (GI) tract within 3 days without incident. If the tooth is located in the tracheobronchial tree, it must be retrieved, even if it means a thoracotomy. A tooth in the tracheobronchial tree is a sure source of lung infection. A dentist may reimplant an avulsed permanent tooth under certain circumstances. Primary teeth should not be reimplanted under any circumstances. Reimplantation of primary teeth will likely harm the permanent tooth bud that is immediately below in the tooth socket.

Perioperative Anesthetic Management

After speaking with the dental practitioner about the procedures, an anesthetic plan may be formulated. Many dental procedures may be performed with MAC. As an example, complete oral rehabilitation, which includes dental prophylaxis plus dental caries removal and restoration, may be accomplished with intravenous sedation and local anesthesia. However, in the case of young children or noncommunicative patients, the use of local anesthesia may be problematic. On one hand, the perioperative analgesia reduces the need for parenteral or inhaled agents. On the other hand, however, local anesthetics may create dysphoria. Also, the potential exists for soft tissue maceration when children or handicapped adults bite their tongue or adjacent soft tissues.

Premedication of uncooperative patients may be easily accomplished with oral midazolam (0.5 mg/kg, 15 to 20 mg maximum) with or without acetaminophen (10 to 15 mg/kg). Reasonable sedation and separation from a parent or caregiver may occur within 15 minutes of administration. Patients with a history of poor response to midazolam or of combative behavior may benefit from adding ketamine (3 to 5 mg/kg) to midazolam. Intramuscular midazolam (100 µg/kg) plus ketamine (3 mg/kg) plus atropine (10 µg/kg) is a satisfactory alternative. Transnasal spray of midazolam (250 µg/kg), with or without ketamine, and 1 to 3 mg/kg is a third alternative for premedication. The addition of ketamine to the premedication will likely prolong the patient's time of discharge. However, the risk-to-benefit ratio in the combative patient suggests that the addition of ketamine far outweighs any disadvantage. Rectal premedication with these drugs is possible, but today it is not necessary; it is messy, unpleasant for everyone, and has an unpredictable onset and duration.

If intravenous cannulation is needed prior to inhalation induction of anesthesia or if a MAC technique is the primary goal, then the application of topical lidocaine or lidocaine-prilocaine creams may be prudent. However, in order for these topical anesthetics to be effective, one must plan for their application prior to use and they must be properly applied to the selected sites. Caregivers can be instructed on how to apply a topical anesthetic so that it will be effective upon arrival of the patient at the surgical facility. Patients at risk for removing or chewing the bio-occlusive dressing that covers the topical anesthetic should have an additional protective dressing covering the bio-occlusive dressing.

Although the placement of local anesthetic creams at home may be reasonably safe, the practice of administering a sedative premedication at home and then transporting a child to the facility is dangerous and should be actively discouraged! The risk of sedation and subsequent airway obstruction is significant, especially if a small child is confined to an automobile safety seat.

After satisfactory mask induction of anesthesia, intravenous cannulation is performed. If needed, neuromuscular blockers are administered to facilitate intubation of the trachea. Administration of an antisialagogue, especially glycopyrrolate, may be very helpful in maintaining a dry mouth since the use of a rubber dam barrier is inconvenient. Since the incidence of postoperative nausea and vomiting is higher in this patient population, the administration of antiemetic medication is often helpful. Currently, topical fluorides are applied with a concentrated gel on a cotton-tipped applicator. Therefore, patients are less likely to swallow fluoride and endure subsequent emesis than they are with older preparations, which required a large amount of topical fluoride. Useful antiemetics include dexamethasone (200 to 500 μg/kg, with a ceiling of 10 mg) plus any one of the available 5-HT3 antagonist drugs.

Maintenance of anesthesia may be accomplished with total intravenous anesthesia (TIVA), inhalation anesthesia, or, more commonly, a combination of both agents. Depending upon availability and necessity, any of the inhalation agents is satisfactory. Common agents include sevoflurane, desflurane, isoflurane, and, in increasingly rare instances, halothane. The use of nitrous oxide is optional and is a provider preference. However, since nitrous oxide has been associated with increased postoperative nausea and vomiting, providers may not use it for that reason alone. Neuromuscular blockade is rarely necessary except to facilitate intubation of the trachea. If facial nerve monitoring is necessary for excision of facial masses or similar procedures, its use must be discussed with the dentist prior to anesthesia.

Perioperative fluid management should be guided by the patient's overall clinical condition since intraoperative fluid losses are rarely an issue. The use of a balanced salt solution or normal saline in adults or children is usually quite satisfactory. Dextrose-containing solutions should only be used when underlying clinical conditions warrant dextrose supplementation. Dental or oral surgery patients who require blood transfusion therapy are not usually satisfactory ambulatory candidates.

Airway Management

Prior to management of the airway, a discussion should take place between the anesthesiologist and the dentist as to whether nasotracheal intubation is necessary. An intranasal spray of a vasoconstrictor such as oxymetazoline will likely reduce the possibility and severity of epistaxis if nasotracheal intubation is performed. Alternatives to oxymetazoline include phenylephrine and cocaine. Hypertensive responses from topical phenylephrine are unpredictable, and potentially dangerous patient reactions to cocaine make both alternatives unwise choices for nasal vasoconstriction.

A flexible suction catheter or nasogastric tube may be placed through the lumen of the nasotracheal tube before gently being inserted into the nares. This technique will reduce the possibility or severity of epistaxis when using a nasotracheal tube. Frequently, the patient

who requires dental care under general anesthesia has a congenital syndrome that involves the craniofacial matrix. Such a patient may have a high and narrow palatal vault with severe malocclusion. Consequently, direct laryngoscopy may be difficult due to inability to properly position a laryngoscope blade. In this situation, the anesthesiologist should have a flexible fiberoptic laryngoscope, an assortment of rigid laryngoscope blade styles, and several sizes of Magill forceps available.

Small children can be intubated through the nasotracheal route with greater ease using a small curved laryngoscope blade with a Magill forceps. This is especially true in the child with a narrow palate and dental malocclusion. A small curved blade creates a greater airway space within which to manipulate a Magill forceps. Keep in mind, however, that the use of a curved blade in a small child is not common among most pediatric anesthesiologists.

The drawbacks to using nasotracheal intubation in the ambulatory patient are no different than those in the inpatient. The important complications include epistaxis, mucosal excoriation and dissection, fracture of the nasal turbinates, and sinusitis. The use of a precurved nasotracheal tube will usually afford dentists a better view and greater access to the patient's mouth. It may be inadvisable to anesthetize patients who have known or potentially difficult airways or who have syndromes involving the head and neck in locations outside of a surgicenter or hospital.

If nasotracheal intubation is not desired or warranted, the placement of a flexible supraglottic airway device is a reasonable alternative. Due to its flexibility and its long history of successful use, the flexible laryngeal mask airway is the preferred supraglottic device for most anesthesia providers. The advantages of the flexible laryngeal mask airway (LMA) include a relatively low profile, the ability of the flexible conducting tube to be turned in any direction to improve surgical access, and its availability in both disposable and reusable forms. Midline dental procedures may require vertical or oblique displacement of the LMA tube. Inexperienced anesthesiologists and dentists who have not used the LMA under these circumstances find that successful use of the LMA has a very short learning curve (Box 12-3).

The Goldman nasal mask has been used for the administration of nitrous oxide in dental offices. However, it is not really a good choice for the administration of either volatile agents or nitrous oxide. It lacks the ability to provide positive pressure ventilation and, in addition, lacks the ability to scavenge waste anesthetic gases. It is noteworthy that there are little data on nitrous oxide pollution of the dental operator, as to whether it is greater with an uncuffed endotracheal tube or with a nasal mask and an open mouth. Nonetheless, nitrous oxide analgesia through the nasal mask, with or without parenteral sedation, is an alternative to the use of general anesthesia in the appropriately selected patient. In fact, nitrous oxide alone may have a significant depressant effect on the psychomotor activity of children.

General dentists and pediatric dentists will frequently use a fluid barrier on a U-shaped frame to isolate the teeth from the oral cavity so that saliva and blood do not contaminate the operative field. Barriers may keep oral fluids from reducing the adhesiveness and tensile strength of restorative materials. Additionally, endodontists routinely use this same barrier to block the oropharyngeal migration of dental instruments, which are thin and exceedingly sharp. The potential for aspiration, ingestion, and subsequent perforation of the aerodigestive tract is real and quite dangerous.

The use of a fluid barrier has a consequence that is not well known to the medical community. The barrier is often generically called a "rubber dam." Most rubber dams are actually manufactured from natural latex products. In an increasingly latex-free environment, the operating room (OR) staff must be cognizant of the nature of this device and switch to a non-latex material. Dentist should be made aware of any suspicion of patient latex allergy so they do not bring any latex products into the operating room.

Oral Surgery

Oral surgery is frequently performed on an ambulatory basis. Most of the cases are for exodontia (i.e., tooth pulling), but biopsies, preprosthetic surgery, implantology, orthognathic surgery, and cosmetic surgery are also

part of this type of practice. Many oral surgeons have medical degrees with advanced training beyond oral surgery. This may include plastic surgery fellowships, which then permit them to branch beyond traditional procedures. Procedures that may be performed in the modern oral surgery office include rhinoplasty, cosmetic blepharoplasty, botulinum toxin injection, lip augmentation, and similar facial cosmetic surgeries. With reimbursement for advanced orthognathic procedures decreasing or refused by primary carriers for inpatient procedures, many of these procedures are now performed in the oral surgery office or surgicenter. Consequently, mandibular advancement procedures, rapid palatal expansion, and other potentially hemorrhagic procedures are planned and carried out in the dental office setting. Communication between the anesthesiologist and the surgeon is imperative in order to allow all providers to be comfortable and prepared prior to these procedures.

Ambulatory surgery care changes, to a certain degree, when performing these procedures. The patient will often require a prolonged postoperative and postanesthetic recovery of up to 4 to 6 hours. These procedures are usually amenable to airway management with nasotracheal intubation. However, cases such as rapid palatal expansion may be performed with an LMA. Either TIVA or inhalation anesthesia is acceptable for any of these procedures.

Perioperative analgesia for oral surgical procedures primarily involves local anesthesia. However, as previously explained in this chapter, very young patients may become dysphoric when unable to feel their oral structures, and they may also bite their tongue or cheek. Supplemental analgesia may be begun using preoperative acetaminophen or ibuprofen if significant hemorrhage is not predicted.

Postoperative Care

Postoperative recovery of the ambulatory dental patient rarely requires extraordinary measures. Postoperative nausea and vomiting (PONV) is not usually difficult to treat. Because PONV is more likely after these procedures, prophylactic administration of an antiemetic may be quite helpful. Dexamethasone and a 5-HT3 antagonist (i.e., ondansetron, granisetron, or dolasetron) are quite helpful in preventing or reducing any episodes of PONV. Administration of parenteral diphenhydramine, dimenhydramine, or a small dose of propofol as rescue antiemetics is usually quite successful. Unlike 5-HT3 antagonists, these rescue agents have one significant drawback—the patients will sleep for at least ½ to 1 hour longer prior to meeting discharge criteria.

Postanesthetic care unit (PACU) nurses should discourage these patients from spitting if exodontia has occurred. Spitting generates enough force to dislodge any maturing clots from the tooth socket and will renew surgical site hemorrhage. If the patients feel such an urge to rid themselves of blood or secretions, they should be allowed to have secretions passively drain from the mouth. Any dental packing should be left in place with sufficient force to compress the area for approximately 1½ to 2 hours. After this time, the clot will have matured sufficiently to prevent adherence to the gauze pack mesh and can be removed without further risk of hemorrhage. If ice packs are recommended at home, a simple remedy may be suggested to the patients and their families: frozen peas and corn, available in 1-pound bags, are far more comfortable to any region of the body than plastic bags containing ice cubes or crushed ice. The frozen peas and corn easily conform to the body, including the facial region, and are far less expensive than the medically specific ice bags.

Postoperative analgesia may be facilitated with ketorolac if it is not used during the intraoperative period. Commonly, standard postoperative oral analgesics include oxycodone, hydrocodone, and nonsteroidal anti-inflammatory drugs (NSAIDS). Intraoperative injection of ketorolac and dexamethasone (or methylprednisolone) will aid in perioperative analgesia. Ketorolac (500 µg/kg) is an especially effective analgesic medication for dental, oral, and maxillofacial surgery in both children and adults. The dose should not exceed 30 mg in the adult patient. Its use in patients under 2 years of age should be done with caution since renal maturation does not occur until 6 months to 1 year of age. It is important to confer with the oral surgeon prior to its use since there may be surgical reasons not to give it. Fentanyl (1 to 4 µg/kg) may also aid in postoperative analgesia without causing severe respiratory depression or delaying discharge to home. Fentanyl is an especially helpful medication when a longer-acting agent such as morphine has been used intraoperatively. Dosing may need to be modified in patients with known drug sensitivity or obstructive sleep apnea.

AMBULATORY ANESTHESIA FOR OFFICE-BASED SURGERY

Office-based anesthesia and surgery were once largely dental surgery. However, during the years of the twentieth century, there was an increase in patient and surgeon acceptance of simple procedures performed away from the hospital setting. In 1919, Waters[2] described his solo office practice, emphasizing its convenience, safety, and personal remuneration. One decade before Waters' article, Nicoll,[3] in Scotland, described the variety of pediatric surgical procedures that he performed on an outpatient basis. He noted that the patients recovered well at home. Visiting nurses examined wounds and changed the dressings to facilitate recovery.

Reasons for Surgery Shifting to the Office

Modern office-based anesthesia started within the past decade as hospital and surgicenter remuneration waned. Until then, most office-based practitioners performed only minor procedures: biopsies, dilatation and curettage, termination of early pregnancy, and similar types of procedures that had supposed minimal surgical and anesthesia morbidity. Plastic surgery offices frequently had body-sculpting activities including liposuction, breast augmentations and reductions, face-lifts, and nasal recontouring. Depending upon the plastic surgeon, voluntary participation in the American Association for Accreditation of Ambulatory Surgical Facilities (AAAASF) demonstrated a commitment to safe office-based surgery and anesthesia.

By the mid 1990s, with the shift of many procedures to the office environment, safety regulations that already existed were beginning to be enforced. Simply put, adverse outcomes coupled with public outcry yielded more stringent control over office-based surgery. Procedures such as total body liposuction had little regulation over how much fluid could be removed in the presence of a tumescent technique. In 1997, the Accreditation Association for Ambulatory Health Care (AAAHC) decided to accredit office-based anesthesia practices. In the ensuing years, AAAASF, the American College of Surgeons (ACS), and the Joint Commission on Accreditation of Healthcare Organizations (JCAHO) examined and revamped their standards to include issues of office-based anesthesia. The Society for Ambulatory Anesthesia (SAMBA) and the American Society of Anesthesiologists (ASA) also educated their membership through national meeting lectures, regional lectures, and publications. Combined SAMBA and ASA committees made joint efforts to formulate recommendations and to publish guidelines for their membership. In addition to national society and organization input, state legislatures and their state boards of medicine have also promulgated rules and regulations to promote patient safety. However, there is wide variability in the state-specific rules and regulations. Some states still have no requirements.

In order for anesthesiologists to provide services in the office-based environment, they have to redirect their thinking. Patients who may be satisfactory candidates for a hospital or surgicenter operating room may be inappropriate candidates for the office-based surgical environment. For instance, a patient who requires 24-hour continuous nasal oxygen and presents for partial mastectomy is a poor candidate for an office-based environment; yet, the patient may be a perfectly acceptable

Box 12-4   Surgeons and Procedures Suitable for Office Surgery

Gastroenterologist: Colonoscopy, upper endoscopy, and biopsy

General surgeon: Mastectomy, herniorrhaphy, excision of soft tissue masses, and hemorrhoidectomy

Gynecologist: Ovum retrieval, laparoscopy, cone biopsy, termination of pregnancy, and excision of perineal lesions

Ophthalmology: Cataract surgery, scleral buckle surgery, probing and irrigation, and ophthalmic plastic surgery involving the eyelids and adnexal tissues

Oral surgeon: Exodontia, palatal expansion, implantology, tuberosity reduction, and preprosthetic surgery

Orthopedic surgeon: Arthroscopy, hand surgery, and dislocation reduction

Otolaryngologist: Myringotomy, functional endoscopic sinus surgery (FESS), septorhinoplasty, uvulectomy, and biopsy

Plastic surgeon: Breast surgery, facial cosmetic surgery, and liposuction

Podiatrist: Hammer-toe correction, bunionectomy, screw removal, plantar fasciotomy, and osteotomy

Urologist: Cystoscopy, vasectomy, varicocelectomy, needle ablation of the prostate, and urethral dilation

candidate for a surgicenter environment. See Box 12-4 for the types of surgeons and procedures that are suitable for office surgery.

In general, candidates for office-based surgery should be ASA physical status I or II. Less commonly, ASA III or IV patients may be satisfactory candidates, provided the procedures are brief and minimally invasive (e.g., an upper GI endoscopy or a colonoscopy). The office environment is a very poor choice for risky patients undergoing risky procedures. Despite the risk, these patients may well be routine patients in the oral surgeon's or dentist's office.

The extent of surgical invasiveness, also known as *pushing the envelope,* will increase over time until several factors have been reached that will inhibit the patient, the anesthesiologist, or the surgeon's staff from voluntarily participating in the procedure. These include regulatory restrictions, insufficient equipment, extensive blood loss, or extreme duration of surgery. A 6 to 8 hour surgical procedure is likely extended by a prolonged recovery in the office environment. Patients may well remain in the office recovery area for many hours, long after the surgeon has left the facility, leaving the anesthesiologist and office staff to care for the patient.

Lapses in vigilance may occur during the postoperative and recovery period. Early data from the *American Society of Anesthesiologists Closed Claims Study* suggest that claims from the office-based anesthetics were judged to be largely preventable in the postoperative

period. The study suggested that quality improvement should direct efforts on improving postoperative care and monitoring. The early data also suggest that payouts were greater in the office environment than in the ambulatory surgicenter. In contradistinction, recent data from the oral surgery closed claims analysis suggest that there were fewer adverse outcomes in the oral surgery office.

Getting Started and Being Safe

What are the prerequisites prior to instituting an office-based practice? All necessary safeguards should be in place prior to embarking upon office-based care (Box 12-5). In 1999, and reaffirmed in 2004, the American Society of Anesthesiologists[4] developed *Guidelines for Office-Based Anesthesia.* In 2000, the ASA[5] published *Office-Based Anesthesia: Considerations for Anesthe-*

Box 12-5   Suggested Guidelines for Establishing a Safe Office-Based Anesthesia Practice

ADMINISTRATION AND FACILITY

Includes accreditation and governance, provider qualifications and credentials, and records and documentation including quality improvement, equipment safety, infection control and occupational safety, and controlled substance regulation.

CLINICAL CARE

Patient and procedure selection are mandatory. Preoperative, intraoperative, and postoperative care must be carefully planned and documented. Which physician will discharge the patient from the facility must be established and documented. Uses of ASA's *Monitoring Standards* and *Definition of Anesthetic Depths* are quite useful. In addition, ASA's *Guidelines for Ambulatory Anesthesia and Surgery* and *Nonoperating Room Anesthetizing Locations* are very helpful.

SPECIAL CONSIDERATION FOR PEDIATRIC PATIENTS

Acceptability of patient and procedure types should be known prior to scheduling these patients. Additional considerations include nothing-by-mouth (NPO) issues, premedication and induction techniques, and maintenance techniques. Guidelines for uses of analgesics and fluid management as well as for recovery and discharge are all helpful.

EMERGENCY AND TRANSFER TO AN ALTERNATIVE CARE FACILITY

Total management plans and possible algorithms should be in place prior to the events. Emergencies include cardiopulmonary resuscitation (CPR) and malignant hypothermia (MH).

(Full Guidelines located in Appendices 1 and 2)

siologists in Setting Up and Maintaining a Safe Office Anesthesia Environment. This is an excellent reference manual and starting point: every novice and experienced office-based anesthesiologist is encouraged to study and use it! The full ASA *Guidelines for Office-Based Anesthesia* and portions of *Office-Based Anesthesia* are located in the appendices of this book.

In addition to accounting for compliance issues with all regulatory issues for the office-based practice, the anesthesiologist should visit the office several times prior to agreeing to participate in patient care in the office. Familiarity with the office layout, the anesthesia and resuscitative equipment, the recovery area, and patient care flow will only aid in good patient outcomes. Can an ambulance stretcher or wheelchair fit in the doorway of each office room as well as the front and back door of the entire facility? How powerful is the backup electrical supply? Inspection of the flow of the office in relation to the affability of the staff and their interpersonal skills will go a long way in convincing the office-based anesthesiologist or group that their relationship will be mutually satisfactory. Simple issues, such as inspection of the policies and procedures book, access to regulatory licenses, evidence of continuing education, or means of disposal of biohazardous materials, will also be key indicators of the same.

What arrangements will be made to cover you or your practice when you are ill or on vacation? Is your group or service large enough to cover personal absence contingencies? Will the anesthesia coverage provider be comfortable with the surgical practice, and will they be comfortable with the anesthesiologist?

Potential areas of contention exist for both the anesthesiologist and the surgeon. Issues include deciding who is responsible for purchasing or providing the anesthesia equipment; who maintains the equipment; and how these charges are figured into reimbursement for anesthesia services. An additional area of concern includes the acquisition, storage, and security of medication, especially controlled substances. If this area is the anesthesiologist's responsibility, then he or she will need to have a separate Drug Enforcement Administration (DEA) Form 222 for dispensing the medication as well as the standard DEA form for prescribing and administering the medication. A separate DEA Form 222 is needed for each office location. Some states require a separate controlled substance permit. These permits must be obtained prior to caring for patients.

Emergencies occur irrespective of the location of patient care. They may occur in the hospital, the ambulatory surgical center, or the office-based environment. How these emergencies are handled is key to success. Since emergency transfer agreements must be in place prior to opening an office-based anesthesia and surgical practice, has the facility also alerted the emergency medical service (EMS) and the local police and fire departments of the nature of the office?

Each office that performs office-based anesthesia and surgery should have laminated copies of algorithms for the treatment of emergencies. Laminated copies of the Basic Life Support (BLS), Advanced Cardiac Life Support (ACLS), Pediatric Advanced Life Support (PALS) guidelines, as well as the ASA Difficult Airway Algorithm and MH Guidelines would aid in the rapid treatment of such problems. Unless these crises are simulated on a frequent, ongoing basis, most clinicians tend to forget the algorithms over time. In some cases, these laminated cards are included with the books provided by the American Heart Association or can be purchased from various organizations. Despite the pressures of time and economics, regularly scheduled drills of office crises may well help to improve patient outcome. Continuing medical education can easily be accessed on-line at all hours of the day.

Anesthesia Techniques and Equipment for the Office-Based Environment

The key to a successful office-based anesthetic practice is to have an awake, comfortable patient at the termination of the procedure. A good working relationship between the surgeon and the anesthesiologist is one that will emphasize the judicious use of local and regional anesthesia to aid in intraoperative and postoperative comfort. In many cases, successful local or regional block techniques will dramatically reduce the need for large amounts of anesthetic agents.

Nevertheless, the office-based anesthesiologist will utilize a variety of medications that permit the patient to emerge rapidly with minimal pain and minimal postoperative nausea and vomiting. Anesthesia providers utilize both inhalation and intravenous agents to accomplish this. Techniques such as propofol boluses and propofol infusions, with or without ketamine, are popular for many procedures. Small doses of ketamine, opiate boluses with fentanyl, or infusions with remifentanil work well for patient comfort without prolonged sedation or adverse side effects. However, the cost of prolonged infusions with propofol and remifentanil may be fiscally daunting. The use of level-of-consciousness monitors may aid in more accurate titration of medication. The anesthesiologist must be mindful of prolonged and high concentrations of propofol since there is a small risk of propofol-induced metabolic acidosis. Additional useful medications are midazolam, ketorolac, and clonidine. Antiemetics of the 5-HT3 class are relatively expensive. However, the cost of patient dissatisfaction, discomfort, and a prolonged stay in the facility makes investment in this class of medication wise. Rescue antiemetics such as dimenhydramine or diphenhydramine are very cost-effective in terms of acquisition but invariably cause patients to fall asleep in the recovery area for at least 30 minutes before they awaken and feel better. As a result, patients spend more time in the office, possibly hindering the schedule. Neuromuscular blockers of the intermediate variety are useful in the office environment for longer procedures. However, they may require reversal, which may be associated with PONV. Mivacurium and cisatracurium have the advantage of ester hydrolysis to hasten their offset. Unfortunately, they do not obviate the need for available reversal medication. Residual neuromuscular blockade may delay patient recovery and discharge.

When an anesthesia machine is not available or practical in the office-based practice, TIVA is frequently the anesthetic technique of choice. For instance, gastroenterology procedures such as colonoscopy or endoscopy rarely require more than propofol or midazolam with fentanyl. A small bolus of propofol or methohexital will facilitate the pain of a regional block by an ophthalmologist, otolaryngologist, or oral surgeon. Even blocks for herniorrhaphy may be satisfactorily administered with a prior bolus of propofol or methohexital. It is important to emphasize that the presence of running intervenous (IV) solution throughout many of these procedures is not always necessary. A patent IV catheter with a T-connector and a saline flush may be all that is necessary for the procedure. Significant volume shifts or blood loss are not seen in cataract surgery, varicocele repair, or ovum retrieval.

The administration of supplemental oxygen does not require the availability of an anesthesia machine. Supplemental oxygen may be administered by nasal cannula or blow-by from a wall outlet or tank with the appropriate flowmeter. However, as part of the mandatory safety equipment, the ability to provide positive pressure ventilation with bag and mask is fundamental. Equipment for full resuscitation, including a defibrillator and an external pacemaker, needs to be available. The anesthesiologist needs to inspect this equipment, irrespective of ownership.

Anesthesiologists who practice in office-based facilities may bring their own favorite or special equipment—use of a tackle box for storage is common—in addition to the available equipment in the office. The tackle box may contain specialized laryngoscope blades, rescue airway devices such as intubating LMAs (i.e., the Fastrach), cricothyrotomy kits, flashlights, and other equipment that an anesthesiologist finds necessary for patient care and safety.

If longer procedures require the presence of an anesthesia machine, single vaporizer machines with a limited number of flowmeters exist. Machines with interchangeable vaporizers may be a wiser alternative if widely varying procedure times exist. Sevoflurane is a common choice for an all-around inhaled agent. It per-

mits inhalation inductions for both children and needle-phobic adults. It has the advantage of rapid emergence due to its low solubility. It does not require a more complex heated vaporizer, whereas desflurane does. Both agents are, however, more expensive compared to isoflurane.

Anesthesia machines exist that are sufficiently small enough to fit on a counter or small table and that have limited accessories. They are affordable, portable, and, most importantly, useful for the office-based practice. Because anesthesia ventilators are not always available on the anesthesia machine designed for the office environment, they require additional space and power and add considerable cost to the purchase. Refurbished full-sized anesthesia machines are a wise choice for the fixed office-based practice that has a full-sized operating room. New anesthesia machines may average $50,000 or more to purchase!

Syringe pumps are a cost-effective means of administering propofol with or without ketamine. There are a number of manufacturers who have created syringe pumps that are amenable to the office-based practice. If a syringe pump is too costly, the use of a mini-drip IV administration set may work just as well.

The office-based anesthesiologist may be required to perform a variety of regional blocks, including blocks for upper-extremity and lower-extremity surgery. Even spinal or epidural blocks may be necessary. The choice of local anesthetic should be appropriate for the duration of surgery with, if possible, sufficient residual analgesia without motor impairment. The use of head and neck blocks for oral and extraoral surgery or facial cosmetic surgery is not only helpful but also adds an element of versatility to the anesthesiologist's skills. These skills translate into favorable patient outcome and help to maintain a good relationship with the surgeon.

Recovery of the patient may occur in the operating location, the waiting room, or a separate recovery location. It is the responsibility of the anesthesiologist to oversee that the patient is continuously observed during the recovery period. Who observes the patient and where that recovery occurs varies from office to office. It may be a luxury to have a dedicated PACU nurse in the office. Multifunctional nurses who handle the preoperative, intraoperative, and postoperative care are more likely to be present in this practice. Recovery time may not be prolonged when the patient receives an anesthetic that results in the patient being sufficiently enough awake during emergence that he or she can walk with assistance to the recovery area. Despite the rapidity of recovery, the cautions about driving, working, and performing certain tasks remain important irrespective of the patient's own wishes and desires.

The Business Side of Office-Based Anesthesia

Taking a cue from Waters'[2] famous treatise "The Downtown Anesthesia Clinic," the office-based anesthesia practitioner should have all financial arrangements made prior to embarking upon the venture. A number of questions are worthy of consideration. What arrangements need to be made with the surgeon, the patient, or the third-party payer? If a third-party payer covers the procedure, what documentation is needed prior to anesthetizing the patient? What payer mix is necessary to financially survive and thrive during the vicissitudes of a single surgical provider agreement? Should the anesthesiologist provide services to a variety of practitioner types, such as plastic surgeons, gastroenterologists, general surgeons, podiatrists, and radiologists, to assure a continuous cash flow? See Box 12-6 for a variety of financial questions that should be addressed prior to working in the office-based environment.

Cost containment in terms of drugs and disposables needs to be discussed with both the surgeon and the supplier. Frequent reviews of any contracts should be negotiated and renegotiated as prices change. If the anesthesiologist engages in a solo practice, the ability to negotiate lower prices may be difficult. Joining forces with other solo practitioners, surgeons, or groups with purchasing power may be quite helpful. There are Web-based organizations that can provide the solo practitioner with that purchasing power as well.

Cost containment also applies to the surgeon-client relationship with the anesthesiologist. Low-volume, low-profit surgical practices should be carefully scrutinized in relationship to more profitable ventures. However, the caveat for abandoning low-profit practices today is the reality that they become highly profitable tomorrow! Continually evaluating all aspects of the office-based practice is a must. The anesthesiologist would need a crystal ball to predict the best financial trends in his or her region.

Box 12-6   Business and Reimbursement Questions to Answer Prior to Providing Anesthesia Services

Do you have an attorney and an accountant who are knowledgeable in health care finance and law as it relates to anesthesia billing?

Are you a single entity, an S corporation, a limited liability company (LLC), or a professional corporation (PC)?

If you use a billing service, are they knowledgeable in the area of office-based anesthesia?

Is the anesthesia fee included in the surgical fee, or is it a separate fee (as might happen in a plastic surgery office)?

Has your practice sought or been accredited by any of the national accrediting bodies such as AAAASF, AAAHC, or JCAHO?

Have you created any questionable *quid pro quo* arrangements with the surgeon or the facility for equipment and service?

Have you created an unrealistic expense-to-revenue ratio, such as using more costly equipment than you need or purchasing more medications and disposables than are necessary for a reasonable time period?

If you are a solo practitioner, have you formulated coverage plans while you take vacation? Is your substitute as competent and as ethical as you?

SUMMARY

Anesthesia for ambulatory dental patients requires careful and specific communication between the anesthesiologist and the dentist. Discussion of anticipated case duration, the type of procedure, the use of specialized equipment, and the requirements of airway management will prevent needless changes or mistakes in the anesthetic plan at the time of surgery. Rarely will postoperative analgesia be difficult to manage. Primarily, however, the most common problem for patients is postoperative nausea and vomiting. Depending on the specific patient and previous experiences, PONV prophylaxis may be a preferred option over rescue treatment in order to improve overall patient satisfaction after dental procedures.

Office-based anesthesiologists must be affable, affordable, available, and adaptable in order to thrive or even to survive. They must be knowledgeable about business arrangements, regulatory issues, and the competitive market in which they practice. They must also possess the interpersonal skills of an ambassador, the clinical skills of the best clinician anywhere, and the wisdom of a sage. However, none of this knowledge matters unless the anesthesiologist puts clinical care and safety as the primary concern. The ability to balance all of these factors will promote a thriving career.

REFERENCES

1. Bennett CR (ed): Conscious-Sedation in Dental Practice, 2nd ed. St. Louis, Mosby, 1978, pp 1–23.

2. Waters R: The downtown anesthesia clinic. Am J Surg (Suppl) 33:71–73, 1919.

3. Nicoll JH: The surgery of infancy. Brit Med J 753–754, Sept 18, 1909.

4. American Society of Anesthesiologists: Guidelines for Office-Based Anesthesia, 1999.

5. American Society of Anesthesiologists: Office-Based Anesthesia: Considerations for Anesthesiologists in Setting Up and Maintaining a Safe Office Anesthesia Environment, 2000, pp 1-32.

SUGGESTED READING

Chikungwa M, Smith I: Controversial issues in ambulatory anesthesia. Anesthesiol Clin North America 21:313-327, 2003.

Friedberg BL: Propofol ketamine anesthesia for cosmetic surgery in the office suite. Intl Anesthesiol Clin 41:39-50, 2003.

Hall CE, Shutt LE: Nasotracheal intubation for head and neck surgery. Anaesthesia 58: 249-256, 2003.

Herlich A: Anesthesia for Dentistry. In Motoyama EK, Davis PJ: Anesthesia for Infants and Children, 6th ed. St. Louis, Mosby-Yearbook, 1996, pp 677-690.

Herlich A: Dental and Salivary Gland Complications. In Gravenstein N, Kirby RR (eds): Complications in Anesthesiology, 2nd ed. Philadelphia, Lippincott-Raven, 1996, pp 163-174.

Houpt MI, Limb R, Livingston RL: Clinical effects of nitrous oxide conscious sedation in children. Pediatr Dent 26:29-36, 2004.

Koch ME, Dayan S, Barinholtz D: Office-based anesthesia: An overview. Anesthesiol Clin North America 21:417-443, 2003.

Kotob F, Twersky RS: Anesthesia outside the operating room: General overview and monitoring standards. Intl Anesthesiol Clin 41:1-15, 2003.

Krohner RG: Anesthetic considerations and techniques for oral and maxillofacial surgery. Intl Anesthesiol Clin 41:67-89, 2003.

Perrott DH, Yuen JP, Andresen RV, Dodson TB: Office-based ambulatory anesthesia: Outcomes of clinical practice of oral and maxillofacial surgeons. J Oral Maxillofac Surg 61: 983-995, 2003.

Redmond M, Florence B, Glass PSA: Effective analgesic modalities for ambulatory patients. Anesthesiol Clin North America 21:329-346, 2003.

Wat LI: The laryngeal mask for oral and maxillofacial surgery. Intl Anesthesiol Clin 41:29-56, 2003.

Webb MD, Moore PA: Sedation for pediatric dental patients. Dent Clin North Am 46:803-814, 2002.

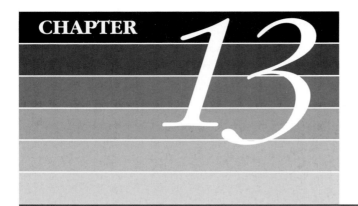

CHAPTER 13

Ambulatory Surgery Accreditation

THOMAS B. KLOOSTERBOER
MOLLY KAY KLOOSTERBOER

Prior to the 1970s, almost all surgical procedures were performed in inpatient facilities. However, due to advances in anesthetic techniques, surgical innovations, and external pressures by insurance providers, many procedures moved to the ambulatory setting by the 1980s. At first, unlike inpatient hospital centers, there was almost no oversight of freestanding ambulatory surgical facilities. Gradually, several accreditation organizations have developed programs for ambulatory surgery centers and office-based surgery facilities. These organizations have general or specific requirements for ambulatory facilities in order to provide safer conditions for both patients and workers. In addition, states and other professional organizations have developed guidelines that may be quite specific regarding either facility or provider responsibilities. Accreditation organization standards can assist ambulatory surgery centers and office-based practices in maintaining safety even while expanding to more complex procedures on sicker patients. The successful completion of a national or regional accreditation process means only that the current requirements or standards have been met. Due to the constantly changing nature of the health care system, accreditation organizations review and update their standards on a regular basis. However, accreditation by itself cannot guarantee a high skill level or good judgment by any particular provider in the facility.

There are three major nongovernmental national ambulatory surgical care accrediting agencies in the United States and several additional regional organizations. The three major national organizations specify facility size, the number of surgeons, or both to differentiate ambulatory surgery center accreditation programs from office-based programs. Some groups, such as the dental and maxillofacial surgeons, have a requirement of an inspection process for their member facilities every 5 years. However, this inspection is not an independent accreditation process, per se.

Although patients often assume that outpatient surgical facilities must have official oversight in order to provide medical care, this is not the case in most states. Only a handful of states currently require accreditation, inspection, or even specific medical practices in freestanding surgical facilities. Many state accreditation agencies, as well as the national accreditation organizations themselves, set forth different requirements for different types of anesthesia. The use of a local anesthetic without sedation requires the lowest level of patient care and facility equipment versus the highest level of care for general and major conduction anesthesia.

ACCREDITATION ASSOCIATION FOR AMBULATORY HEALTH CARE

The Accreditation Association for Ambulatory Health Care (also known as the Accreditation Association or AAAHC) was founded in 1979 as a nonprofit organization in the state of Illinois. Since the organization's founding, it has accredited multiple types of ambulatory organizations including ambulatory surgery centers, college and university health centers, single- and multi-specialty group practices, and health networks. AAAHC currently accredits over 1800 ambulatory care organizations in the United States and Canada. During its survey process,

AAAHC focuses on multiple core standards that it has developed for their practicality and their relevance to the changing health care systems of today. AAAHC also has adjunct standards that are applied based on the services provided by the organization seeking accreditation (Table 13-1).

To become accredited, each organization must meet all eligibility requirements set forth by AAAHC. A variety of ambulatory health care organizations are eligible for AAAHC accreditation, including ambulatory health care clinics, lithotripsy centers, health maintenance organizations (HMOs), multi-specialty group practices, occupational health centers, and urgent care centers. Each organization applying for accreditation must meet the eligibility criteria. However, AAAHC determines an organization's eligibility on an individual basis. If the AAAHC standards cannot be applied to an organization, AAAHC reserves the right to deny an application for an on-site survey (Box 13-1).

AAAHC uses ambulatory physicians, dentists, nurses, and administrators to conduct their on-site surveys. Each survey is specifically adjusted to fit the type, size, and range of services offered by the organization. After detailed analysis of the findings of the on-site accreditation survey, the AAAHC Accreditation Committee determines the acceptance or denial of accreditation status.

Each organization receives one of the following accreditation statuses: 3-year accreditation, 1-year accreditation,

Box 13-1 Accreditation Association for Ambulatory Health Care Eligibility Criteria

Has been providing health care services for a minimum of 6 months prior to the on-site survey (unless the organization is applying for an early option survey).

Is a legally constituted organization or a subunit that primarily provides health care services.

Follows all current federal, state, and local laws and regulations, including provincial laws for Canadian facilities.

Is licensed by the state in which it is located if the state requires licensure.

Provides care under the supervision of a physician or group of physicians, dentists, or doctors of podiatric medicine, optometry, or chiropractic medicine and who accept responsibility for the medical care given.

Shares records, business management, facilities, and equipment among members of the organization.

Is in compliance with the U.S. Equal Employment Opportunity Commission Rules and Regulations.

Submits a completed "Application for Accreditation Survey" and other required documents before the survey.

Pays the appropriate fees.

Provides complete and accurate information to AAAHC during the accreditation or reaccreditation process.

Table 13-1 AAAHC Standards

Core Standards	Adjunct Standards
Rights of patients	Anesthesia services
Governance	Surgical and related services
Administration	Overnight care and services
Quality of care	Dental services
Quality management and improvement	Emergency services
Clinical records and health information	Immediate and urgent care services
Professional improvement	Pharmaceutical services
Facilities and environment	Pathology and medical laboratory services
	Diagnostic imaging services
	Radiation oncology treatment services
	Employee and occupational health services
	Other professional and technical services
	Teaching and publication activities
	Research activities
	Managed care organizations
	Health education and wellness

6-month accreditation, deferred accreditation decision, or denial of accreditation. If an ambulatory surgery center obtains a 3-year term of accreditation, the committee believes the organization is well within compliance standards. A 1-year term of accreditation is awarded when the organization's operations are acceptable but there are areas that need further change to achieve a 3-year term. When an organization is in compliance with standards, yet has not been in operation for 6 months, the surgery center is awarded 6-month accreditation through AAAHC's Early Option Survey program. After the 6 months, another on-site survey is performed to determine a new accreditation decision and term. If an organization does not comply with the standards but demonstrates the commitment and capability to correct deficiencies within 6 months, the Accreditation Committee invokes the deferred accreditation decision. Denial of accreditation occurs when the organization is not in substantial compliance with any one of the standards.

In December of 2002, the Centers for Medicare/ Medicaid Services (CMS) granted the AAAHC renewal of its deemed status for Medicare. The "deemed status" designation means that facilities may simultaneously be accredited by the accreditation organization and achieve

Medicare certification. As a result, ambulatory surgery centers have the option of choosing a survey in which only the standards found in the *Accreditation Handbook for Ambulatory Health Care* will be applied or undergoing an AAAHC-Medicare deemed status survey that includes additional CMS requirements.

AAAHC is unique among the major organizations in that it offers accreditation to office-based anesthesiology groups as well as to surgical facilities. Office-based anesthesiology groups may have their multisite practice approved if they meet all the requirements. So far, only two office-based anesthesiology groups, one on the East Coast and one in the Midwest, have applied for and met the AAAHC standards.

AMERICAN ASSOCIATION FOR THE ACCREDITATION OF AMBULATORY SURGERY FACILITIES

In the 1970s, as office-based ambulatory anesthesia became a more significant aspect of a surgeon's practice, the American Society of Plastic and Reconstructive Surgeons (ASPRS) felt it was necessary to ensure that certain standards were being met in the facilities in which they practiced. In 1980, the Society established the American Association for the Accreditation of Ambulatory Plastic Surgery Facilities (AAAAPSF), a single-specialty accrediting agency. Following inquiries from other ambulatory-surgery-based subspecialties, AAAAPSF formed the American Association for Accreditation of Ambulatory Surgery Facilities, Inc. (AAAASF) in 1992. AAAASF only accredits facilities in which the facility director, as well as all surgeons and anesthesiologists, are board certified or are eligible by a surgical specialty board of the American Board of Medical Specialties (ABMS). Facilities that offer procedures such as dentistry or podiatry services cannot become accredited by AAAASF because they are not recognized by the ABMS. For each specialty, requirements remain constant, including having hospital and transfer privileges for the same procedures being performed within the ambulatory surgery unit and adherence to the appropriate laws and regulations governing ambulatory and office-based surgery units. AAAASF has accredited more than 1100 facilities (Box 13-2).

The accreditation program for outpatient surgery centers is based on aspects of verifiable quality-care standards from nationally recognized guidelines. The accreditation program also provides standardized practice guidelines for a surgeon operating in an ambulatory surgery setting (Box 13-3). Accreditation consists of a three-part review that includes an on-site visit, an AAAASF accreditation committee assessment of site-visit findings, and successful participation in a peer review and quality assurance program requiring on-line reporting

---

Box 13-2   American Association for the Accreditation of Ambulatory Surgery Facilities Quality Care Standards

The facility's general environment
The operating room environment
Policies and procedures
General safety in the facility
Blood and medications
Medical records
Quality assessment and quality improvement
Personnel
Governance

---

to AAAASF semi-annually. Inspections are performed by ABMS Board Certified surgeons who own or direct an accredited surgical facility. The facility has the right to refuse up to three inspectors to avoid issues such as conflict of interest, being reviewed by a competitor, or current or past affiliations. No inspector may review a facility in his or her own community, and reciprocal inspections are not permitted. These rules were put in place to assure a nonbiased, fair review of facilities.

The inspection process verifies compliance with standards and provides an educational opportunity with

---

Box 13-3   American Association for the Accreditation of Ambulatory Surgery Facilities Standardized Practice Guidelines for a Surgeon Operating in an Ambulatory Surgery Setting

Is owned and/or directed by an ABMS board certified surgeon with comparable hospital privileges for all procedures performed in the outpatient center

Has successfully completed the quality assurance and peer review activities established within the facility or developed among other surgeons or by a review organization

Adheres to ethical standards of the appropriate surgical specialty society or the American Medical Association (AMA)

Adheres to the laws and regulations governing the operation of the facility, such as the Occupational Safety and Health Act (OSHA), Bloodborne Pathogens Standards, Hazardous Waste Standards, the Americans with Disabilities Act, state and local laws, and appropriate federal laws

Meets the high standards of the accreditation program

interactions between the inspectors and the facility staff. Specific aspects of the surgical facility are reviewed (Box 13-4). The inspector also assesses the scope of procedures performed in the outpatient center to assure that that the surgeons have comparable core hospital privileges for procedures being performed at the facility. All findings are reviewed by the Association's Accreditation Committee, which issues a full accreditation, a provisional accreditation, or a denial of accreditation.

AAAASF recognized the need for classifying level (i.e., depth) of anesthesia administered in accredited facilities (Box 13-5). Accreditation is a 3-year cycle in which approximately 95% of inspected facilities receive full accreditation. The first year consists of an on-site visit; the second and third years of accreditation include a self-evaluation conducted by the facility director and staff using the same standards and checklist booklet. The results of this self-evaluation are computer analyzed and are returned to the accredited facility for review. Costs of accreditation depend on the number of surgeons and their specialties, as well as the type of anesthesia. The fee runs from $710 to $3885, with Medicare-deemed status adding approximately $500.

JOINT COMMISSION ON ACCREDITATION OF HEALTHCARE ORGANIZATIONS

The Joint Commission on Accreditation of Healthcare Organizations (JCAHO) was founded in 1951 under the sponsorship of the American Hospital Association, the American Medical Association, the American College of Physicians, and the American College of Surgeons to act as an independent accrediting body of hospitals nationwide. Subsequently, the American Dental Association was added. The Canadian Medical Association was one of the original founding members of JCAHO but departed in 1958 to lead development of a national health care accrediting body in Canada. The self-proclaimed mission of JCAHO is to "continuously improve the safety and quality of care provided to the public through the provision of healthcare accreditation

---

Box 13-4 AAAASF Review Areas

Operating room environment
Policies and procedures
General safety
Medications
Medical records
Quality improvement and peer review
Personnel
Governance
Anesthesia

Box 13-5 American Association for the Accreditation of Ambulatory Surgery Facilities Classification of Surgical Center Capability Levels

CLASS A

Surgical procedures are performed in the facility under local or topical anesthesia.
The facility meets every "A" standard.

CLASS B

Surgical procedures are performed in the facility under local or topical anesthesia
and/or
Surgical procedures are performed in the facility under intravenous or parenteral sedation, regional anesthesia, analgesia, or dissociative drugs (excluding propofol) without the use of endotracheal or laryngeal mask intubation or inhalation general anesthesia (including nitrous oxide).
The facility meets every "A" and "B" standard.

CLASS C

Surgical procedures are performed in the facility under local or topical anesthesia
and/or
Surgical procedures are performed in the facility under intravenous or parenteral sedation, regional anesthesia, analgesia, or dissociative drugs (excluding propofol) without the use of endotracheal or laryngeal mask intubation or inhalation general anesthesia (including nitrous oxide).
and/or
Surgical procedures are performed in the facility with intravenous propofol, spinal or epidural anesthesia, endotracheal or laryngeal mask intubation, or inhalation anesthesia by an anesthesiologist or a Certified Registered Nurse Anesthetist (CRNA).
The facility meets every "A," "B," and "C" standard.

---

and related services that support performance improvement in healthcare organizations."[1] Due to the changing health care environment in America, the Joint Commission broadened its scope in 1975 to include ambulatory care. JCAHO accredits a total of 16,000 organizations across eight different health care branches that include, among others, ambulatory care, behavioral health care, home care, and long-term care.

In 2004, JCAHO launched its Shared Visions—New Pathways accreditation process (Box 13-6). The JCAHO periodic performance review (PPR) is a core provision of the Shared Vision—New Pathways program. The PPR requires organizations to review all applicable standards and accreditation participation requirements from the Standards Manual and the National Patient Safety Goals. The completed PPR allows an organization to identify areas in which it may not comply with standards and directs the organization in correcting the areas. The ambulatory center can then submit its plan of action to JCAHO; the plan should include a timetable for specific changes that will be made in the areas of noncompliance. Each plan of action requires "measures of success," quantifiable and data-driven measurements to track the progress toward compliance, followed by the "priority focus process" to convert organization-specific presurvey data into specific steps for improvement. From data attained from the priority focus process, a "tracer methodology" is established. A tracer methodology tracks specific patients throughout their entire experience in the organization, monitoring the services provided to the patient. Within 90 days of the completion of the on-site survey, the organization is then required to file evidence of standards compliance with JCAHO for standards determined to be noncompliant. Evidence of standards compliance includes the data-driven measurements of measures of success and evidence that the organization is in complete compliance with all standards. The organization becomes accredited once JCAHO approves the standards of compliance and the measures of success.

To apply for accreditation through JCAHO, an organization must meet the following eligibility requirements: the organization is not hospital owned or operated, no inpatient care is provided, a quality improvement program is in place, the organization is located within the United States or meets specific criteria for foreign organization eligibility, and all services provided are identified when requesting an accreditation survey (Box 13-7).

When an organization has determined that they are eligible, it uses JCAHO's *Comprehensive Accreditation Manual for Ambulatory Care (CAMAC)* reference guide to prepare for accreditation. The CAMAC is designed to aid in self-assessment by containing all functional standards for the ambulatory surgery setting. The manual is subdivided into two main sections: patient-focused functions and organization functions. The patient-focused

functions portion contains chapters regarding patient rights, provisions of care, medication management, and infection control. The organizational function section includes chapters on performance improvement, leadership, the environment of care, human resources, and information management.

Following the completion of the survey, based on the organization's compliance of standards, the Joint Commission can award an accreditation decision in one of six categories: accreditation, provisional accreditation, preliminary accreditation, conditional accreditation, preliminary denial of accreditation, and denial of accreditation. The Joint Commission requires ongoing self-assessment and corrective actions between 3-year on-site surveys. In addition to the periodic performance review, the Joint Commission randomly selects 5% of accredited ambulatory care organizations for an unannounced survey halfway through the 3-year cycle. The fees for an ambulatory surgery center 3-year accreditation cycle range from $7800 to $14,400, based on patient visits and types of services. For a typical 1-day office-based surgery survey, the fee is $3975. Medicare-deemed status is included at no additional cost.

ADDITIONAL ACCREDITATION OPTIONS

Although AAAHC, AAAASF, and JCAHO are the three primary accreditation organizations in the United States, these are not the only accreditation options. The following organizations also offer accreditation: the Institute for Medical Quality (IMQ), the Academy of Ambulatory Foot and Ankle Surgery (AAFAS), the American Osteopathic Association's Healthcare Facilities Accreditation Program (HFAP), and the Commission on Dental Accreditation (CDA), which operates under the auspices of the American Dental Association. Additionally, in August of 2001, the Federation of State Medical Boards (FSMB) drafted model guidelines and identified three pathways that state medical boards can adopt separately or in combination for oversight of office-based surgery in unregulated settings. The three pathways are adoption of FSMB Model Guidelines, required accreditation by a recognized national or state accrediting organization, or development of individual state standards. The FSMB Model Guidelines describe recommended practices regarding administration, quality of care, clinical practices, and other aspects of outpatient surgery care.

DEEMED STATUS

AAAHC, AAAASF, JCAHO, HFAP, and others have been granted deemed status by Medicare. This designation means that facilities may be simultaneously accredited by the accreditation organization and achieve Medicare certification. To be granted deemed status, the accrediting organizations must demonstrate that their standards meet or exceed the Medicare *Conditions of Participation (COP)* requirements (see Centers for Medicare & Medicaid Services at http://www.cms.hhs.gov/cop/1.asp) as determined by the Centers for Medicare & Medicaid Services (CMS). The deemed status survey option also means that the combined survey must be unannounced. In addition, several states have deemed one or more accreditation organizations as meeting state mandated review requirements.

At the beginning of 2006, TÜV Healthcare Specialists submitted an application for deemed status to the Center for Medicare Services (CMS). If CMS approves the TÜV Healthcare Specialists' National Integrated Accreditation for Healthcare Organizations (NIAHO) accreditation program, it will become an alternative survey program for determining compliance with Medicare's Conditions of Participation and the first new accreditation agency for health care facilities in over 25 years.

CREDENTIALING, PRIVILEGING, AND QUALITY IMPROVEMENT

Credentialing and privileging is the process of identification and confirmation of current medical or technical competence and performance. It evaluates and monitors a clinician's decision-making or procedure expertise and often compares it to some professional standard. The entire process investigates and verifies an individual's license status, clinical experience and judgment, medical certification, education, training, malpractice occurrences, technical capabilities, and overall character. Analysis of these criteria determines the clinician's scope of practice. Ongoing quality improvement and assurance programs verify that the clinician remains within the scope of privileges that are granted and has acceptable clinical outcomes.

Credentialing is a peer review process, using criteria that have been determined by legal, professional, and administrative practices and approved by a formal local consensus process. Peer review decisions must be fair, equally applied, justifiable, confidential, and well-documented. The credentialing process is an ongoing one. After the organization initially approves the clinician's credentials, it must continually add quality-of-care information to the clinician's file. This information is crucial to subsequent reviews and decisions about recredentialing and current privileges.

Although the credentialing and privileging process has a long history and is well-established within hospitals, smaller facilities have variable resources to deal with this issue. Although many clinicians have credentials and privileges in hospitals, increasingly, many practice solely in the ambulatory setting. How, then, should their credentials and expertise be determined? Smaller facilities may band together to share the resources necessary to accomplish this, or they may contract with large medical and business organizations. Significantly, a relatively new development is that some third-party payers may require proof of credentialing or specific procedure expertise before approving reimbursement.

Quality assurance and improvement programs are essential in promoting high-quality patient care regardless of the venue of care. After each clinician's procedures are performed, outcome events and continuous quality indicators should be documented (Box 13-8). These data should be periodically reviewed at the medical facility in which the procedures are performed. However, as ambulatory procedures move more into small office-based anesthesia settings, this process is made much more difficult due to the small number of clinicians available to perform a review. Occasionally, cases can only be reviewed by the clinician who performed the procedure, potentially leading to bias. A possible solution includes the use of accreditation agencies or other third parties to provide quality oversight. Quality improvement data should be used during subsequent recredentialing and repriviliging reviews.

CONCLUSIONS

Currently, many ambulatory surgery centers and office-based practices are not accredited and are not required to have state inspection. Accreditation may improve patient care by examining patient processes, identifying weaknesses, and making changes for improvement, while assuring that certain recognizable standards are met. Some states, including California, Rhode Island, Pennsylvania, and Florida, and some professional organizations, such as the American Society of Plastic Surgeons and the American Society for Aesthetic Surgery, require accredita-

---

Box 13-8   Outcome Indicators for Office-Based and Ambulatory Surgery

OUTCOME EVENTS

Cancellation rates and reasons
Central nervous system or peripheral nervous system new deficit
Need for reversal agents (i.e., narcotics or benzodiazepine)
Reintubation
Unplanned transfusion
Aspiration pneumonitis
Pulmonary embolus
Local anesthetic toxicity
Anaphylaxis
Possible malignant hyperthermia
Infection
Return to operating room
Unplanned postprocedural treatment in a physician's office or emergency department
Unplanned admission to a hospital or an acute care facility
Cardiopulmonary arrest or death

CONTINUOUS QUALITY INDICATORS

Cardiovascular complications in recovery requiring treatment (e.g., arrhythmias, hypotension, and hypertension)
Respiratory complications in recovery requiring treatment (e.g., asthma)
Nausea not controlled within 2 hours of recovery
Pain not controlled within 2 hours of recovery
Postoperative vomiting rate
Prolonged PACU stay (>2 hours)
Medication error
Injuries (i.e., to the eyes or teeth)
Time to return to light activities of daily living (ADL)
Common postoperative sequelae (e.g., sore throat, muscle pain, and headache)
Postdural puncture headache or transient radicular irritation
Discharge without escort or against medical advice
Patient satisfaction
Equipment maintenance

Adapted from ASA Committee on Ambulatory Surgical Care and ASA Task Force on Office-based Anesthesia: http://www.asahq.org/publicationsAndServices/outcomeindicators.pdf

---

tion of their member ambulatory surgery centers and office-based surgery practices. Some third-party payers and Medicare require accreditation for reimbursement of both facility and professional fees. Additionally, accreditation may improve marketing to both patients and surgeons by demonstrating that the facility has met high standards. The only drawback of accreditation is cost, both in actual dollars and in people-hours of preparation.

Sadly, some ASCs and surgery offices will not agree to accreditation and clinical oversight unless required to do so. With the current push for procedures to be performed on more complex patients in an outpatient setting, many believe mandatory accreditation of some type will be required by all states and payers in the future.

Credentialing and privileging remain difficult issues for providers who do not practice in the hospital setting. Accreditation may provide direction, and each facility must decide how best to handle this dilemma. No matter what accreditation, credentialing, or privileging process occurs, collection and analysis of quality improvement data for procedures performed in the ambulatory setting are essential to ensure high-quality care in an arena in which there is considerable emphasis on speed and efficiency.

REFERENCE

1. Joint Commission on Accreditation of Healthcare Organizations. http://www.jcaho.org

SUGGESTED READING

Accreditation Association for Ambulatory Health Care. http://www.aaahc.org

Accreditation Association for Ambulatory Health Care, Inc.: Accreditation Handbook for Ambulatory Health Care, 2003.

American Association for Accreditation of Ambulatory Surgery Facilities, Inc. http://www.aaaasf.org

American College of Surgeons: Patient Safety. http://www.facs.org/patientsafety/patientsafety.html

American Dental Association's Commission on Dental Accreditation. http://www.ada.org/prof/ed/accred/commission/index.asp

American Society of Anesthesiologists: Office-Based Anesthesia Guidelines. http://www.asahq.org/Washington/oba.htm

American Society of Anesthesiologists: State Legislative and Regulatory Activities: Office-Based Anesthesia. http://www.asahq.org/Washington/rulesregs.htm

Federation of State Medical Boards: Report of the Special Committee on Outpatient (Office-based) Surgery. http://www.fsmb.org/Policy%20Documents%20and%20White%20Papers/outpatient_surgery_cmt_rpt.htm

Outpatient Surgery Magazine Editors: Accreditation Roundup: What's in Store for 2004? Outpatient Surgery Magazine, 28–33, January 2004.

Saufl NM, Fieldus MH: Accreditation: a "voluntary" regulatory requirement. J Perianesth Nurs 18:152–159, 2003.

Taylor D: Weighing the Pros and Cons of Accreditation. Outpatient Surgery Magazine, 54–59, January 2003.

TÜV Healthcare Specialists. www.tuvhs.com

Ambulatory Surgery Facility Design and Construction

DOROTHY S. FRYER

In the last 2 decades, the number of freestanding ambulatory surgery centers (ASCs) has increased sevenfold. Approximately 3700 Medicare-certified outpatient centers currently exist. This increase has occurred due to physician demands, patient preference, changes in requirements for certificates of need, new policies of third-party payers, and availability of capital. The success or failure of these freestanding units depends on multiple factors, but rests largely on the quality of the facility, the type of services it offers to the physician and the patient, and its competitiveness with other health care providers in the community.

Typically, anesthesiologists are not participants at the beginning of the planning and development of an ambulatory surgery center, perhaps from the perception that input from anesthesia providers would not result in attracting patients (which increases profitability) to the center. However, attracting patients into the center is not the only determinant of a center's profitability. In fact, the anesthesiologist's insight into operating room (OR) efficiency can greatly increase the productivity of an ASC, resulting in positive effects on the center's daily operations, thereby increasing its profitability significantly.

This chapter broadly outlines the development of an ASC, beginning with the origin of the concept: assessing the feasibility of the project, hiring the necessary people, and designing the facility. Knowing how ambulatory facilities develop from beginning to end will give anesthesiologists information that can allow them to see how and where they can influence the planning for a facility. There are, of course, specific anesthesia-related topics that should be considered during the planning phases of any ambulatory surgery center. Many of the topics here are also applicable to the development of office surgical facilities, although on a smaller scale. The requirements for an office surgery suite vary greatly, depending on local and state regulation of office practice.

PREDESIGN

Goals of Predesign

The plan to construct an ambulatory surgery facility is developed in response to some unmet health care need in the community or, usually, because of physician desire for more autonomy or increased profitability. Or perhaps there are an insufficient number of operating rooms or inefficient care in operating rooms of existing facilities. Whatever creates the idea for developing an ASC, the surgeon/developer now has a goal: providing efficient, cost-effective, and profitable health care. However, before an ASC is constructed, there are many areas to research and much preparation to be done. One of the key issues before even beginning is a consideration of any local requirement for a certificate of need (CON). CONs give local government a way to limit medical facility construction. There has been a recent resurgence in CON interest by government as a way to limit the growth of health care costs.

Management Team

No matter what the specific goal for the center, the same initial steps should be followed. A business plan must be developed, and this critically important business plan drives the selection of a development plan. The surgeon/developer should enlist the help of others who will be participating in the ambulatory center. Those who agree to help should be totally committed to the project. They must be made aware that serious demands will be made on their time, energy, and finances.

Once the physicians who will be involved are identified, a management team should be selected from among their ranks. This management team will have multiple functions. They will be involved in planning the development of the ASC from beginning to end. When the building is completed, they will ensure that the proper program elements are in place to keep the facility operating smoothly. The management team should select a manager who will assume many of the day-to-day activities as the ASC is planned, constructed, and becomes operational.

Partnership Structure

There are four options for partnership structure commonly used in developing an ambulatory surgery center (Table 14-1). Most often, a partnership is formed consisting only of physicians who fully own and operate the ASC.

This type of ASC is referred to as an "independent" ASC. Although more financial risk is involved, more profits are seen for the investors (i.e., the physicians) involved. The second partnership structure is a "corporate partnership," in which physicians partner with a for-profit ASC corporation. Most of the investment is provided by the partnering corporation; therefore, its greatest advantage is the limited investment risk for the physicians involved. The corporation will also provide a management team to assist in the center's development. The drawbacks here are sharing profit and less autonomy for the physicians. For the third kind, occasionally a hospital will partner with a physician group to form a "hospital-physician partnership." Again, there is sharing of contract negotiations and investment risk, but also sharing of profits and control. The fourth kind, a "joint venture" ASC, is formed by a hospital, a for-profit ASC firm, and a physician group. This partnership approach combines all three groups—physicians, ASC corporations, and hospitals—and is the least common partnership structure.

Business Plan and Feasibility Study

The business plan and feasibility study are a very crucial part of the predesign phase and should be done with extraordinary care. Surgeons who will use the facility should be asked to provide relevant statistics for the business plan, which evaluates the type and volume of cases that these surgeons can bring to the ASC. This caseload review should realistically estimate the potential number

---

Table 14-1 Partnership Models

Type of Partnership	Pros	Cons
Independent	• Controlled and managed by physicians/owners • Autonomy for physicians • 100% of the profits shared by physicians/owners	• Higher investment risk (physicians provide all the capital) • Risk of underutilization • Low facility fee payment • Physicians negotiate all contracts • Shared profits
Corporate	• Reduced physician risk • Professional management • Contracting expertise • Higher revenues and facility fees • Accessible capital	• Shared control
Hospital	• Convenient location • Hospital provides capital • Hospital negotiates contracts • Certificates of need are easier to acquire • Good facility fees	• Physicians lose leverage • Competing uses for capital • Hospital usually wants majority ownership
Joint Venture	• Three parties to provide capital • Lowered risk for all • Balanced and less adversarial • Managed like an ASC • Good facility fees	• Profit split three ways • Less ownership by physicians

and type of patients in order to determine the practicality of going forward with development.

It should be stressed that the past caseload data that are evaluated should only come from surgeons who are committed to using the new facility. Information collected from physicians who are not committed to the project can result in faulty data that will yield inaccurate and overly optimistic projections. The final product could be a facility that is unable to support itself.

The caseload data can be gathered on forms such as the one shown in Figure 14-1. These forms are sent to the physicians who will be involved in the ambulatory center. They can be filled out by the office manager or by any employee who has access to his or her caseload. As noted in the figure, the caseload should be separated into Medicare and non-Medicare cases. The cases should then be categorized according to a nationally accepted coding and billing system. Information on surgical cases, reimbursement codes, and facility fees may be found in the *Federal Register* and has been compiled into several commercially available manuals. The codes and fees that are contained in these manuals are essential in computing an accurate total facility fee. The income generation potential of a new ASC can be determined by cataloging patients according to their proper status (e.g., Medicare,

Medicaid, or other third-party payer); assigning case-specific diagnostic-related group (DRG), current procedural terminology (CPT), international classification of disease (ICD), and Health Care Financing Administration (HCFA) common procedure coding system (HCPCS) codes; and deriving exact facility fees. Analysis should take into account current proposed changes in government outpatient reimbursement.

Once the caseload data are collected from the surgeons, the total number of cases per year available to be performed in the ASC can be calculated using the form in Figure 14-2. Notice that once the total number of cases is compiled, it is then reduced, or discounted, somewhat. Not all the cases that could be done in the ASC will actually be done there. There are several reasons for this. Some managed care providers will not allow patients to use a particular ASC, some patients will prefer not to be cared for there, and some patients will not be suitable freestanding surgery center candidates. It is important to consider increased competition from hospitals or other ASCs. Figure 14-3 shows an example of what a projected caseload might look like.

The next part of the feasibility study is determining the number of operating rooms required, thereby determining the size of the facility. To accomplish this task, an

Enclosed is the *Federal Register*, with procedures listed and the procedure payment group number. Please enter the total number of each procedure your physician(s) has performed in the last 12 months onto this chart. This chart must be filled in or the five-year cash flow analysis will not be able to be computed.

_____ **Percentage of procedures performed as outpatient**

Group number	Number of cases per 12-month period
Group 1	_____
Group 2	_____
Group 3	_____
Group 4	_____
Group 5	_____
Group 6	_____
Group 7	_____
Group 8	_____
Group 9 (50590 renal extra corporeal shockwave lithotripsy)	_____
Misc.	_____
(please also list misc. reimbursement fee)	$_____

_____ **Percentage of Medicare reimbursement**

_____ **Percentage of third-party reimbursement**

Please include on another sheet any major procedures and their respective reimbursement fee that are not listed in the register (e.g., tonsillectomies, vasectomies, etc.)

Figure 14-1 Surgery preprogramming form. (Redrawn from Billig HE 3rd: The Ambulatory Surgery and Outpatient Services Manual. New York, McGraw-Hill, 1997, p 13.)

	Medicare Groupings									Total	% Medicare	% Third-Party Payer
	I	II	III	IV	V	VI	VII	VIII	IX			
Physician 1	——	——	——	——	——	——	——	——	——	——	——	——
Physician 2	——	——	——	——	——	——	——	——	——	——	——	——
Physician 3	——	——	——	——	——	——	——	——	——	——	——	——
Physician 4	——	——	——	——	——	——	——	——	——	——	——	——
Physician 5	——	——	——	——	——	——	——	——	——	——	——	——
Total	——	——	——	——	——	——	——	——	——	——		
Discount 15%	——	——	——	——	——	——	——	——	——	——		
Total anticipated caseload	——	——	——	——	——	——	——	——	——	——	——	——

Future anticipated caseload*

*Increase caseload from 3% to 10% per year.

Figure 14-2   Caseload analysis form. (Redrawn from Billig HE 3rd: The Ambulatory Surgery and Outpatient Services Manual. New York, McGraw-Hill, 1997, p 14.)

1995												
	Medicare Groupings									Total	% Medicare	% Third-Party Payer
	I	II	III	IV	V	VI	VII	VIII	IX			
Physician 1	160	94	96	213	26	18	46	0	0	653	12%	88%
Physician 2	0	23	60	18	53	23	0	0	0	177	15%	85%
Physician 3	0	0	0	45	24	19	0	230	0	318	80%	20%
Physician 4	0	18	87	88	65	40	39	0	0	337	20%	80%
Physician 5	180	80	270	190	50	14	54	0	0	838	16%	84%
Total	340	215	513	554	218	114	139	230	0	2,323		
Discount 15%	51	32	77	83	33	17	21	34	0	348		
Total anticipated caseload	289	183	436	471	185	97	118	196	0	1975	24%	76%

Future anticipated caseload

1996*	2,073
1997*	2,177
1998*	2,286
1999*	2,400
2000*	2,520
2001*	2,646

*Assume 5% increase per year.

Figure 14-3   Sample caseload analysis. (Redrawn from Billig HE 3rd: The Ambulatory Surgery and Outpatient Services Manual. New York, McGraw-Hill, 1997, p 15.)

operating room utilization chart, shown in Figure 14-4, should be used. This will establish the number of cases that can be performed in one operating room per day. This information, combined with the total number of cases to be done each year, will tell you how many operating rooms will be needed in the facility. Figure 14-5 shows a sample of the operating room utilization chart.

The final form needed to complete the feasibility study is shown in Figure 14-6. It represents a typical form itemizing all the rooms that will be needed in the ASC. The *40% circulation* number represents space allotted for hallways and walls. Decreasing this number significantly may hamper the flow of personnel and patients within the facility.

Figure 14-7 is a form calculating the land requirements for the ASC, including parking space. Parking will be a very significant issue for any ASC. Unlike a hospital, where some patients enter the facility and remain for several days, every patient who enters the outpatient facility will be leaving the same day. This will produce considerably more traffic than an inpatient facility. In order to avoid congestion and traffic jams, which will be time-consuming and frustrating for the patients and doctors, careful planning must go into designing the parking area. The parking lot needs to have about four parking spots for every preoperative space in the facility. Some use estimates of four to five parking spaces per 1000 square feet. This ratio accommodates a reasonable estimate of the needs of doctors, nurses, and patients. It is essential to have smooth parking lot ingress and egress, as well as

easy patient drop-off and pick-up. Poor parking and congested traffic patterns would be a major drawback for any ASC.

The careful and precise quantification of the facility's program requirements will result in a facility that is not overbuilt. Doing so will avoid incurring unnecessary rent and maintenance costs, which could be the difference between profit and loss at the end of a year.

CLINICAL CAVEAT: INADEQUATE FEASIBILITY STUDY

- To predict ASC needs, all participants must be surveyed—patients, physicians, investors, and city officials.
- To predict ASC size, the caseload data need to be accurately collected. Factor in the proper adjustment for current caseload and how needs will change in the future.

Design and Construction Options

If the project is deemed viable after all the data are collected and examined, the management team can then continue to the design and construction phase. There are three basic options for the *design, bid, build* process. The management team can hire an architect to design

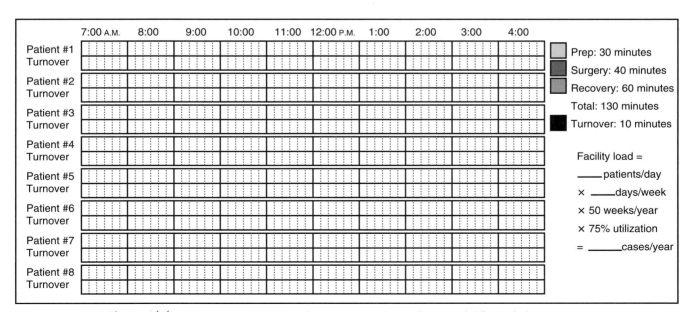

Figure 14-4   Operating room analysis form. (Redrawn from Billig HE 3rd: The Ambulatory Surgery and Outpatient Services Manual. New York, McGraw-Hill, 1997, p 15.)

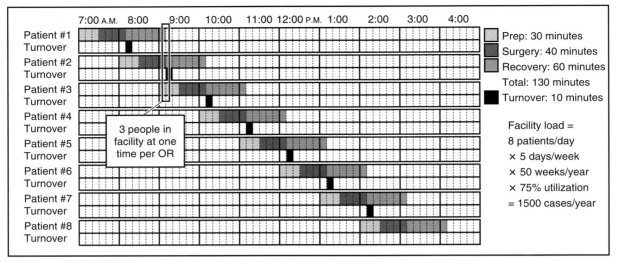

Figure 14-5   Sample operating room utilization chart. (Redrawn from Billig HE 3rd: The Ambulatory Surgery and Outpatient Services Manual. New York, McGraw-Hill, 1997, p 17.)

the ASC, to prepare construction documents, to bid the project, and then to begin construction. This has been the traditional way, even though it is time-consuming and the potential exists for the actual bids to exceed the estimated construction costs.

A second construction method that has become popular is for the management team to hire both an architect and a construction firm. This shifts some risks to the owner but can be faster and can establish parallel phasing. The construction firm has the responsibility of providing a construction manager who coordinates the project. This manager bids out, hires, and oversees all of the subcontractors. He or she manages the project entirely, from beginning to end. The success or failure of the facility's construction is heavily dependent on the construction manager. If the manager has much experience in the development of ASCs, this method may be acceptable, but if he or she has little experience, there are likely to be many problems.

The third method of construction involves hiring an ASC consultant group to provide a turnkey process. These groups have substantially multiplied in number in the last decade. Locating one can be as simple as looking in the yellow pages or in any of the outpatient surgery journals. When a consultant group is hired, it expects to be involved as early as possible. They want to establish a team, to do the feasibility study, and to advise on partnership formation, in addition to designing and constructing the facility. They have total control over the facility's development. This method has the advantage of requiring less decision-making on the part of the management team. It can also be very efficient and cost-effective. The tradeoff can mean giving up control and not having input into the project, which could result in owning a facility that is not exactly what the

management team or the owners had envisioned. It is essential to have an open-book arrangement to monitor and control costs.

Selecting a construction method that will ultimately result in the desired ASC depends on careful research, planning, and adherence to strict and objective criteria. The architect, construction firm, or health care consultant should have considerable experience in working with health care and ambulatory care facilities. Conducting interviews with the prospective candidates will help establish their experience level, professionalism, ability to communicate, and current workload. Paying visits to sites that are under construction or completed allows assessment of the quality of their workmanship. Talking to former clients will elicit information about their overall satisfaction with the final product. The physicians should ask about the candidate firm's dependability and overall integrity, responsiveness to their clients, and ability to meet deadlines and to stay within a budget. Persistent questioning should lead to selecting a partner who will perform well.

The team should not forget that, in addition to the usual building codes, the state and federal government have guidelines and regulations specifically for health care facilities. The design firm should research and consider these. If Medicare certification is desired, they, too, have rigorous stipulations that must be heeded. Make sure that the ASC complies with any state licensure laws. Medicare also mandates meeting the requirements of federal and state safety codes, conditions of participation (COP) from the Centers for Medicare and Medicaid Services (CMS), the National Fire Protection Association, and the American Institute of Architects (AIA).

	Single-Specialty, Attached to Practice			Multispecialty Freestanding		
		Subtotal	Total		Subtotal	Total
A. Vestibule*	80 to 120 SF		____ SF	80 to 120 SF		____ SF
B. Waiting						
1. Seats	6 Seats × # of ORs @ 18 SF/seat =	____ SF		6 Seats × # of ORs @ 18 SF/seat =	____ SF	
2. Nourishment/TV	1 @ 15 SF =	____ SF	____ SF	1 @ 15 SF =	____ SF	____ SF
C. Waiting room toilet*	1 @ 55 SF =		____ SF	1 @ 55 SF =		____ SF
D. Business area						
1. Positions						
• Reception/scheduler	60 SF/person	____ SF		60 SF/person	____ SF	
• Transcription	40 SF/person	____ SF		40 SF/person	____ SF	
• Billing/collection	40 SF/person	____ SF		40 SF/person	____ SF	
2. Files	40 SF/OR	____ SF		40 SF/OR	____ SF	
3. Work/computer	30 to 50 SF =	____ SF	____ SF	30 to 50 SF =	____ SF	____ SF
E. Family room*	1 per OR @ 80 SF =		____ SF	1 per OR @ 80 SF =		____ SF
F. Patient dressing						
1. Toilet/dressing	1 per OR @ 55 SF =	____ SF		1 per OR @ 55 SF =	____ SF	
2. Patient lockers/gowns	3 per OR @ 55 SF =	____ SF	____ SF	3 per OR @ 55 SF =	____ SF	____ SF
G. Control station	80 to 120 SF		____ SF	100 to 150 SF		____ SF
H. Prep/recovery						
1. Curtained stations	2 per OR @ 80 SF =	____ SF		2 per OR @ 80 SF =	____ SF	
2. Enclosed stations	1 per OR @ 80 SF =	____ SF		1 per OR @ 80 SF =	____ SF	
3. Recovery lounge	3 per OR @ 80 SF =	____ SF		3 per OR @ 80 SF =	____ SF	
I. Operating rooms	350 to 400 SF		____ SF	350 to 400 SF		____ SF
J. Soiled utility	60 to 80 SF		____ SF	80 to 120 SF		____ SF
K. Clean utility/sterilization	60 to 80 SF		____ SF	80 to 120 SF		____ SF
L. Sterile storage	60 to 80 SF		____ SF	80 to 150 SF		____ SF
M. Scrub sink	1/OR @ 10 SF =		____ SF	1/OR @ 10 SF =		____ SF
N. Clean storage	30 to 50 SF		____ SF	40 to 80 SF		____ SF
O. Soiled holding	30 to 50 SF		____ SF	40 to 80 SF		____ SF
P. Anesthesia/work/storage	40 to 80 SF		____ SF	40 to 80 SF		____ SF
Q. Staff dressing						
1. Male dressing	80 to 120 SF	____ SF		100 to 150 SF	____ SF	
2. Female dressing	100 to 150 SF	____ SF		120 to 180 SF	____ SF	
3. Toilet with shower	2 @ 65 SF =	____ SF		2 @ 65 SF =	____ SF	
4. Break room*	80 to 100 SF	____ SF	____ SF	100 to 120 SF	____ SF	____ SF
R. General storage	80 to 100 SF		____ SF	100 to 250 SF		____ SF
S. Equipment storage	60 to 120 SF		____ SF	100 to 250 SF		____ SF
T. Janitor's closet	20 to 30 SF		____ SF	20 to 30 SF		____ SF
U. Gas storage	30 to 50 SF		____ SF	30 to 50 SF		____ SF
V. UPS room	30 to 50 SF		____ SF	30 to 50 SF		____ SF
W. Mechanical space	80 to 100 SF		____ SF	80 to 120 SF		____ SF
X. Miscellaneous areas						
1. Laser room*	80 to 120 SF		____ SF	80 to 120 SF		____ SF
2. Dark room*	30 SF		____ SF	30 SF		____ SF
3. Director's office*	80 to 120 SF		____ SF	80 to 120 SF		____ SF
4. Endoscopy rooms*	180 to 220 SF		____ SF	180 to 220 SF		____ SF
5. Endoscopy utility*	60 to 80 SF		____ SF	60 to 80 SF		____ SF
Total net area	Sum of A through X		____ SF	Sum of A through X		____ SF
40% circulation	40% of total net		____ SF	40% of total net		____ SF
Total gross area	Total net + circulation		____ SF	Total net + circulation		____ SF

SF, Square feet.
*Not required by Medicare.

Figure 14-6   Surgery area space form. (Redrawn from Billig, HE 3rd: The Ambulatory Surgery and Outpatient Services Manual. New York, McGraw-Hill, 1997, p 20.)

1. Building footprint from space program		____ SF
2. Parking	4 stalls per pre-op/post-op station 350 SF/Stall	____ SF
Subtotal		____ SF
3. Green area	(1 + 2) × .5	____ SF
Total land area		____ SF

SF, Square feet.

Figure 14-7   Surgery area land requirements form. (Redrawn from Billig HE 3rd: The Ambulatory Surgery and Outpatient Services Manual. New York, McGraw-Hill, 1997, p 22.)

DESIGN

Once the preplanning phase is complete, the design phase of the facility can begin. The basic design requirements of the facility are already determined by the nuber of surgeons involved, their specialties, the expected patient load, and the general needs of any ambulatory surgery center.

The first phase in facility design is to locate a site. We already know the space needs of the facility based on the outcome of the feasibility study. If a site is located that is adequate in size, the next criterion it must meet is visibility. Patients must be able to recognize the facility easily. A facility that is difficult to locate will ultimately result in lost time and clients. Once the ASC is recognized, it should be accessible to all those who use it: patients, surgeons, and staff. The final issue regarding the site is the cost. Not only must the location of the facility be large enough, visible, and accessible, but it must also be affordable.

The overall design of the ASC should emphasize ease of patient flow and efficiency. When ease of patient flow and efficiency are compromised, patients will spend a longer amount of time in the ASC, ultimately resulting in smaller volumes of patients per facility. This will defeat the basic purpose of the ASC. How will entry access, patient entrance design, and patient exit requirements affect the final physical plan? Are there needs for future expansion?

The design of the facility is accomplished in two phases. The first phase is the rough draft or schematic design. This produces the basic size and outline of the building, its rooms, and its general area. Once agreement is reached on the schematics, the hard work begins on a detailed design development plan. Close cooperation is essential among the designers, the construction firm, and the facility owners and users to work out the very specific details of each room.

A sample schematic design of an ambulatory surgery facility is seen in Figure 14-8. All ambulatory surgery facilities have certain basic requirements. The precise function of the facility will further delineate the design and layout. Familiarity with design requirements will aid those involved in their development to make certain all requirements are met, without omissions or oversights. It may also yield insight into the management and functioning of the ASC once construction is concluded.

The basic layout of ASCs can be divided into three areas: the reception area, the perioperative area, and the storage area.

Reception Area

The reception area will include a reception desk, a waiting area for escorts, a business office, a conference room, and public restrooms. Because the reception area is the first area the patient will see, it sets the tone for the patient's outpatient experience. The facility should be designed and decorated with the expected clientele in mind. If there has been insufficient attention to detail, the patients and their escorts may feel the ASC is substandard. Over-the-top reception areas may create a feeling of unnecessary expense to the patient, and they will not want to pay for this aspect of their medical care.

Upon entering the ASC, patients should automatically walk toward a reception desk where they register. The registration area should provide privacy and a comfortable chair to sit upon while the patient completes forms, answers questions, and listens to instructions. The patient and the escort can then be directed to the adjacent waiting area.

The waiting area should be quiet and friendly. Patients who are about to undergo surgery will be experiencing increased emotional stress. A relaxed atmosphere in the waiting area will go a long way toward reducing their tension. Comfortable chairs should be arranged in small groupings. The waiting area should have a television with appropriate entertainment channels, a refreshment area for family and friends of the patient (clearly marked "not for preoperative patients"), a table or desk where writing might be done, and possibly an Internet hookup. Restrooms should be located conveniently, but discreetly, nearby.

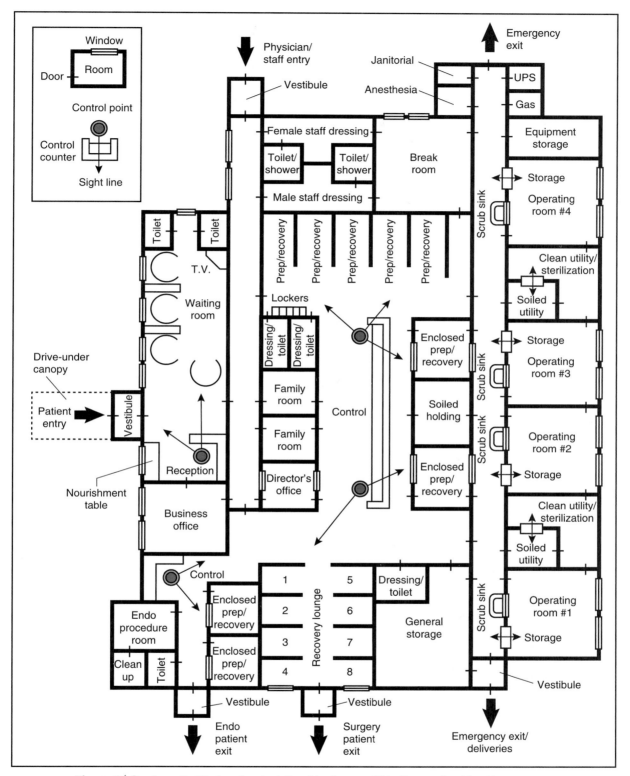

Figure 14-8   Large facility functional relationship diagram. This diagram should not be construed as a floor plan. (Redrawn from Billig, HE 3rd: The Ambulatory Surgery and Outpatient Services Manual. New York, McGraw-Hill, 1997, p 47.)

In centers where plastic surgery is frequently performed, patients may feel more comfortable with a separate entrance into the facility and a private waiting area prior to their surgery, or they may go directly to an enclosed preoperative cubicle. There are multiple ways that this situation can be handled, but a private entrance should be considered during the initial planning stages of the design layout. Adding it later could be strategically difficult and very expensive.

The business office will also be in the reception area. Its size and function will vary depending on the facility. Some facilities may want to outsource much of their billing and record keeping, and then there is no need for a large billing office. Alternatively, if the billing is done primarily onsite, a separate office for the business manager of the facility may be included. Office space for the facility's medical director should also be situated nearby and, ideally, would be accessible to both the business office and the perioperative area.

Perioperative Area

The perioperative area contains the patient changing rooms, the physician and staff locker rooms, a physician and staff lounge, preoperative slots, Phase I and Phase II postoperative slots, a control desk, and the operating rooms.

At the appropriate time, patients will be led from the waiting room to the perioperative area. They will first be taken to a changing area where they will remove their clothes, put on a surgical gown, and store their belongings. The precise configuration of this space can be arranged in a variety of ways. It should provide a large enough area for the patient to comfortably undress, have seating so that patients can remove their shoes, and have a place for patients to securely store their belongings. The changing area also should have at least one restroom nearby.

The staff should have a changing area and a lounge in this section of the ASC. Most states require separate changing areas for male and female staff, with separate restrooms and showers. These changing areas should be located so that staff and physicians can enter the ASC from a nonsterile environment, change into their scrub attire, and then proceed to their destinations within the center. The changing areas need adequate locker space to store the clothes and belongings of staff and physicians. It is tempting to conserve space in this area. However, this may result in alienating physicians who are frustrated by a cramped locker room.

Once patients have changed into hospital garb, they are led to a preoperative slot where further assessment can be conducted. Here nurses, anesthesia providers, and surgeons can obtain necessary information from patients. Three types of preoperative slots are possible in an ASC design: curtained, partially enclosed, and fully enclosed. Curtained areas have curtains on three sides, require the least amount of space, and are the most cost-effective to build. They also have the least amount of privacy and are the least customer-friendly design. Facilities usually should provide more privacy for patient interviews, surgical marking, and the performance of procedures such as nerve blocks. Partially enclosed cubicles are separated by a solid wall on the sides and are curtained off at the door. Private cubicles are fully enclosed and should have a window in the door to allow observation by those at the control desk. Minimum space requirements for the kind of slots selected are predetermined by AIA regulations.

The heart of the perioperative area is the control desk. The control desk needs to have a central location so that people staffing the control desk have a view of patients in both the preoperative and postoperative recovery areas (Fig. 14-8). Since the desk needs to serve multiple functions, it should contain areas for charting, cleanup, medicine preparation, and refreshment, as well as a utility area. It should also be a place in which the surgeons can freely discuss patient-care plans with nurses without being overheard by patients and families. Either in this area or close by should be an area where surgeons can dictate reports of their procedures.

Anesthesia personnel should also have a presence at the control desk. The control desk is where the daily schedule is orchestrated. Both anesthesia providers and nurses will be responsible for managing the daily schedule and its changes; a central control desk can be the appropriate place for such a function. The control desk should also provide easy viewing of patients coming in and out of the operating rooms as well as the areas for pre- and postoperative patients. There may be a video monitor at the control desk that connects to all of the ORs. This allows the progress within each OR to be tracked from the control desk in order to expedite the schedule.

As the day progresses in the ASC, patients will no longer fill the preoperative slots as they move on to the OR. At some point in time, the predominant activity will shift from preoperative care to postoperative care. The most efficient way to utilize space within the perioperative area, therefore, is to also designate the preoperative slots as postoperative Phase I recovery slots. Newer designsmake this a natural transition. This is a very efficient use of space and personnel. As the busy time in the preopertive area decreases, the activity in the postoperative areas increases. The preoperative nurses can now move over to the recovery area and take charge of the patients there, which optimizes manpower. The only caution would be not to place a preoperative patient too close to a postoperative patient who may have disconcerting postoperative complications such as retching and vomiting. These usually upset a patient waiting for surgery.

When preoperative patients have completed the necessary preoperative requirements, they proceed to the operating room. The design of the operating room is critical. It needs to be located close to the preoperative area. The corridors leading to the OR must be uncluttered and large enough to make transport smooth. Transport gurneys must be placed in a convenient, out-of-the-way storage area for the time the patient is in the OR. Attention to these details ensures that delays are minimized.

The size of the OR should not be excessive, but it needs to be large enough to accommodate the surgery that must be done. The room's layout has to be carefully planned so that each square foot available is used to maximum advantage. The placement of electrical, communication, and gas lines and outlets must be considered. Proper orientation of the door to the OR, the OR table, and the OR equipment allows for the easy flow for nurses, surgeons, anesthesia, and patients. Many of the design decisions will be mandated by building codes, but advice from nurses, surgeons, and anesthesia providers should be elicited. Every effort should be made to avoid a setup that creates time-consuming movement. The goal of the design is to optimize efficiency and flow. It is also important to consider using materials that are easy to clean and maintain.

Once the surgery has been completed, the patient is returned to the postoperative recovery area. An example of a postoperative area location can be seen in Figure 14-8. The recovery process is divided into Phase I, the initial phase of recovery when the patient first comes out of the operating room, and Phase II, the period when the patient approaches discharge home. The Phase II area can be furnished with lounge-style chairs and may be curtained off so that patients can change back into their own clothes.

Storage and Utility Area

The last area to be considered is the storage and utility area. This area has predetermined functions that must be included. The area itself can be divided into two groups (Fig. 14-8). The first group of rooms is directly associated with the operating rooms. These rooms consist of the soiled utility area, the clean utility area, and the sterilization and storage area. Close attention needs to be paid to the location of this utility area. The movement of the instruments and other equipment traveling from the operating rooms to the soiled utility area and to reprocessing or disposal is a key determinant of the turnover time of operating rooms. The storage area may require

variable amounts of space. "Just-in-time" inventory techniques can reduce bulk storage requirements and can be a cost-effective management tool.

The second grouping of rooms in the storage and utility area consists of a soiled holding area, a clean storage area, the janitors' closets and equipment storage area, a mechanical storage room, and an anesthesia storage room. This second group of storage and utility rooms needs to be accessible to the control area.

Although not present in Figure 14-8, ambulatory centers that perform certain procedures will want laboratory facilities. General surgeons performing breast biopsies, for example, will need the specimens examined immediately. Office space is another convenience that busy surgeons appreciate, and may possibly demand, if they bring their patients in to the ASC.

The description above presents a very broad outline of the design process of an ASC facility with an attempt to stress features that should not be overlooked in the design process. The architects or health care consultants that are steering the project, along with any mandatory building guidelines, will provide additional details.

ANESTHESIA

Anesthesia services are an integral part of most outpatient facilities, and because of this, anesthesiologists should be involved in the design process as early as possible. For example, anesthesia providers must decide how medications will be managed. If a pharmacy is used, choose its location so that it is easily accessible. If, instead, only a drug storage area is used, it should be in an efficient location. Additionally, there are government regulations for accountability of controlled drugs and requirements for the secure construction of a storage room. These issues should be addressed early in the planning process so that a satisfactory system can be established.

Anesthesia for outpatients may involve the extensive use of regional anesthesia. Decisions have to be made about where these procedures will be performed. They can be performed in the preoperative cubical, in a separate block area, or in the operating room itself. If a block cart is used, determine where it should be stored. Each facility should use a method that presents the most efficient system, and only an anesthesia provider can help answer these questions.

Anesthesia personnel should be involved in the administration and the daily operations of any ASC. Their input is also crucial when making decisions about ASC design. They can offer advice about layout of operating rooms, specifying anesthesia equipment, the contents and location of the resuscitation cart, and many other operational details. A large ASC may require a sophisticated communications system to control traffic in the ASC efficiently, and anesthesia providers can greatly help this workflow design. At the earliest ASC planning stages, attention to detail by anesthesia providers can improve the efficiency of the facility.

CURRENT CONTROVERSY: CAN INCREASED MONETARY EXPENDITURE LEAD TO INCREASED EFFICIENCY?

Major equipment purchases, consultants for feasibility studies, and high-tech communications systems are all expensive. Can these high-ticket items result in increased efficiencies and yield significant monetary returns?

OCCUPANCY AND STARTUP

Although there are many issues that must be attended to before a medical facility can begin caring for patients, one of the most important is arranging for a certificate of occupancy. Local building code authorities must assure themselves and the public that the facility is suitable for habitation. Assuring that this process goes smoothly is the responsibility of the construction manager. During the stages of construction, there should be periodic walk-through events attended by representatives of the architectural, construction, and management teams. It is during these tours that the true physical layout of the facility becomes apparent. In addition, government building inspectors are required to sign off at various stages of the construction process before the next phase can begin. Construction mistakes or misunderstandings among the groups may be identified and corrected by means of these walk-through events.

Prior to occupancy, and even after, the owners will review and comment on the construction manager's punch-list, the to-do list of all corrections and changes that remain to be performed. Once the designers, builders, and owners are satisfied that local, state, and federal regulations concerning occupant safety have been addressed, inspectors arrive to give the final permission for occupancy by caregivers. At that time, medical and administrative staff can begin the process of moving, unpacking, and storing the supplies and equipment needed for the ultimate goal: caring for patients.

EXPANSION

In performing the initial ASC feasibility study, an attempt should have been made to plan for future expansion. It is entirely possible that the use projections will be inaccurate and that the center may have to be enlarged later. This option can and should be planned for in the initial design phase of the center. To include extra space in the initial plans would incur unnecessary costs, but the building can be planned in a modular style that will make future additions easier. Deciding where an addition might be placed could spare much time and expense in the future. The location of the building mechanical systems, patient flow patterns, and parking will all influence future expansion.

SUMMARY

Understanding facility design is essential, not only when planning new ASCs, but also in examining existing facilities, in order to improve their function. The emphasis on workflow and efficiency for doctors, patients, and staff is critical. Familiarity with the elements involved in the actual design stages of a center is also useful. The goal should be to develop an ASC that is the right size, that has the right number of rooms, and that is properly configured, ensuring the center's ability to provide the safest, fastest, and most efficient perioperative care possible.

SUGGESTED READING

2006 Manager's Guide to Surgical Construction. Outpatient Surgery Magazine. Herrin Publishing Partners, 2006.

American Institute of Architects: Guidelines for Design and Construction of Hospital and Health Care Facilities. Washington, D.C., American Institute of Architects, 2001.

Apfelbaum JL, Schreider BP: Outpatient Facility and Personnel. In White P (ed): Outpatient Anesthesia. New York, Churchill Livingston, 1990, pp 57–81.

Bell KA: Planning ahead: Practical hints for designing ambulatory care facilities. J Ambul Care Manage 22:74–88, 1999.

Billing HE 3rd: The Ambulatory Surgery and Outpatient Services Manual. New York, McGraw-Hill, 1997.

Kane DA: Innovation and customer service drive successful ambulatory care programs. J Ambul Care Manage 22:50–57, 1999.

Pinker LD: A physician's perspective on development of ambulatory care business. Woodrum Ambulatory Systems Development, Article 8, 1998–2003, http://www.woodrumasd.com

Pyrek KM: Master planning helps avoid mishaps in healthcare construction. Today's Surgicenter 6:14–17, 2003.

Roark J: SAMBA makes its mark. Today's Surgicenter 6:3–8, 2004.

Snyder DS, Pasternak LR: Facility Design and Procedural Safety. In White PF, Apfelbaum JL (eds): Ambulatory Anesthesia and Surgery, 2nd ed. Philadelphia, W.B. Saunders, 1997, pp 61–76.

Staunton EW, Vick JC: ASC business models: which one is right for you? Outpatient Surgery, Manager's Guide to Surgical Construction Issue: 8–10, 2004.

Taylor ED: 5 top tips for construction success. Outpatient Surgery, Manager's Guide to Surgical Construction Issue: 12–14, 2004.

Zasa RJ: Trends in the development of ambulatory care centers. Today's Surgicenter 6:18–21, 2003.

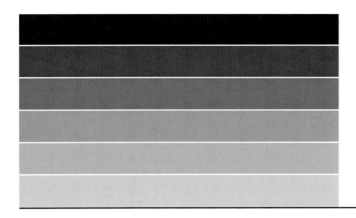

Appendix 1: Guidelines for Office-Based Anesthesia

(By permission of the American Society of Anesthesiologists. Approved by ASA House of Delegates on October 13, 1999; last affirmed on October 27, 2004.)

Administration and Facility
  Quality of Care
  Facility and Safety
Clinical Care
  Patient and Procedure Selection
  Perioperative Care
  Monitoring and Equipment
  Emergencies and Transfers

These guidelines are intended to assist American Society of Anesthesiologists (ASA) members who are considering the practice of ambulatory anesthesia in the office setting: office-based anesthesia (OBA). These recommendations focus on quality anesthesia care and patient safety in the office. These are minimal guidelines and may be exceeded at any time based on the judgment of the involved anesthesia personnel. Compliance with these guidelines cannot guarantee any specific outcome. These guidelines are subject to periodic revision as warranted by the evolution of federal, state, and local laws, as well as technology and practice.

ASA recognizes the unique needs of this growing practice and the increased requests for ASA members to provide OBA for health care practitioners (defined herein as physicians, dentists, and podiatrists) who have developed their own office operatories. Since OBA is a subset of ambulatory anesthesia, the ASA "Guidelines for Ambulatory Anesthesia and Surgery" should be followed in the office setting as well as all other ASA standards and guidelines that are applicable.

There are special problems that ASA members must recognize when administering anesthesia in the office setting. Compared with acute care hospitals and licensed ambulatory surgical facilities, office operatories currently have little or no regulation, oversight, or control by federal, state, or local laws. Therefore, ASA members must satisfactorily investigate areas taken for granted in the hospital or ambulatory surgical facility, such as governance, organization, construction, and equipment, as well as policies and procedures, including fire, safety, drugs, emergencies, staffing, training, and unanticipated patient transfers.

ASA members should be confident that the following issues are addressed in an office setting to provide patient safety and to reduce risk and liability to the anesthesiologist.

ADMINISTRATION AND FACILITY

Quality of Care

The facility should have a medical director or governing body that establishes policy and is responsible for the activities of the facility and its staff. The medical director or governing body is responsible for ensuring that facilities and personnel are adequate and appropriate for the type of procedures performed.

Policies and procedures should be written for the orderly conduct of the facility and reviewed on an annual basis.

The medical director or governing body should ensure that all applicable local, state, and federal regulations are observed.

All health care practitioners and nurses should hold a valid license or certificate to perform their assigned duties.

All operating room personnel who provide clinical care in the office should be qualified to perform services commensurate with appropriate levels of education, training, and experience.

The anesthesiologist should participate in ongoing continuous quality-improvement and risk-management activities.

The medical director or governing body should recognize the basic human rights of its patients, and a written document that describes this policy should be available for patients to review.

Facility and Safety

Facilities should comply with all applicable federal, state, and local laws, codes, and regulations pertaining to fire prevention, building construction and occupancy, accommodations for the disabled, occupational safety and health, and disposal of medical waste and hazardous waste.

Policies and procedures should comply with laws and regulations pertaining to controlled drug supply, storage, and administration.

CLINICAL CARE

Patient and Procedure Selection

The anesthesiologist should be satisfied that the procedure to be undertaken is within the scope of practice of the health care practitioners and the capabilities of the facility.

The procedure should be of a duration and degree of complexity that will permit the patient to recover and be discharged from the facility.

Patients who by reason of pre-existing medical or other conditions may be at undue risk for complications should be referred to an appropriate facility for performance of the procedure and the administration of anesthesia.

Perioperative Care

The anesthesiologist should adhere to the *Basic Standards for Preanesthesia Care, Standards for Basic Anesthetic Monitoring, Standards for Postanesthesia Care,* and *Guidelines for Ambulatory Anesthesia and Surgery,* as currently promulgated by the American Society of Anesthesiologists.

The anesthesiologist should be physically present during the intraoperative period and should be immediately available until the patient has been discharged from anesthesia care.

Discharge of the patient is a physician responsibility. This decision should be documented in the medical record.

Personnel with training in advanced resuscitative techniques (e.g., advanced cardiac life support [ACLS] and pediatric advanced life support [PALS]) should be immediately available until all patients are discharged home.

Monitoring and Equipment

At a minimum, all facilities should have a reliable source of oxygen, suction, resuscitation equipment, and emergency drugs. Specific reference is made to the ASA *Guidelines for Non-Operating Room Anesthetizing Locations.*

There should be sufficient space to accommodate all necessary equipment and personnel and to allow for expeditious access to the patient, anesthesia machine (when present), and all monitoring equipment.

All equipment should be maintained, tested, and inspected according to the manufacturer's specifications.

Back-up power sufficient to ensure patient protection in the event of an emergency should be available.

In any location in which anesthesia is administered, there should be appropriate anesthesia apparatus and equipment that allow monitoring consistent with ASA *Standards for Basic Anesthetic Monitoring* and documentation of regular preventive maintenance as recommended by the manufacturer.

In an office where anesthesia services are to be provided to infants and children, the required equipment, medication, and resuscitative capabilities should be appropriately sized for a pediatric population.

Emergencies and Transfers

All facility personnel should be appropriately trained in and should regularly review the facility's written emergency protocols.

There should be written protocols for cardiopulmonary emergencies and other internal and external disasters such as fire.

The facility should have medications, equipment, and written protocols available to treat malignant hyperthermia when triggering agents are used.

The facility should have a written protocol in place for the safe and timely transfer of patients to a prespecified alternate care facility when extended or emergency services are needed to protect the health or well-being of the patient.

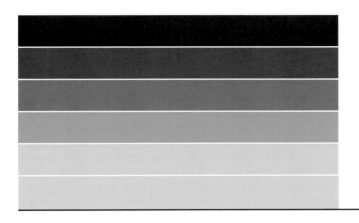

Appendix 2: Excerpt from *Considerations for Anesthesiologists in Setting Up and Maintaining a Safe Office Anesthesia Environment*

An informational manual compiled by the ASA Committee on Ambulatory Surgical Care and the ASA Task Force on Office-Based Anesthesia, 2000
Chair: Rebecca S. Twersky

ADMINISTRATION AND FACILITY

I. Facility Governance

The facility should have a medical director or governing body that establishes policy and is responsible for the activities of the facility and its staff. It should be a legal entity that may include a solo practitioner, partnership, corporation, or limited-liability corporation (LLC).

The medical director or governing body is responsible for ensuring that facilities and personnel are adequate and appropriate for the type of procedures performed. Policies and procedures should be written for the orderly conduct of the facility and should be reviewed on an annual basis. All applicable state and federal regulations, local laws, codes, and regulations pertaining to fire prevention, building construction and occupancy, accommodations for the disabled, occupational safety and health, and disposal of medical waste and hazardous waste should be observed.

II. Facility Accreditation

Several states already require or will be requiring accreditation of office surgical facilities as a means of objectively evaluating practices where state resources cannot provide inspections. Accreditation of office-based practices are currently conducted by the three major accrediting bodies: Joint Commission on Accreditation of Healthcare Organizations (JCAHO), Accreditation Association for Ambulatory Health Care (AAAHC), and American Association for Accreditation of Ambulatory Surgery Facilities (AAAASF). JCAHO, AAAHC, and AAAASF

181

are accreditation organizations that have received "deemed status" from Medicare. Developed to assure verifiable quality care with definable standards, these three accrediting organizations address, in a similar fashion, aspects of office-based surgery: the facility's physical layout, patient and personnel records, peer review and quality assurance, operating room personnel, equipment, operations and management, and environmental safety. Anesthesia requirements for accreditation are very generalized. Despite this, the classification of the surgical facilities used by the accrediting organizations focuses on the level of anesthesia provided. However, the classifications are not standardized. ASA has the following:

Class A: Minor surgical procedures performed under topical, local, or infiltration block anesthesia without preoperative or intraoperative sedation.

Class B: Minor or major surgical procedures performed in conjunction with oral, rectal, parenteral, or intravenous sedation or under analgesic or dissociative drugs.

Class C: Surgical procedures that require general anesthesia or major conduction blocks and support of vital bodily functions.

JCAHO and AAAHC will not accredit a freestanding surgery center unless it is also licensed in the state if that state has licensure of surgery centers. AAAASF does not require state licensure. This difference can result in AAAASF physical plant requirements that are not as stringent as those of the other two accrediting organizations. All three organizations will accredit an office-based surgery facility. JCAHO and AAAHC have traditionally focused their efforts on hospital-based and freestanding surgical facilities, respectively; AAAASF has focused primarily on the office-based center.

The standards for JCAHO are incorporated into generic statements for all types of services and patient care activities. Specific standards for office-based surgery are currently under development by JCAHO. AAAHC has delineated five additional standards specific for office-based anesthesia. Additionally, they have the capability to formally accredit anesthesia office practices that practice solely office-based anesthesia. With AAAASF, the focus of the standards is office-based surgery, and the requirements are aligned with that limited focus.

III. Provider Credentials and Qualifications

All health care practitioners (defined herein as physicians, dentists, podiatrists) and nurses should hold a valid license or certificate to perform their assigned duties. All operating room personnel who provide clinical care in the office should be qualified to perform services commensurate with their level of education, training, and experience.

A physician who administers or supervises the administration of anesthesia services in an office shall have credentials reviewed by the medical director or governing body of the office surgical facility. ASA believes that anesthesiologist participation in all office-based surgery is optimally desirable as an important anesthesia patient safety standard. However, regulations of many states contemplate that where anesthesiologist participation is not practicable, nonphysician anesthesia providers must, at a minimum, be directed by a licensed physician or by the operating practitioner. The health care practitioner providing direction should perform a preanesthetic examination and evaluation, prescribe the anesthesia, assure that qualified practitioners participate, remain physically present and immediately available for diagnosis, treat and manage anesthesia-related complications or emergencies, and assure the provision of indicated postanesthesia care. The supervising licensed physician or operating practitioner should be specifically trained in the office-based surgery being performed as well as sedation, anesthesia, and rescue techniques appropriate to the type of sedation being provided. It is recommended that anesthesiologists and surgeons practicing in an office-based setting maintain current advanced cardiac life support training. All other medical personnel, at a minimum, must maintain training in basic cardiopulmonary resuscitation.

IV. Records and Documentation

All patient records, including anesthesia records, must be available for review and kept on file by both the office-based practice and the anesthesia care provider (anesthesia records). These records should be kept according to state regulation: they should be maintained from the time the facility is opened and for the number of years thereafter as mandated by state regulations. The individual anesthesia care provider should also maintain the anesthesia records in a similar manner. Evidence of preoperative and postoperative evaluations must be documented in the patient record. Any necessary laboratory reports, including electrocardiogram or radiographs, medical consultation, and telephone contact with the patient, should be documented and available on the patient record.

Any forms signed by the patient (including consent, living wills, release of medical records permission, or others) should be kept in the file.

V. Quality Improvement Activities

The anesthesiologist should participate in ongoing continuous quality improvement and risk management activities of each particular office practice.

A. A written plan should be in place to continually assess, document, and improve the outcome of the anesthesia care provided.

B. Quality improvement activities are the ultimate responsibility of each facility or the administrative and economic entity responsible for providing patient care. The quality improvement plan itself is the responsibility of the owner or governing body of the office facility. This facility may include one or multiple sites.

C. Each anesthesiologist or anesthesiology group providing services in an office-based facility is responsible for evaluating and improving the care they provide as part of the overall facility effort.

D. An anesthesiologist or an anesthesiology group that provides anesthesia care at multiple facilities may form its own quality improvement unit to evaluate the total anesthesia care it provides.

E. The quality improvement plan should specify the individual who is responsible for performing each element of the plan.

F. The quality improvement plan should include anesthesia and surgical issues and consider the following elements:

1. Review of morbidity and adverse or sentinel events. Examples include the following.
    a. Death, cardiac, or respiratory arrest
    b. Unplanned reintubation
    c. Central nervous system or peripheral nervous system deficit appearing within 2 days of anesthesia
    d. Myocardial infarction within 2 days of anesthesia
    e. Pulmonary edema within 1 day of anesthesia
    f. Aspiration pneumonia
    g. Anaphylaxis or adverse drug reactions
    h. Post-dural puncture headache within 4 days of spinal or epidural anesthesia
    i. Dental injury
    j. Eye injury
    k. Surgical infection rate
    l. Excessive blood loss
    m. Unplanned admission to a hospital or other acute care facility

2. Review of quality indicators, to include measures of patient satisfaction.

3. The quality improvement plan should include at least an annual review and check of anesthesia equipment to ensure compliance with current safety standards and the standards for the release of waste anesthetic gases.

4. For each office facility at which anesthesia is provided on a regular or ongoing basis, facility quality improvement reviews should be conducted. The reviews should be performed by a group that includes, at a minimum, the medical director, a representative of the anesthesiologists currently providing patient care, and a representative of the operating room or recovery nursing staff. The frequency of the reviews

would be appropriate for the number of procedures performed, but they should be conducted at least annually and result in written minutes and conclusions.

VI. Continuing Education

Anesthesiologists participating in an office-based practice and the nonphysicians they medically direct should engage in regular and current courses of study of medical, ethical, and safety issues relevant to that office practice.

A. The continuing education should:
1. Be eligible for recognition as Category 1 credit by the American Medical Association or meet the equivalent requirements of the accrediting agency appropriate to the nonphysician provider.
2. Meet or exceed the requirements for continuing medical education to maintain state licensure.
3. Meet or exceed the requirements either:
    a. Established for office-based anesthesia in the state in which the anesthesia is administered, if such standards exist, or if not,
    b. Established by acute care hospitals in that local area for the administration of comparable types of anesthesia.

B. Written records of continuing medical education meeting these requirements should be maintained for at least 3 years by each anesthesiologist who administers or directs anesthesia.

VII. Professional Liability

It is essential that the individual practitioner not take liability coverage for granted and should also carefully examine the policy and all its declarations, amendments, attachments, and qualifications. It is common for insurers to require specific performance criteria for anesthesiologists, often citing ASA standards or guidelines and making adherence to these a condition of coverage. Such issues as mandatory oxygen saturation measurement, end-tidal CO_2 monitoring, constant presence in the operating room, and, increasingly, temperature measurement may well be part of policy requirements. It is vitally important that these provisions be understood and followed.

There are potential differences between hospital and office-based liability coverage. A few specific areas of difference are:

1. Insurers may lack an established peer-review structure to examine the quality of the exclusively office-based practitioner.
2. Insurers may lack a facility accreditation system to assess risk related to adequacy of the equipment,

supplies, and protocols and procedures in place for patient protection.

3. Office-based providers will frequently work only 1 or 2 days a week at a given office, so multiple sites complicate underwriting calculations.

4. Practices may cross state lines, giving rise to how multistate coverage is written.

5. Vicarious liability—the legal liability that may exist for others involved in the same incident—takes on a different perspective when considered in an office setting where the surgeon is the determinant of both the surgical risk and the risk associated with ownership and management of the facility and equipment.

Insurers may or may not consider entity coverage of the office-based site, covering surgeon, anesthesiologist, and facility in a single policy.

SUGGESTED PRACTICES OR OPTIONS

A. Information gained from several regional and national professional liability insurance agents and underwriters reveals some consistent requirements but a variety of approaches to this market. Among the information considered by one very conservative company prior to issuing a policy to an office-based surgeon or anesthesiologist are:

1. Clinic ownership and practitioner list;
2. Existence of policy and procedure manuals for routine and emergency situations, record review, and outcome analysis;
3. Types of anesthesia to be administered;
4. A description of equipment and monitoring capabilities;
5. Evidence that all patients give informed consent to both surgeon and anesthesiologist;
6. Evidence of adherence to a formal credentialing policy;
7. Procedures for resuscitation and arrangements for transport to an emergency or tertiary facility and that such a facility be within close proximity to the office;
8. Assurance of adherence to all applicable ASA standards;
9. Assurance that all patients will be discharged with a responsible adult;
10. Presence of a defibrillator if general anesthesia, regional anesthesia, or parenteral sedation/analgesia is to be administered;
11. Onsite inspection by the company's consultant anesthesiologist;
12. Compliance with all applicable federal and state statutes; and
13. Evidence that any voluntary accreditation is obtained.

B. Insurers appeared to have no bias against the exclusive office-based practitioner otherwise, however. One can postulate that the increased risk associated with the isolation of a surgical office is offset by the overall decreased ASA risk categorization of the typical office-based population. However, this may change as the medical complexity of the office-based patient increases.

C. There are concerns regarding the assumption of vicarious liability of others in the office-based surgical situation. It is vital that the anesthesiologist practicing in an office be absolutely certain of the license status, training qualifications for the procedures performed, and professional liability insurance of the operating surgeon and all assisting personnel. The anesthesiologist should personally examine all liability insurance policies for limitations or restrictions on the type of surgery to be performed and inquire of the state medical board for any limitations placed on the operating surgeon's license.

D. It is advisable to compare coverage limits with the surgeon. A wide disparity in coverage in which the anesthesiologist has significantly higher limits of coverage could invite disproportionate accusations of liability; in other words, the "deep-pocket" phenomenon. Assure also that any state requirements for liability insurance are met by all in the operating team.

E. Few sources indicated any demand for entity insurance. This is most likely due to the current "cottage industry" nature of office-based practice. As it becomes more prevalent and office surgical groups coalesce to be able to hire or contract for the full-time services of an anesthesiologist, increased demand will occur, and the clinic entity, including the anesthesiologist, is likely to be covered by a single insurance policy.

VIII. Facility and Safety

While state regulatory control is increasing, in the majority of office-based practices there will be no specific state regulatory authority; only general health, fire, and safety provisions will therefore apply. Voluntary organizations may offer guidelines or some degree of oversight. Ultimately, enforcement of any safety codes is up to the local, state, or federal authorities having jurisdiction.

A. Fire Safety

1. Both patient and anesthesiologist assume greater challenges with office-based anesthesia in a facility that does not meet the standards described in the National Fire Protection Association (NFPA) 99 Health Care Facilities document. The medical or commercial office building is built with the idea of an orderly evacuation in the event of a fire or similar disaster. In contrast, most hospitals follow a plan of "defend in place," with lateral evacuations if needed. Within an elevator building, there must be adequate capacity in an elevator to allow transport of a ventilated patient on a stretcher, either because of medical necessity or because the building must be evacuated. In all cases, protocols for fire drills and other emergencies will have to be developed and practiced.

2. Air handling within a commercial building in the event of a fire may be a problem. Long before heat or flames from a fire elsewhere in the building reach the office-based site, there may be toxic fumes. In contrast to the classic hospital operating room with its individualized ventilation and exhaust, an office building may separate rooms only by drywall partitioning below suspended ceilings. Several rooms may share a single ventilation system. Windows or window air-conditioning units that allow air intake from outside the building may make it more difficult to achieve adequate ventilation.

3. The guidelines of some surgical organizations speak to the use of ether and other flammable compounds for skin preparation; however, these are best avoided to eliminate noxious fumes and the risk of fires and explosions.

4. Office-based anesthesia often involves plastic surgery of the head and neck with the use of electrocautery. The use of supplemental oxygen during these procedures increases the risk of fire.

5. The disposal of waste anesthetic gases should also be assessed, both from an environmental and fire code perspective.

B. Medical Gases

NFPA has described gas supplies at health care facilities as Level 1, 2, or 3. Level 1 is the state in which patients are dependent on mechanical ventilation; Level 2 signifies that the medical, surgical, or diagnostic intervention is dependent on the piped system; and in Level 3, patients are not on critical life support equipment. It must be acknowledged that NFPA standards are not required in the office setting unless accrediting organizations indicate this. The Level 1 standard is the most comprehensive and one that most anesthesiologists are familiar with from the hospital setting. Each level has requirements with regard to piped or cylinder supplies as well as monitoring and capacity expectations. A full description can be found in the NFPA 99 *Standards for Health Care Facilities* (1999 edition), available from the NFPA (1-800-344-3555). If one seeks accreditation conforming to NFPA 99 regulations, then facilities conducting procedures on intubated patients on a ventilator will need to meet Level 1 requirements, whereas maximum allowable concentration (MAC) procedures may only require a Level 2.

In an office-based anesthesia practice, the anesthesiologist should evaluate the gas system to see if it is adequate for clinical needs and patient safety in that office. One may encounter medical gas systems that range from portable tanks on the anesthesia machine to sophisticated medical gas storage and distribution systems that meet NFPA specifications.

In any case, tanks need to be stored properly, and an adequate volume of gas must be on hand to meet the day's needs. Storage must conform to NFPA guidelines. Tanks should be transported and stored safely. When transporting gases, special attention should be given to ensuring that tanks are well secured in the vehicle and protected from puncture. Regulators attached to tanks must be protected. The tanks should be in a well-ventilated area of the vehicle (to prevent leaks from overwhelming the driver or causing an explosion risk). Smoking around gas cylinders is prohibited. Before transporting compressed gases, one should check to see if there are applicable local regulations (e.g., transporting gases in a tunnel).

Information and regulations that address the transportation of compressed or liquefied gases come primarily from the Compressed Gas Association (CGA) and the Department of Transportation (DOT), although local and state regulations may also apply. When transporting gas cylinders by motor vehicle, requirements of Title 49 of the Code of Federal Regulations (49 CFR: 171, 177) apply. In addition, the DOT regulates the driver and vehicle carrying the compressed gases (49 CFR: 390–397). The CGA has many publications that may be of interest to the physician who is handling gases (e.g., CGA P-1, P-2, P-12, and PS-6).

Compressed air and vacuum sources should also be evaluated. Compressed air in a Level 1 facility such as a JCAHO-approved hospital comes from a compressor that will not introduce lubricating hydrocarbons into the air stream. Cleanliness of the office's compressed air source should be ascertained. In a modern acute care hospital (Level 1), vacuum pumps have back-ups and emergency power provision; this may not be found in the typical office-based setup. In the event of a power failure, it is likely the vacuum will be lost, and another source must be available.

Options for anesthesia waste gas disposal are limited. Halogenated hydrocarbons or ethers and nitrous oxide are the primary anesthetic concerns for operating suite air pollution. Hospital or ambulatory surgery facilities make use of either active waste gas scavenging (with a piped vacuum system) or a passive system (with waste gases directed into the facility ventilation exhaust system). An office may utilize these standard methods or could opt for other methods to use. An exhaust hose may be run to an outside window; however, due care should be taken to ensure that the flow of waste gas does not re-enter that, or any other, living space. Another option is adsorption of hydrocarbons or ethers by activated charcoal. If this method is used, the manufacturer's instructions concerning system capacity and replacement should be followed. For an in-depth description of OSHA's advisory guidelines for anesthetic gas exposure, see http://www.osha-slc.gov/dts/osta/anestheticgases/index.html.

C. Equipment Safety

If the anesthetic is conducted in typical medical arts or commercial buildings, there may be no source of back-up electrical power unless specific provisions have been made with the practice. In such buildings, emergency lighting is only required to allow a safe and orderly exit from the building. Monitoring equipment with trickle-charged battery back-up might provide some capability for 1 or more hours. Battery life, however, is dependent on many factors, not the least of which is adequate preventive maintenance as prescribed by the manufacturer.

In a JCAHO-approved acute care hospital, the essential electrical distribution system must be a Type 1 electrical system that has both an emergency component (lighting and communications, etc.) and a critical component (bedside power to operating rooms and intensive care units, etc.). Electrical service is assured through the use of an emergency generator or an alternate source of power. In the simplest essential electrical system installation allowed by NFPA (Type 3), the system is capable of supplying only a limited amount of lighting and power necessary for life safety and the orderly termination of a procedure during a time that normal electrical service is interrupted. The emergency system must have an alternate source of power separate and independent from the normal source that failed. The alternate source must be effective for a minimum of 1.5 hours.

All equipment needs to be maintained, tested, and inspected according to the manufacturer's specifications. Electrical shock hazard is a concern. The office-based site will not likely be provided with isolated power supplies and therefore will not have line isolation monitors. At best, one may find ground fault circuit interrupters (GFCIs). If the GFCI is triggered by an errant current, all current flow will cease until the fault is corrected and the device is reset.

D. Infection Control

Poor infection control poses a risk of wound infection to patients and possible cross-contamination among patients. The infection rate should be reviewed on a regular basis.

SUGGESTED PRACTICES OR OPTIONS

1. The facility must have an area for cleaning, high-level disinfection, and sterilization of surgical equipment and supplies, with appropriate quality control procedures/indicators.
2. A procedure for cleaning and disinfecting procedure rooms must be in place, as should procedures to document training or qualifications of personnel in aseptic technique.
3. Protective clothing, appropriate to the procedure, must be worn by health professionals when surgery is in progress.

E. Occupational Safety

Office surgical procedures pose risk to personnel (and patients) due to exposure to hazardous/infectious body fluids and/or hazardous materials.

SUGGESTED PRACTICES OR OPTIONS

1. The facility must comply with OSHA Standard 1910.1450 to protect patients and personnel from toxic exposure.
2. Policies and procedures must exist to address chemical spills when hazardous chemicals are in use (e.g., formaldehyde and mercury).
3. The facility must comply with OSHA Standard 1910.1030 to protect patients and personnel from exposure to biohazardous waste.
4. Universal precautions shall be instituted and observed.
5. Policies and procedures must exist for handling biohazardous waste (sharp and nonsharp, including containers, labels, transport, and disposal).
6. Policies and procedures must exist for management of employee exposure to biohazardous fluids (e.g., needlestick).
7. Hepatitis B vaccination must be offered to personnel at employer's expense.

IX. Controlled Medications

Physicians are empowered by individual states to administer or prescribe specific types of medications to patients. States may have varying rules and requirements. Controlled medications (Schedule II, III, IV, and V) are commonly used in the course of providing sedation, analgesia, and anesthesia. Policies and procedures are required to comply with laws and regulations pertaining to controlled drug supply, storage, and administration. In addition, all medications used in anesthesia care need to be controlled, and regular inspection of the medication supply ensures safe and effective administration to patients. There are separate federal Drug Enforcement Administration (DEA) registration certificates for manufacturing, distributing, dispensing, and administering controlled medications. A separate state-controlled drug registration

SUGGESTED PRACTICES OR OPTIONS

The use of any medication in the office setting must be under the direction of state-licensed medical providers. These individuals should assume professional, organizational, and administrative responsibility for the use of prescriptive medications. It should be clear in the office policies and procedures who are responsible for various medications and how issues such as drug outdating or recall are handled.

Anesthesiologists are in an excellent position, by virtue of training, knowledge, and experience, to develop and oversee policies and procedures governing anesthesia-related medications, including controlled and resuscitation drugs.

The anesthesiologist must ensure that the transport, storage, and use of all medications supplied by him or her comply with applicable local, state, and federal laws and regulations. The anesthesiologist should ensure that each office surgery location attended has policies and procedures that address controlled (and other) drug use. These should include:

Drug Supply

An individual anesthesiologist working in the office setting may supply the controlled drugs used for anesthesia care or may use the supply provided by the surgeon's office. If there are multiple office locations where controlled medications may be administered/dispensed, a separate registration number is needed for each one.

These "dispensing entities" must obtain controlled drugs from a medication supplier using DEA form 222.

Occasionally, a pharmacy may dispense controlled medications to individual physicians to administer, using a 222 order form.

Periodic Full Drug Inventory

For a physician or office acting as a "dispenser" of controlled drugs, an inventory must be taken on the date of DEA registration and every 2 years thereafter. The inventory must include:

1. The name, address, and DEA number of the registrant
2. The date/time of inventory
3. The name and signatures of the person(s) taking inventory

The inventory must be kept on file for 2 years (some states require longer time periods). There must be a separate record for Schedule II drugs.

Daily Drug Use Inventory

Records must be maintained that account for the use and wastage of all controlled medications on each patient for each date. DEA regulations should always be followed. Records must be kept for at least 2 years (some states require longer time periods) and are subject to DEA inspection. The recording method and any back-up media should be specified.

Drug Security

Controlled drugs must be kept in a locked cabinet or safe. Any loss or theft of drugs must be reported to the regional DEA office (Form 106). Any theft or loss of a DEA Controlled Drug Order Form 222 must be reported immediately to the DEA. If controlled drugs are transported to the office site, security is essential to protect the drug supply, to protect the public from lost or stolen medications, and to protect the anesthesiologist from physical harm during attempted theft. For this reason, it may be easier to have the office location order and stock controlled drugs.

Other noncontrolled medications should be kept in designated locations and, when patients are not being anesthetized, maintained in a place secure or locked, away from potential tampering or theft. Other medications, although not on the DEA schedule list, can be abused. These include sympathomimetic stimulants and any of the potent anesthesia vapors or nitrous oxide. Sufficient safety precautions must be taken to prevent accidental or intentional misuse.

Glossary

Administer: to directly cause a medication to be applied externally or internally to a patient.

Controlled drugs or medications: Clinical drugs that are under the jurisdiction of the Controlled Substances Act. These are stratified into Schedule II, III, IV, and V based on presumed abuse potential.

DEA Form 223: The DEA Controlled Substances Certificate issued to the physician or business.

DEA Form 224: Application for certificate. Renewed every 3 years on form 224a. The address on the form is important. DEA registrations are issued for controlled substance administration at a specific location. If there are multiple office locations where controlled medications may be administered/dispensed, a separate registration number is needed for each one. To have controlled

(Continued)

CLINICAL CARE

I. Procedure Selection

Procedure selection defines the types of surgical procedures that can be performed under office-based anesthesia. A review of existing state regulations and professional recommendations reveals a wide variation as to how much the state or regulating body assumes the responsibility for defining the complexity of case that can be performed and how much is left to the practitioner to define for himself or herself. For example, the regulations governing office-based anesthesia in some states have defined the level of surgical complexity based on the extent to which sedation or anesthesia is required. This ranges from Level l surgery, such as excision of moles, warts, and cysts, requiring minimal preoperative tranquilization, to Level 3 surgery, which includes procedures that would reasonably require general anesthesia or major conduction anesthesia. In other states, health care practitioners themselves establish written policies governing the specific surgical procedures that may be performed in their office. Some procedures have specific physiologic needs that the anesthesiologist should be aware of. These include, but are not limited to, tumescent liposuction, hysteroscopy with glycine, and oral reconstructive surgery.

Scheduling of procedures should take into account both the need to have patients recover adequately and the desire to avoid discharge delays. This may require that patients who undergo longer procedures or who need longer observation are scheduled early, with shorter procedures to follow.

Notwithstanding these definitions of surgical complexity, the anesthesiologist should satisfy him- or herself that the procedure to be undertaken is within the scope of practice of the health care practitioners and the capabilities of the facility. Procedures involving significant blood loss, major intra-abdominal, or intrathoracic or intracranial cavities are not appropriate for the office setting. Furthermore, the procedure should be of a duration and degree of complexity that will permit the patient to recover and be discharged from the facility within a reasonably short period of time. The procedure to be performed should be agreed upon by the patient, anesthesiologist, and surgeon before the procedure is undertaken and before sedative medication is administered to the patient.

II. Preoperative Patient Selection

Each office should establish guidelines that describe criteria for determining patient selection for office procedures. These guidelines will take into account:
1. Patient's medical status
2. Degree of stability of that medical status
3. Patient's psychological status
4. Patient's support system at home (i.e., social evaluation)

(Continued)

SUGGESTED PRACTICES OR OPTIONS—CONT'D

4. The choice of preprocedure laboratory tests, chest x-ray (CXR), and electrocardiogram (ECG) should be guided by the patient's underlying medical condition and the likelihood that the results will affect the anesthetic plan.

5. The following is a partial list of specific factors that should be taken into consideration when deciding whether anesthesia in the office setting is appropriate:
   a. Abnormalities of major organ systems and stability and optimization of any medical illness,
   b. Difficult airway,
   c. Previous adverse experience with anesthesia and surgery,
   d. Current medications and drug allergies,
   e. Time and nature of the last oral intake,
   f. History of alcohol or substance use or abuse, and
   g. Presence of an adult who assumes responsibility specifically for caring for and accompanying the patient from the office.

6. The anesthesia preoperative evaluation (as defined in "ASA Basic Standards for Preanesthesia Care") shall consist of determining the medical status of the patient, developing a plan of anesthesia care, and acquainting the patient or the responsible adult with the proposed plan. The patient or guardian must consent to anesthesia after a discussion of the anesthetic plan, risks, and benefits with the anesthesiologist.

III. Perioperative Care

The anesthesiologist providing patient care in an office setting should adhere to standards and guidelines adopted by the American Society of Anesthesiologists in an effort to assure the same measures of safety and comfort to all patients regardless of the location of their surgery.

A. Preoperative Preparation

An appropriate fasting protocol and medications to take or withhold before surgery shall be explained to the patient or guardian. For patients not at risk for aspiration, the *ASA Practice Guidelines for Preoperative Fasting* indicate that patients may drink clear liquids until 2 hours prior to surgery. Clear liquids include water, fruit juices without pulp, carbonated beverages, clear tea, and black coffee; this does not include alcoholic beverages. An anesthesiologist will conduct a preanesthesia evaluation and examine the patient prior to anesthesia and surgery. In the event that nonphysician personnel are utilized in this process, the anesthesiologist must verify the information obtained and repeat and record essential key elements of the evaluation. Pertinent laboratory data and consultations shall be reviewed. The informed consent process will include discussion and documentation of the risks and benefits of anesthesia and an explanation of alternatives.

B. Intraoperative Care

Anesthetic techniques used in the office setting range from local infiltration and sedation to general anesthesia. Sedation is recognized as a continuum from anxiolysis, to moderate sedation/analgesia (conscious sedation), to deep sedation/analgesia, to general anesthesia.

The following are definitions from the ASA document *Continuum of Depth of Sedation: Definition of General Anesthesia and Levels of Sedation/Analgesia* (approved by House of Delegates, October 13, 1999):

Minimal sedation (i.e., anxiolysis) is a drug-induced state during which patients respond normally to verbal commands. Although cognitive function and coordination may be impaired, ventilatory and cardiovascular functions are unaffected.

Moderate sedation/analgesia (i.e., conscious sedation) is a drug-induced depression of consciousness during which patients respond purposefully to verbal commands, either alone or accompanied by light tactile stimulation. No interventions are required to maintain a patent airway, and spontaneous ventilation is adequate. Cardiovascular function is usually maintained.

Deep sedation/analgesia is a drug-induced depression of consciousness during which patients cannot be easily aroused but respond purposefully following repeated or painful stimulation. The ability to independently maintain ventilatory function may be impaired. Patients often require assistance in maintaining a patent airway, and spontaneous ventilation may be inadequate. Cardiovascular function is usually maintained.

General anesthesia is a drug-induced loss of consciousness during which patients are not arousable, even by painful stimulation. The ability to independently maintain ventilatory function is often impaired. Patients often require assistance in maintaining a patent airway, and positive pressure ventilation may be required because of depressed spontaneous ventilation or drug-induced depression of neuromuscular function. Cardiovascular function may be impaired.

Because sedation is a continuum, it is not always possible to predict how an individual patient will respond. Hence, practitioners intending to produce a given level of sedation should be able to rescue patients whose level of sedation becomes deeper than initially intended. Individuals administering moderate sedation/analgesia should be able to rescue patients who enter a state of deep sedation/analgesia, while those administering deep sedation/analgesia should be able to rescue patients who enter a state of general anesthesia.

The depth of sedation/analgesia achieved varies from patient to patient in the amount of drug required and the rapidity of the induction. Major conduction anesthetics may result in cardiovascular collapse, respiratory insufficiency, or a failed block requiring supplementation or general anesthesia. It is imperative for the office practitioner to be prepared with all needed equipment, drugs, and skills for rescue and resuscitation, including oxygen, positive pressure ventilation, airway aids, resuscitation medications, and continuous anticipation of potential untoward events. The most important clinical aspects of giving anesthesia remain the training, experience, continuing education, and vigilance of the anesthesia personnel.

C. Postoperative Care

The issues regarding recovery relate to which aspects of a patient's recovery need to be monitored and by whom, how many phases of recovery are needed, when the patient can be safely discharged, and whether the recovery criteria are any different following office surgery and anesthesia. These are issues that are relevant to all locations of anesthesia care in the ambulatory setting. Proper postanesthesia recovery care in the office includes an environment that ensures that the medical aspects, the design, the equipment, and the staffing of the postanesthesia care are met.

The purpose of this section is to identify appropriate standards and guidelines for postanesthesia care in the office-based setting. Although office-based settings can offer unique and challenging environments for recovering a patient from anesthesia, well-established ASA standards and guidelines on postanesthesia care are readily available to all practitioners. These standards and guidelines include the following:

1. Standards for postanesthesia care
2. Guidelines for office-based anesthesia
3. Guidelines for ambulatory anesthesia and surgery
4. Practice guidelines for sedation and analgesia by nonanesthesiologists

The attention to patient safety issues provided by these standards and guidelines should apply to all postanesthesia care regardless of facility location. Structural and support differences among surgical facility sites present unique challenges to successful postanesthesia care.

SUGGESTED PRACTICES OR OPTIONS

1. Anesthesia for office-based surgery can be accomplished using a variety of approaches. Induction and maintenance of sedation or anesthesia can include intravenous and inhalational techniques. Short-acting agents are most appropriate. Central and peripheral regional anesthetic techniques can also be valuable.

2. More important than the choice of specific agents or techniques, the anesthesiologist must focus on providing an anesthetic that will give the patient a rapid recovery to normal function, with minimal postoperative pain, nausea, or other side effects.

3. Continuous clinical observation and vigilance are the basis of safe anesthesia care. Specific requirements for basic anesthesia monitoring are addressed in another section. In addition, positioning care and patient protection should be individualized according to patient needs and type of surgery. Adjunctive care for selected office-based surgery procedures may include active warming measures, blankets, eye protection during laser surgery, Foley catheter, and antiembolic stockings.

4. The intraprocedure record must document anesthetic agents, medications and supplemental oxygen used, vital signs, oxygen saturation, ECG interpretation, and end-tidal carbon dioxide, inspired oxygen, and temperature measurements when required. Vital signs should be monitored at least every 5 minutes. The volume and type of fluids administered, along with blood loss and urine output, when measured, should be recorded.

5. A proactive approach to pain management is critical. Local infiltration with long-acting local anesthetics by an anesthesiologist or surgeon should be paired with systemic narcotics and nonsteroidal anti-inflammatory drugs (NSAIDS) to provide postoperative pain control. Long-acting regional blocks can provide excellent postprocedural analgesia. Both of these should be combined with patient education to clarify appropriate regimens for oral analgesia and to establish appropriate expectations.

6. The individual administering the anesthetic or monitoring the patient should accompany the patient to the postanesthesia area and remain with the patient until vital signs are evaluated and a complete oral report is given to the nurse or other qualified personnel responsible for the patient's recovery and that nurse or other qualified personnel accepts responsibility for the nursing care of the patient. In an office in which the anesthesia provider monitors initial recovery, the recovery location is often the original procedure room. Care may be transferred to qualified health care personnel when criteria for advancement to the next level of observation are met and documented.

Office-based practitioners should identify differences in structure and support systems and should design postanesthesia care policies and procedures that address the unique features of each office facility. Office-based practitioners should refer to the above-referenced standards and guidelines when designing policies and procedures that ensure the safest recovery of their patients in an office-based setting.

Specifically, Standards for Postanesthesia Care, approved by the ASA House of Delegates, includes:

Standard I—All patients who received general anesthesia, regional anesthesia, or monitored anesthesia care shall receive appropriate postanesthesia management.

In an office environment, the area designated for postanesthesia care can be highly variable. Wherever the recovery of the patient is to occur, the area designated must provide an environment that ensures that space, equipment, and staffing adequately meet the intent of current postanesthesia care guidelines and standards. Policies and procedures specific to the postanesthesia care of the patient should be developed and routinely reviewed by all office staff members.

Standard II—A patient transported to the postanesthesia care unit (PACU) shall be accompanied by a member of the anesthesia care team who is knowledgeable about the patient's condition. The patient shall be continually evaluated and treated during transport with monitoring and support appropriate to the patient's condition.

Standard III—Upon arrival in the PACU, the patient shall be reevaluated and a verbal report provided to the responsible PACU nurse by the member of the anesthesia care team who accompanies the patient.

The surgical office environment can present unique challenges for patients recovering from anesthesia. In many offices, patients recover in the surgical or procedure room without transport to a postanesthesia recovery area. In other offices, when transport to a postanesthesia recovery area is necessary, doorways and hallways may not have been constructed to ensure easy transport of patients. Policies and procedures specific to the characteristics of each surgical office should be in place, addressing issues such as transport, documentation of patient status, staffing, and responsibility of care at the beginning of and through the entire postanesthesia care period.

Standard IV—The patient's condition shall be evaluated continually in the PACU.

Regardless of facility site, all patients shall be observed and monitored by methods appropriate to the patient's medical condition by appropriately trained staff. Particular attention should be given to monitoring oxygenation, ventilation, circulation, and temperature. A quantitative method of assessing oxygenation, such as pulse oximetry, should be employed. Accurate documentation of the patient's status in the postanesthesia care period should be maintained. The anesthesiologist should remain in the facility and should be immediately available until the patient has been discharged from anesthesia care.

Standard V—A physician is responsible for the discharge of the patient from the PACU.

Regardless of where a patient may recover from anesthesia in an office-based setting, discharge of the patient from the initial postanesthesia care period is a physician responsibility. Personnel with training in advanced resuscitation techniques (e.g., ACLS, PALS) should be immediately available until all patients are discharged home.

Documentation of the patient's condition at the time of discharge should be noted in the medical record and can be facilitated by using recognized discharge criteria. Verbal instructions understood by the patient and confirmed by written instruction should be provided to each patient at discharge. In addition, the following should be included in the instructions:

1. Procedure performed and information about complications that may arise
2. Telephone numbers and names of medical providers if complications or questions arise
3. Instructions for any medication prescribed
4. Instructions for pain management, if appropriate
5. Date, time, and location of the follow-up or return visit
6. Predetermined place(s) to go for treatment in the event of emergency

D. Discharge Criteria

Patient discharge is a physician responsibility. Appropriate written criteria for discharge should be applied and should conform to any specific state regulations that govern the provision of office anesthesia.

IV. Monitoring and Equipment

The purpose of this section is to identify appropriate standards and guidelines for monitoring and equipment in the delivery of anesthesia care in the Suggested Practices or Options box on p 192.

The following documents already approved by the ASA House of Delegates appropriately address these issues:

A. Standards for basic anesthetic monitoring,
B. Guidelines for office-based anesthesia,
C. Guidelines for ambulatory anesthesia and surgery, and
D. Guidelines for nonoperating room anesthetizing locations. (Full text in source document.)

SUGGESTED PRACTICES OR OPTIONS

Patients should be evaluated for discharge from the office operating room suite by the anesthesiologist or physician responsible for the patient's anesthesia care, using written criteria that allow the patient to either be transferred to a "recovery area" or ambulate directly to a chair with reclining abilities. While traditional Phase 1 and Phase 2 criteria for discharge need to be met, the process and location of these phases are frequently combined.

The office frequently does not have a specially designated area for recovering patients. Space limitations and insufficient nursing personnel have catalyzed the concept of fast-tracking patients, even more so than in the traditional ambulatory surgical setting. This has become feasible through the use of short-acting anesthetics, judicious use of local anesthesia infiltration, and prophylactic multimodal analgesics and antiemetics when anticipated. Often the anesthesiologist will observe the patient in the operating room until the patient has recovered from anesthesia and is ready to walk out in the lounge area and be discharged. If several cases are scheduled to follow, nurses or other qualified personnel trained in postanesthesia care should assist the physician with patient recovery and subsequent discharge from the office. While in the operating room, the patient is evaluated to determine whether criteria have been met for Phase 1 recovery using standardized criteria such as the Modified Aldrete Score or Fast-Tracking Criteria. In addition to the scoring criteria in the Modified Aldrete Score, Fast-Tracking Criteria use the same scoring criteria with two additional assessments: postoperative pain and postoperative emetic symptoms. Phase 1 recovery may take place in the operating room or in a recovery area and is completed when the patient achieves a Modified Aldrete Score of >9 or Fast-Tracking Criteria score >12. A dedicated postanesthesia care nurse can conduct this assessment, or, under the circumstances in which the anesthesiologist is not engaged in the administration of another anesthetic, the anesthesiologist can observe the patient during recovery and continue the Phase 1 assessment until completed. The anesthesiologist should be physically present during the intraoperative period and immediately available until the patient has been discharged from anesthesia care.

The Phase 2 portion of the recovery includes assessment and evaluation of the patient to determine when the patient is suited to be discharged home. Ambulatory Discharge Criteria include that the patient's vital signs be stable; that the patient is fully orientated; that the patient can ambulate without dizziness; that the patient has minimal pain, nausea, vomiting, and bleeding; and that the patient has a responsible vested adult escort. Personnel with training in advanced resuscitation techniques should be immediately available until all patients are discharged home.

V.   Special Considerations for Pediatric Patients

Since office-based anesthesia is an extension of freestanding ambulatory practice, all applicable management guidelines should apply equally to both practice locations. One of the major requirements for safe management in either location is the anesthesiologist's high level of comfort, which is based on both training and experience, with the child's age, medical condition, and proposed surgical procedure. The other is the availability of an environment that is designed and equipped to promote the safety and well-being of children.

A.   Acceptable Patients

The child should be in good health; if not, any systemic disease must be under good control. Although an absolute minimal age for otherwise healthy infants cannot be rigidly suggested, it is probably prudent to limit the selection of infants to those who have successfully transitioned from the neonatal period (i.e., age 4 to 6 months). The ex-premature infant is probably not a good office candidate for an even longer period. The risk of postoperative apnea mandates a longer period of observation and monitoring, which is not practical in an office setting.

B.   Acceptable Procedures

Brief and superficial procedures such as herniorrhaphy, myringotomy, dental procedures, and circumcision are selected most often. Since most procedures on children require general anesthesia or a deep level of sedation and since most children prefer a technique that does not involve "needling" when they are awake, the availability of an anesthesia gas machine is an important factor in determining the type of pediatric procedure (e.g., bilateral myringotomy and tubes) that can be readily performed in the office without increasing the complexity of the anesthetic technique.

C.   Preoperative Considerations

Preoperative screening and preparation is usually done in association with the surgeon and his or her office staff. It is very desirable to have the anesthesiologist contact the parents in advance of the day of surgery by telephone or any other convenient way to introduce him- or herself, to get a good history, to explain the need for preoperative fasting, and to discuss the anesthetic and recovery plans.

D. Premedication/Preinduction Choices

Although many children do not need preoperative sedation (provided that they have established a good rapport with the anesthesiologist), some do. Midazolam (0.5 mg/kg) can be administered orally 20 to 30 minutes before induction to decrease preoperative anxiety, to facilitate separation from the parents, and to improve the child's cooperation during induction without significantly delaying recovery and discharge. Alternatively, the parents may be allowed to stay with the child during the induction of anesthesia.

E. Inhalational Techniques

Inhalation induction has long been favored by children and pediatric anesthesiologists. The only limiting factor is the need for anesthesia machine and vaporizers and scavenging devices that may not be universally available.

F. Total Intravenous Anesthesia (TIVA) in Children

Intravenous techniques are often chosen in many older children, especially when topical local anesthetic cream (such as eutectic mixture of local anesthetics [EMLA]) is used to perform a painless venipuncture, and may be the only available option if an anesthetic machine is not available. Efforts to have this applied at home by parents should be encouraged, especially with the current availability of prepackaged patches.

G. Postoperative Analgesia

Regional blocks or local infiltration should be used whenever possible to supplement general anesthesia and to limit the need for narcotics during recovery. Acetaminophen is the most commonly used mild analgesic for pediatric ambulatory patients. For young children, the initial dose is often administered rectally (40 mg/kg) following induction of anesthesia so that the peak effect may coincide with recovery. Onset time to full effect is 60 to 90 minutes. Supplemental doses are given orally (10 to 15 mg/kg every 4 to 6 hours, not "as needed"). The total daily dose should not exceed 100 mg/kg.

H. Perioperative Fluid Management

Preoperative fasting should be minimized according to the current ASA guidelines. The need for routine administration of intravenous fluids during pediatric office surgery is controversial. Children undergoing very brief surgical procedures (e.g., myringotomies) may not need any parenteral fluid administration as long as they are not excessively starved preoperatively and are expected to be able to ingest and retain oral fluids soon after they are awake. For most other children, intraoperative maintenance fluid administration can be calculated based on the child's body weight according to standard formulae.

I. Recovery and Discharge Issues

Rapid recovery and early ambulation are key objectives in the office setting. Most facilities provide a single area for the total recovery period, and the parents are usually invited to stay with their children during this period. In order to provide uniform care and to ensure a complete legal record, specific criteria for discharge must be met before these children are released to go home. Recent studies suggest that as long as the children are well hydrated, they should not be required to drink before discharge from the hospital.

VI. Emergencies

A. Emergency Medications and Supplies

A physician who administers or supervises the administration of medication in office-based anesthesia settings must be prepared to handle emergencies as they occur. Although complications in the delivery of sedation and anesthesia for surgical procedures are rare, emergency situations occur that make it mandatory for certain types of equipment and medications to be readily available. Cardiac dysrhythmias and/or arrest, anaphylactic reactions, and malignant hyperthermia (which is covered in another section of this document) are emergencies that need immediate attention. The medications and equipment in an office-based setting for such emergencies should not be any different than those that are necessary in a hospital or outpatient surgical center. An emergency cart with the necessary medications and equipment to resuscitate an apneic and unconscious patient or one who has experienced a cardiac arrest must be readily available.

In an office where anesthesia services are to be provided to infants and children, the required emergency equipment should be appropriately sized for a pediatric population and personnel should be appropriately trained to handle pediatric emergencies.

A practitioner who is qualified in resuscitative techniques and emergency care should be present and available until all patients have been discharged from the office setting.

Resources for determining appropriate drug dosages and usage should be readily available. The emergency supplies and equipment should be maintained and inspected regularly to ensure that the equipment is present and functional and that drugs have not expired.

Box 1   Emergency Equipment

Suction apparatus
Cardiopulmonary resuscitation (CPR) equipment (i.e., crash cart with medications or equivalent and defibrillator)
Oxygen source
Rigid pharyngeal suction catheter (e.g., Yankauer)
Pulse oximeter
ECG monitor
Means of giving positive pressure ventilation (e.g., Ambu-bag)
Standard intubation tray with variety of blades, endotracheal tubes, laryngeal mask airways (LMAs), and oral airways appropriately sized for the population being served.
Equipment necessary for implementation of ASA Difficult Airway Guidelines
Equipment to treat MH, including ice and cold saline and monitoring capability

The purpose of this section is to give a list of medications and equipment available should an emergency arise. (See Box 1 for a list of emergency equipment.) Appropriate emergency supplies, equipment, and medications should be provided in accordance with the scope of surgical and anesthesia services provided in office-based anesthesia.

In the event of medical complications, emergencies, or other untoward events, personnel should be familiar with the procedures and the plan to be followed and should be capable of taking necessary action. There should be a documented plan and procedure for the safe and timely transfer of patients to a nearby hospital, and all personnel should be familiar with it. Such a plan should include arrangements for an emergency ambulance service or 911 and, when appropriate, escort of the patient to the hospital by an appropriate practitioner. When advanced cardiac life support has been initiated, the plan should include a provision to immediately contact the ambulance service or 911.

B. Emergency Procedures

Disasters may happen. It is important that the office-based practice have written policies about what to do and who is to do it. Considerations include:

1. Who will determine when the disaster plan goes into effect?
2. Who will coordinate information and direct personnel?
3. What are the roles of the various personnel in a disaster?
4. What happens in the case of internal disaster, including fire, bomb, explosion, loss of power, equipment malfunction, loss of oxygen, a hostage situation, or an emotionally disturbed employee or patient?
5. What happens in the case of external disaster, including tornado, hurricane, flood, earthquake, or war?
6. How will communication work internally and externally?

SUGGESTED PRACTICES OR OPTIONS

A specific disaster manager designee must immediately assume responsibility for the implementation of the disaster plan. The designee sees that the police and fire departments are notified. The designee will determine if evacuation of patients is required. The evacuation plan will be part of the policy. This plan should include:
- Horizontal Evacuation: Relocation to a safe area through smoke barrier doors on the same floor.
- Vertical Evacuation: Evacuation to a safe area on a different floor by means of stairwells. All access to exit stairwells is marked by illuminated signs that are on emergency power.

The order of evacuation will be as follows:
1. First priority: Patients who are in imminent danger shall be moved first.
2. Second priority: Ambulatory patients and visitors shall be moved next.
3. Third priority: Wheelchair patients shall be evacuated next.
4. Fourth priority: Nonambulatory patients shall be moved with stretchers. If stretchers are unavailable, use blankets to drag patients.
5. Fifth priority: Patient records, drugs, supplies and equipment. Designate a staging area outside the building.

The designee and/or physician will evaluate patients to determine those who can be discharged and those who will require transfer to a medical facility. Those patients who may be discharged will wait in a designated relocation area for families to escort them home. A list of telephone numbers for local medical facilities and ambulance companies should be kept readily at hand.

7. How will patients be transported to safety? What are the evacuation routes?
8. Where are the fire extinguishers? Alarm pulls?
9. Is evidence of education on file?

C. Malignant Hyperthermia

This section addresses both the management of a malignant hyperthermia (MH) crisis and the management of anesthesia for a MH-susceptible (MHS) patient in an office-based facility.

MH Preventive Measures

One way to markedly decrease the likelihood of treating a malignant hyperthermia episode in an office facility is to obtain an adequate medical history from the patient and the patient's family. If patients themselves have a positive history of an episode that may be MH, their anesthesia should probably be performed in the hospital setting. If the patient cites a family history of MH, unexplained perioperative hyperthermia, perioperative "cardiac arrest," or a myopathy, then the patient should be considered MHS. The management of an MHS patient is discussed below.

Diagnosis and Treatment of MH
(Full text in source document.)

Anesthesia for the MHS Patient

It is not advisable to anesthetize an MHS patient with triggering agents. Emergency equipment, near access (less than 15 minutes away) to blood gas/electrolyte measurements, an MH treatment plan, and medications (including dantrolene) should be available, even if non-triggering agents are used in an MHS patient. (Full text in source document.)

VII. Transfer to Alternate Care Facilities

An office that provides anesthesia services must have a plan in place to transfer patients to an alternate care facility when the services available in the office are not adequate to protect the health of or to treat the patient. It is the responsibility of the physician in charge of anesthesia services to verify that the office has a written transfer agreement with a nearby hospital or only permits elective surgery by physicians with admitting privileges at a nearby hospital before initiating anesthesia. The office location must have a detailed procedural plan for handling the emergency transfer of patients. This plan must include:

1. A means of emergency transportation to a hospital; in areas with 911 service, this is acceptable. In areas without 911 service, an agreement to provide emergency ambulance transportation for patients must be arranged with a provider. Ambulance coverage must be available during the entire period that the patient is in the office.
2. The telephone number of the emergency transportation provider should be prominently displayed in the recovery area of the office and at any other location where an emergency surgical or anesthetic condition is likely to develop.
3. Details of how responsibility for patient care is shifted to the new setting.
4. The mechanism of transferring medical information to the receiving facility.
5. Requirements for appropriate personnel to accompany the patient to the new facility; this should include the operator and/or anesthesiologist if the patient is unstable.

Conditions that warrant transfer to a hospital may include but are not limited to:

1. An expected or actual period of more than 23 hours for recovery from the surgery or anesthesia.
2. Clinical pathology, laboratory, or radiographic services needed to ensure patient well-being that are not available in the office setting.
3. Excessive blood loss requiring transfusion or other blood bank products.
4. Uncontrolled postoperative pain.
5. A new clinical problem requiring hospital diagnosis or treatment.
6. The unanticipated need for specialized surgical or anesthetic equipment or skills not available in the current practice location.
7. The development of perioperative complications that pose a threat to the patient's well-being.
8. A patient's request to be admitted to a hospital.
9. Inability of the office to provide adequate personnel, equipment, or other resources to safely provide for the perioperative care of its patients.
10. The surgeon's and/or anesthesiologist's desire to have the patient transferred to a facility that can provide a higher level of care.

All new employees need to be in-serviced on the transfer policy before assuming patient responsibilities. The transfer policy should be evaluated and updated at least annually.

Patients have the right to know the details of the transfer policy so they can weigh appropriate insurance and personal preference concerns when giving informed consent to undergo an office procedure and anesthetic.

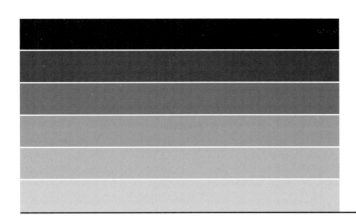

Index

A

Sevoflurane
  advantages and disadvantages of, 45–46, 47
  advantages and disadvantages of inhaled, 47, 47b, 47t
  nephrotoxicity and, 46
Short-acting intravenous anesthetics, 34–41
Sinus surgery, pediatric anesthesia for, 127
  risk of retrobulbar hemorrhage during, 127
Sleep apnea, 115. *See also* Obstructive sleep apnea
Smoking, 120, 130b
Society for Ambulatory Anesthesia (SAMBA), 5
Spinal-epidural, 76–78
Spitting (patient's), 154
Stent, drug-eluting coronary, elective surgery and, 12b
Surgeon
  cardiologist consulting, 26
    regarding patient with implantable cardioverter/defibrillator, 26. 12–13
  credentialing and privileging of, 165
  educated by anesthesiologist, 31
  selecting of, 9, 43, 146, 165, 189
    for dentistry, 149, 154–155, 155b
Surgical procedure selection, 9, 43, 146, 189
Surgicenter. *See* Ambulatory surgery center
Swedish National Registry, on danger to fetus, 14

T

Tachycardia, 98
Target-controlled infusion (TCI), for intravenous anesthetics, 40
Target-controlled infusion (TCI) system, 40–41, 41f
TCI. *See* Target-controlled infusion
TCI system. *See* Target-controlled infusion system
Temperature loss, during geriatric anesthesia, 143
TENS. *See* Transcutaneous electrical nerve stimulation

Testing, preanesthesia, 26–27, 26t, 27b, 28b
  guidelines on
    American Society of Anesthesiologists', 27, 28b
    National Institute for Clinical Excellence's, 27, 28b
  routine "screening" tests, 26–27, 26t
    for pregnancy, 14, 27, 123, 123b
    of adolescents, 27
  routine tests versus "indicated," 26, 26t
TIVA. *See* Total intravenous anesthesia
TNS. *See* Transient neurologic symptoms
Tonsillectomy, pediatric anesthesia for, 125b, 126
Tooth anatomy, 150–151
  fracture or avulsion of, 151
  roots, 151
Topical analgesia, 151
Total intravenous anesthesia (TIVA)
  cost-effectiveness of, 39–40, 40b
  for ophthalmologic procedures, 40b
  for orthopedic and general surgery, 40b
  for plastic surgery, 40b
  propofol as
    adverse effects of, 37–38
    antiemetic action of, 37
    desirable effects of, 37
    dosing
      for elderly, 38
      for lean body mass versus total body mass, 38
      for pediatric patients, 38
    other sedative-hypnotics versus, 38f
    pharmacokinetics of, 37
    reduced residual sedation with, 37
  propofol-opioid infusion as
    induction and maintenance, 39, 40t
    infusion rate, 39, 40t
    neuromuscular blockers with, 39
    recovery time factors, 39
    synergistic interaction of, 38–39
  propofol-remifentanil as
    for postoperative analgesia, 39, 40t
    synergistic interaction of, 36, 37f
    wake-up conditions with, 39

Total intravenous anesthesia (TIVA) (*Continued*)
  remifentanil as
    distinguishing features of, 35, 35f
    for children, 36
    for elderly patients, 36
    for obese patients, 36
    therapeutic and adverse effects of, 35
  using target controlled infusion, 40–41, 41f
Transcutaneous electrical nerve stimulation (TENS), 65
Transient neurologic symptoms (TNS), 75, 75b, 104

U

Upper respiratory illness (URI), 15–16, 16b
Upper respiratory tract illness (URTI), 29
URI. *See* Upper respiratory illness
Urinary retention, 105. 105t. *See also* Genitourinary tract
Urologic procedures, pediatric anesthesia for, 128, 128b
URTI. *See* Upper respiratory tract illness

V

Ventricular septal defect (VSD), 119
VSD. *See* Ventricular septal defect

W

Waste gas, 187
White and Song's patient discharge criteria, 111t

X

X-rays, danger to fetus of, 14